E. JAMES POTCHEN, M.D., *Consulting Editor*

Professor of Radiology
The Edward Mallinckrodt Institute of Radiology
Washington University School of Medicine
St. Louis, Missouri

Published

GASTROINTESTINAL ANGIOGRAPHY
   Stewart R. Reuter, M.D., and Helen C. Redman, M.D.

Forthcoming Monographs

RADIOLOGY OF THE ILEOCECAL AREA
   Robert N. Berk, M.D., and Elliot C. Lasser, M.D.

RADIOLOGY OF THE PANCREAS AND DUODENUM
   S. Boyd Eaton, Jr., M.D., and Joseph T. Ferrucci, Jr., M.D.

THE RADIOLOGY OF VERTEBRAL TRAUMA
   John A. Gehweiler, M.D., and Richard R. Six, M.D.

THE RADIOLOGY OF RENAL FAILURE
   Harry J. Griffiths, M.D.

FUNDAMENTALS OF ABDOMINAL AND PELVIC
ULTRASONOGRAPHY
   George R. Leopold, M.D., and Michael Asher, M.D.

THE HAND IN RADIOLOGIC DIAGNOSIS
   Andrew K. Poznanski, M.D.

PEDIATRIC RADIOLOGY OF THE ALIMENTARY TRACT
   *Edward B. Singleton, M.D., Milton L. Wagner, M.D., and
   Robert V. Dutton, M.D.*

ARTHROGRAPHY: PRINCIPLES AND TECHNIQUES
   Tom W. Staple, M.D.

CLINICAL PEDIATRIC AND ADOLESCENT UROGRAPHY
   Alfred L. Weber, M.D., and Richard C. Pfister, M.D.

CORONARY ARTERIOGRAPHY
   Lewis Wexler, M.D., and Ivo Obrez, M.D.

Volume 2 in the Series
SAUNDERS
MONOGRAPHS
IN CLINICAL
RADIOLOGY

THE
RADIOLOGY
OF
JOINT
DISEASE

D. M. FORRESTER, M.D.

Associate Professor of Radiology,
University of Southern California School of Medicine,
Los Angeles County-University of Southern California Medical Center,
Los Angeles, California;
Consultant Physician in Rheumatology,
Long Beach Veterans Administration Hospital,
Long Beach, California

JOHN W. NESSON, M.D.

Instructor in Radiology,
University of Southern California School of Medicine,
Los Angeles County-University of Southern California Medical Center,
Los Angeles, California

W. B. SAUNDERS COMPANY • *Philadelphia* • *London* • *Toronto*

W. B. Saunders Company: West Washington Square
Philadelphia, Pa.   19105

12 Dyott Street
London, WC1A   1DB

833 Oxford Street
Toronto, Ontario M8Z 5T9, Canada

The Radiology of Joint Disease   ISBN   0-7216-3817-1

Print No.:   9   8   7   6   5   4

To
George Jacobson
and
Lucy Frank Squire
with affection

The winds . . . have suck'd up from the sea
Contagious fogs. . . .
Therefore the moon, the governess of floods,
Pale in her anger washes all the air
That rheumatic diseases do abound.

William Shakespeare
A Midsummer Night's Dream

EDITOR'S FOREWORD

With continuing advances in the diagnosis and treatment of the variety of disorders known collectively as arthritis, it becomes more and more important that the radiologist understand and be able to recognize and differentiate rheumatic diseases. This is not an altogether simple task. The pathologic process in a joint may be inflammatory or degenerative, acute or chronic. Acute arthritis may evolve to a chronic form, and chronic arthritis may have acute episodes. The patient may present with a fundamental pathologic change at varying points in a wide spectrum. In addition, there are conditions known as nonarticular rheumatism, which produce symptoms by changes in structures contiguous to or related to the joints but not in the joints themselves. And of course the etiology of many arthritic diseases remains unknown.

The accurate interpretation of joint radiographs continues to represent a formidable challenge to many practicing radiologists. To help correct this situation, THE RADIOLOGY OF JOINT DISEASE provides a systematic radiographic approach to the arthritides based on the patient's symptoms and pathologic correlation. This approach is uniquely organized about the patient's problems as presented to the physician—that is, as regional joint symptoms and not as established diagnoses. Application of the concepts explained and illustrated in the work will enable the physician to approach any joint film with much greater confidence.

Dr. Forrester has devoted much time as a radiologist to the study and teaching of arthritis, receiving training and experience in radiology at Massachusetts General Hospital and Harvard Medical School, and at Los Angeles County–USC Medical Center. Dr. Forrester is now on the faculty of the University of Southern California School of Medicine. Dr. Nesson, a colleague in the Department of Radiology at USC, is an accomplished photographer, as evidenced by the remarkable illustrations in this book. Together the authors have prepared a highly readable and finely organized text that truly teaches its subject. This book therefore, fills a significant void in a most important area of radiologic diagnosis and will prove highly useful to radiologists, rheumatologists, and all others concerned with diseases of the joints.

E. JAMES POTCHEN, M.D.

PREFACE

This monograph is intended to present a systematic approach to the interpretation of radiographs in rheumatic disorders. Our method is designed to permit an orderly assessment of film findings in order to diagnose pathologic processes and evaluate the course of a disease and its response to treatment. The approach that is suggested can be applied to any joint and any arthritis. It enables the reader to identify clinical and diagnostic features that might otherwise elude the non-specialist.

The principles outlined are intended to serve as building blocks with which to construct an understanding of pathophysiologic processes and the significance of their radiographic manifestations. Whenever possible, pathologic specimens are included to define the precise abnormality. Microscopic preparations of whole joints are rare, and their contribution to an understanding of the radiographic changes is invaluable. That the radiograph *is* the in vivo gross specimen becomes evident when one appreciates the similarity between the microscopic appearance and the film.

The text is limited to problems of joints and is primarily designed as a teaching method for those who face diagnostic dilemmas in this area. It is not a bone book and excludes such major areas as bone tumors and dysplasias. Neither is it a comprehensive atlas, but rather a collection of illustrative examples of the frequent presentations of rheumatic disorders, and it includes specific observations which the authors have found useful.

Part I deals with the basic components of the film: soft tissue, bone and joints. By use of a technique for the radiographic dissection of a joint, the reader may avoid the common pitfall of allowing prominent pathologic changes to mask more subtle ones. In order to facilitate the teaching of basic principles and to dramatize *differences* between radiographic features of various arthritides, the examples in Part I are limited to abnormalities as they appear in the hands.

Part II illustrates the same diseases as they affect joints other than those of the hand. Since anatomic and mechanical forces of different joints impose changes on the basic underlying process, similarities and differences in the radiographic manifestation of the same disease in different areas are emphasized. This allows application of the *principles* described in Part I and permits the reader to compare and analyze specific features of various diseases as they affect each joint.

Organization by region rather than by disease, and by the predominant radiographic abnormality (i.e., soft tissue calcification, periostitis, ankylosis), provides a useful source of reference for the physician faced with a specific clinical dilemma.

One of the exciting benefits of preparing a manuscript involves the logarithmic increase in "here's a great case for your book." We enthusiastically share the 50 greatest of these "great cases" with the reader, as they were shared with us: as "unknowns," at the end of each anatomic section. To each of our co-authors in this endeavor — student, resident, or colleague — our many thanks.

D. M. FORRESTER, M.D.
JOHN W. NESSON, M.D.

ACKNOWLEDGMENTS

The work entailed in translating into book form one's daily experience is far greater than ever anticipated, and unexpected stumbling blocks are numerous. During this time a few people became very special to us because of their generosity:

Yale B. Bickel and John J. Calabro, for their advice and criticism of the manuscript.

Sherwin Levy, who offered the podiatrist's point of view of Chapter 5.

Roger Terry and The Arthritis Foundation, for their unique preparation of pathologic material and their generosity in allowing its publication in this monograph.

John Heller, for his expertise in producing the photographic prints.

Sue Games, whose tireless effort in indexing and case retrieval makes finding "the perfect example" a possibility.

Ramona Payne, Peggy Stokes and Barbara Chapman, for their long hours of hard and accurate work in typing the manuscript.

Jack Hanley, for his enthusiasm and encouragement and his steady supply of innovative ideas.

Jeffrey and Brent, who waited patiently for *their* ABC's while this one was being written.

D.M.F.
J.W.N.

CONTENTS

PART I   THE ABC'S OF ARTHRITIS

PART II   ARTHRITIS FROM HEAD TO FOOT

Part I

THE
ABC'S
OF
ARTHRITIS

INTRODUCTION

Students of medical disciplines hardly need to be informed of the value of an organized approach to diagnosis. Nonetheless, it is apparent that most physicians approaching a joint film employ an organization reminiscent of a Katzenjammer Kids' picnic. This lack of a systematic approach does not entirely preclude an accurate diagnosis but does require greater stores of good fortune or genius than most of us possess. Why, then, is an organized approach to evaluation of joint films uncommon? The answer, of course, is that no systematic method has been taught or recommended either by rheumatologists or radiologists. Although any single method employed to analyze joint films is arbitrary, the necessity for a systematic approach is essential.

The method employed in this monograph, as expressed in the subtitle of Part I, "The ABC'S of Arthritis," uses a step-by-step procedure to indicate the features on the film to be assessed and the sequence in which they are examined. The approach involves serial evaluation of:

A — Alignment
B — Bony mineralization
C — Cartilage space
S — Soft tissue

The mnemonic ABC'S (with a bit of literary license in rearranging the sequence) has several distinct advantages: it is easy to remember and helps the physician quickly isolate unusual findings in a logical order and, most important, usually leads to the correct diagnosis.

Thus, when initially analyzing a film, an overview of general pathologic changes is obtained prior to "coning down" on specific localized abnormalities. This is accomplished by first observing the soft tissues, then noting the alignment of the bones and finally assessing the bony texture or its state of mineralization. Only after this general evaluation is methodically conducted should each joint or cartilage space be visually dissected.

When multiple joints are included on a single film, an orderly assessment is essential. For example, in the hand, beginning proximally with the radius and ulna and proceeding systematically to the distal phalangeal joints prevents overlooking any abnormality revealed on the film.

Chapter 1

SOFT TISSUES OF THE HAND

The systematic analysis of radiographic abnormalities begins with the soft tissues, as would a physical examination. A small but important percentage of films contain the definitive clue to diagnosis in the skin, muscles, tendons and the regions of the joint capsules. These soft tissue structures are all of "water density" and normally blend into each other on the film. Despite this homogeneous shadow, knowledge of the anatomic relationship of each component part allows an accurate localization of an abnormality.

There are two categories of soft tissue change. There may be changes in tissue *mass* (either too much or too little) or in tissue *density* (radiolucency or calcification). Both types of abnormality may be *diffuse* or *localized*. The type of abnormality and the pattern of its distribution are frequently suggestive of a specific disease. Therefore, evaluation of the soft tissue is an important and critical first step in the assessment of a joint.

Early in a disease, the change from normal may be subtle. Often the boundaries of normal overlap the minor degrees of abnormal change, and a single film representing the anatomic features of a joint at any one point in time may appear unremarkable when it is, in fact, abnormal for that individual. It is obvious that possibilities for early detection of pathologic processes may be greatly enhanced by the availability of a previous film of the same area for comparison. Since this is frequently unobtainable, as a joint is first filmed after the onset of the disease, a radiograph of the contralateral part must serve the same purpose.

GENERALIZED INCREASE IN SOFT TISSUE

Generalized or diffuse increase in soft tissues is caused by overgrowth, infiltration or swelling and is more easily detected clinically than radiographically. As with the physical findings, the range of normal is wide; distinction between normal and abnormal amounts of soft tissue on a single film in any given patient may be difficult. Previous films are invaluable to verify a generalized increase when the abnormality is bilateral. If the pathology is confined to only one hand, the opposite hand can act as a base line of normal. Important guides to evaluating soft tissue structures are illustrated in the Figure 1–1, a normal hand.

Normal Hand. A normal hand of a 25 year old woman (Fig. 1–1) illustrates the relationship of the soft tissue to bone and demonstrates the bulge of tissue seen in the areas of the thenar and hypothenar compartments, which provide the bulk of the shadow of the palm. Also shown is a slight increase in density cast by the knuckle pads over the proximal interphalangeal joints. This frequently mimics periarticular soft tissue swelling, but transverse lines cast by the furrows distinguish the normal shadow from the fusiform configuration of a pathologic swelling.

There is very little excess tissue in the region of the wrist, as reflected by the position of the distal radius and ulna just beneath the subcutaneous tissues. Because of the superficial position of these bones, this area is a sensitive radiographic indicator of swelling of the wrist.

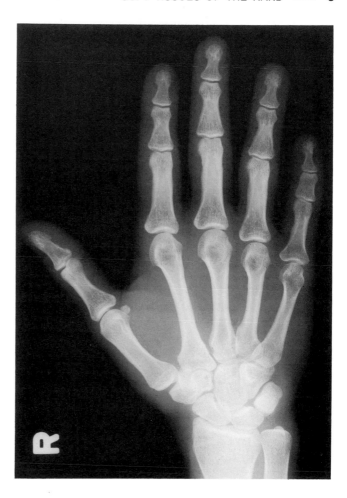

Figure 1-1. Normal hand.

OVERGROWTH

Overgrowth of the soft tissues occurs secondary to excessive growth hormone levels in acromegaly and causes a generalized increase in the thickness of the skin and subcutaneous tissues of the hand. It is indistinguishable radiographically from the infiltration of the skin by edema and fibrous tissue in idiopathic osteoarthropathy (pachydermoperiostosis). Hence, other parameters than soft tissue must be evaluated to distinguish the two entities (see Chapter 3).

Acromegaly. By comparison with the normal hand, the slight generalized increase of soft tissue in a woman with acromegaly (Fig. 1–2) is subtle but real. The prominent convex bulge of the interdigital webs (arrow), which normally cast a concave shadow, is suggestive of an increase in soft tissue of the palm. The muscles of the thenar and hypothenar compartments extend further beyond the margins of the first and fifth metacarpals than normal, again suggesting an increase in bulk. These minor soft tissue findings are critical to the diagnosis of acromegaly in this patient, since there are no other supportive radiographic changes in the bones or cartilage space. The difficulty in detecting diffuse change becomes apparent by this example. No part of either hand can be used as a "normal" base line. Nevertheless, it is at this stage that one hopes to detect the disease, and the combination of soft tissue changes all point to a pathologic condition.

EDEMA

Diffuse increase in soft tissues of the hand may be seen with a systemic disease (myxedema; cardiac, renal or hepa-

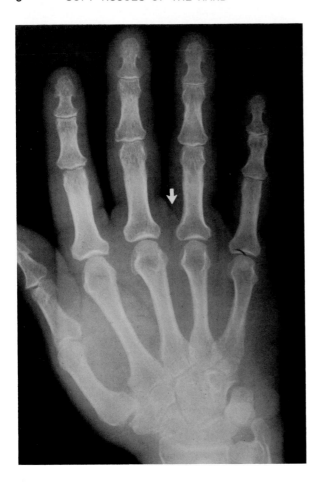

Figure 1-2. Acromegaly.
The overall increase in soft tissue is most easily seen in the palm, as in this patient. Its bulging contour and the fullness of the interdigital webbing (arrow) are striking only when compared to a normal hand.

tic impairment; lymphoreticulosis and malignancy) or localized venous or lymphatic occlusion. Reflex sympathetic dystrophies (Sudeck's atrophy or the shoulder-hand syndrome) and neuropathic disorders may also cause chronic edema. The most common cause of a neuropathic disorder of the hand is syringomyelia. Edema is often a prominent feature of this disorder and may relate to neurovascular instability. The soft tissue enlargement may be contributed to by a superimposed cellulitis which frequently complicates neuropathic joints. Transient edema is commonly seen following a cerebrovascular accident but, although it is bothersome to the personnel responsible for intravenous feedings it is rarely brought to the attention of the radiologist.

Syringomyelia. The earliest change observable in a hand involved by syringomyelia is soft tissue edema. This is demonstrated in Figure 1-3A. The massive distention of the soft tissue is easily recognizable, causing an increase in the bulk of the hand. As in the preceding example, the interdigital webbing is distended and convex in appearance. The most objective and easily evaluated area of abnormality is the soft tissue adjacent to the radius and the ulna, which is swollen to more than twice its normal thickness. The diffuse swelling is even more apparent on the lateral projection (Fig. 1-3B).

GENERALIZED DECREASE IN SOFT TISSUE

Generalized decrease in soft tissues occurs in the presence of muscle atrophy accompanying a variety of diseases. Among the most common causes are rheu-

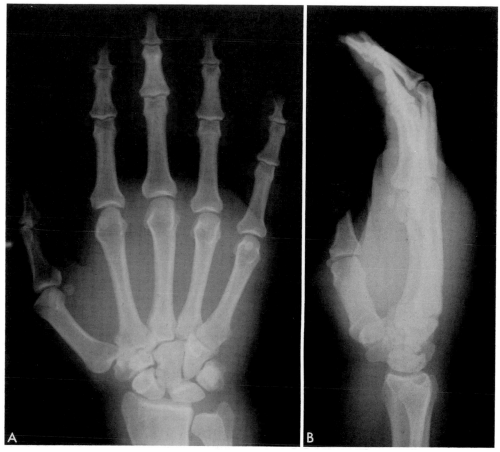

Figure 1–3. Syringomyelia.

   A. Chronic edema characterizes neuropathic conditions, distending the soft tissues diffusely. The generalized increase is best appreciated adjacent to the ulnar styloid process and between the fingers.

   B. The soft tissue increase is much more apparent on the lateral view.

matoid arthritis, dermatomyositis, systemic lupus erythematosus and disuse from muscle or neurologic abnormalities.

   Systemic Lupus Erythematosus. The radiographic appearance of diffuse loss of soft tissue is illustrated by a film of a patient with systemic lupus erythematosus (Fig. 1–4). In this case the muscle loss is so extensive that the lateral borders of the thenar and hypothenar compartments have a concave configuration rather than the normal sloping convex shadow. Other changes frequently seen in the hands of patients with systemic lupus erythematosus are present in this example: hyperextension of the interphalangeal joint

of the thumb and diffuse osteoporosis of the bones. This combination of radiographic findings is so commonly seen in patients with this disease that the film is almost pathognomonic, and will be discussed in more detail in the next two chapters.

LOCALIZED INCREASE IN SOFT TISSUE

   Soft tissue changes that are diffuse and that involve both hands often escape diagnosis until the pathologic condition is extensive. In contrast, a localized ab-

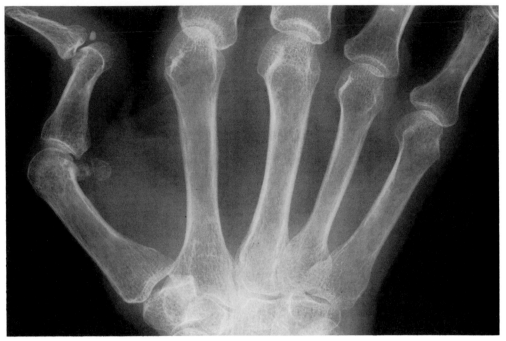

Figure 1–4. Systemic lupus erythematosus.
Soft tissue wasting has altered the normal convexity of the palm. The muscles cast a concave shadow adjacent to the first and fifth metacarpal bones. Diffuse bony demineralization and hyperextension of the interphalangeal joint of the thumb accompany the soft tissue wasting. These changes, and the absence of erosions and cartilage destruction, typify the radiographic picture of lupus.

normality is easily detected very early in the course of a disease, as illustrated by the following examples.

TENDONS, CAPSULES AND BURSAE

Localized inflammation of tendon sheaths, joint capsules and bursae appear *clinically* as swelling. *Radiographically,* swelling manifests itself as a shadow of either increased *density* or increased *width.*

Tenosynovitis. In the patient whose wrists are seen in Figure 1–5, acute onset of pain over the radial styloid process of the right wrist followed an abnormally long session of guitar strumming. The classical "crunch" of De Quervain's tenosynovitis could be detected with a stethoscope. Although films are superfluous when the findings are so typical, they illustrate the ease with which minor localized abnormalities may be detected. The normal width of soft tissue along the radial aspect of the wrist is established

when the opposite hand is filmed (Fig. 1–5A). This demonstrates the sharp delineation of the tissue planes by a black line of fat as well as the normal width of the soft tissue adjacent to the radial styloid process. The inflamed tendon sheath, which contains the extensor pollicis brevis and the abductor pollicis longus tendons, casts a wider shadow in the abnormal wrist (Fig. 1–5B). In addition, tissue planes have been obliterated by the adjacent inflammatory process, and the soft tissues appear as a homogeneous gray shadow.

Rheumatoid Arthritis. The earliest pathologic changes in rheumatoid arthritis are hyperemia and edema of the synovium caused by perivascular inflammation. The inflammatory process results in an effusion within the joint capsule, producing the soft tissue changes of periarticular swelling. Until the subsequent development of pannus leads to secondary erosions in the underlying bone and cartilage destruction, the soft tissue swelling may be the only observable abnormality.

The earliest radiographic manifestations of rheumatoid arthritis in a 25 year old woman are demonstrated in the first film taken following the onset of symptoms of joint pain. The abnormalities are confined to the soft tissues (Fig. 1–6). Swelling adjacent to the ulnar styloid process and distention of the proximal interphalangeal joint capsules are easily detected because they alter the contour of the hand. In the same way, bulging of the second and fifth metacarpophalangeal periarticular soft tissues represents effusion within these capsules. It is far more difficult to detect a similar degree of swelling in the third and fourth metacarpophalangeal joints because the fluid does not distort the outline of the hand. However, these joints are just as severely involved, and the localized increase in soft tissue *density* from the distended capsules casts a definite convex shadow around the joints. This abnormality of soft tissue density is best seen along the ulnar sides of the second, third and fourth metacarpophalangeal joints. Although more subtle than distortion of the *contour* of the hand, the increase in density must be sought in order to assess accurately the distribution of the inflammatory involvement. The usual sites of involvement in rheumatoid arthritis are the wrist, the metacarpophalangeal joints and the proximal interphalangeal joints. The distal interphalangeal joints are generally spared. Recognition of the *pattern of involvement* in this patient enables one to make a tentative diagnosis of rheumatoid arthritis despite the lack of specificity of the pathologic changes on the film.

Monarticular Effusion. Although rheumatoid arthritis tends to involve both hands symmetrically, and all the metacarpophalangeal or proximal interphalangeal joints simultaneously, it is not uncommon for inflammation of the second or third metacarpophalangeal joint to be the initial manifestation of the disease. Eventually, the remainder of the metacarpophalangeal joints may become involved, and the classical symmetry associated with this connective tissue disorder will become apparent in the chronic stage.

This early finding is present in a second young woman with rheumatoid arthritis (Fig. 1–7). When compared to the adjacent finger, capsular distension of the second metacarpophalangeal joint is more obvious, and the spherical increase in tissue density becomes apparent.

Many diseases cause fleeting arthralgias in the hand which are mild and self-limiting. The majority of films taken will be normal. Occasionally a transient capsular distention looking identical to that of Figure 1–7 will be captured. Several gastrointestinal disorders have associated arthralgias: Whipple's disease, ulcerative colitis, Crohn's disease and Henoch-Schönlein purpura. Patients whose small bowel has been bypassed as a treatment for obesity may develop severe arthritis that necessitates therapy with adrenocorticosteroids, yet the film may reveal nothing more than fleeting effusions. One-quarter of patients with sarcoidosis will have pain and swelling of the peripheral joints which disappear spontaneously within several weeks. Any rheumatoid disease early in its course may have radiographic findings that are minimal as compared with the severity of symptoms. This is particularly true of rheumatoid arthritis and systemic lupus erythematosus. Other rheumatic diseases infrequently accompanied by small joint changes, such as ankylosing spondylitis and polymyalgia rheumatica, may occasionally have capsular effusions similar to those shown in Figure 1–7.

Bursae as well as joint capsules are lined with synovium, and edema and pannus formation occur in these areas. The bursa adjacent to the ulnar styloid process is a frequent site of inflammation in rheumatoid arthritis; this is often the only manifestation of a pathologic condition on a hand film taken early in the course of the disease.

Dramatic enlargement of the synovium within the ulnar styloid bursa is seen in Figure 1–8. There is nothing sufficiently characteristic about the soft tissue mass to allow a pathologic diagnosis from the film, but knowledge of the anatomy and

Text continued on page 14

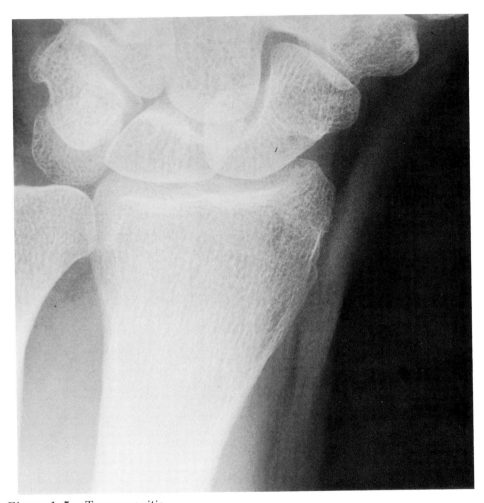

Figure 1–5. Tenosynovitis.
A. Normally a thin layer of soft tissue hugs the radial styloid process and is delineated by a sharp black line of fat.

Illustration continued on opposite page.

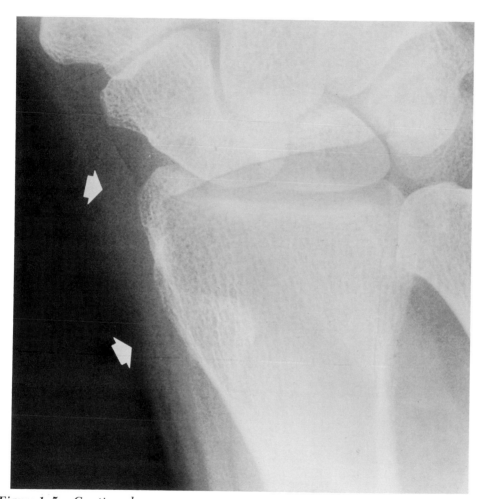

Figure 1–5. Continued.
  B. Acute swelling of the sheath containing the extensor pollicis brevis and abductor pollicis longus tendons occurred after a prolonged guitar playing session. The subtle increase in soft tissue and the obliteration of tissue planes (arrows) are more easily recognized when the normal wrist is available for comparison.

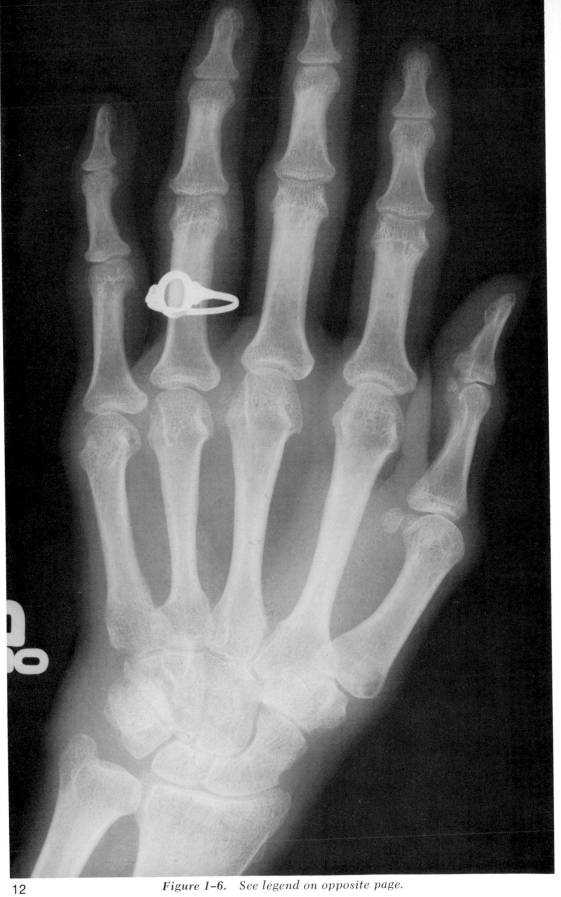

12 *Figure 1-6.* See legend on opposite page.

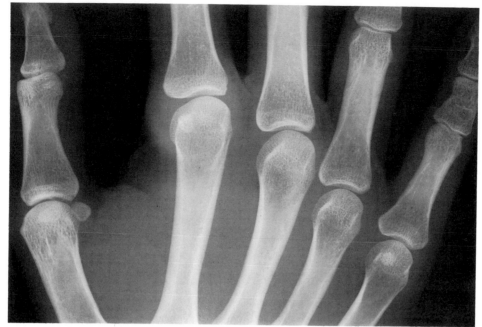

Figure 1–7. Rheumatoid arthritis.
Localized periarticular swelling of the second metacarpophalangeal joint is detectable because of the increased *density* of the image cast by the fluid-filled capsule. Inflammation frequently begins in the second and third metacarpophalangeal joints in rheumatoid arthritis, and asymmetric involvement is not uncommon *early* in the course of this disease.

Figure 1–6. Rheumatoid arthritis.
A specific arthritis may be suggested by the pattern of involvement alone. Periarticular swelling adjacent to the ulnar styloid process and involving all of the metacarpophalangeal and proximal interphalangeal joints with sparing of the distal interphalangeal joints is typical of rheumatoid arthritis. Capsular distension is an early manifestation of inflammation, and it is therefore not surprising to find normal bony mineralization and absence of erosive changes.

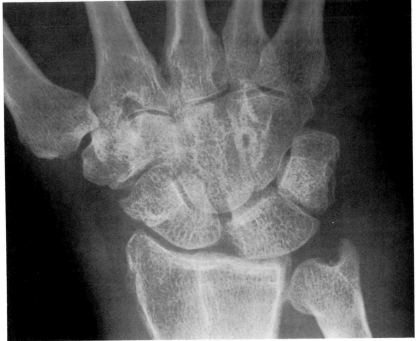

Figure 1–8. Rheumatoid arthritis.
Massive synovial hypertrophy casts a bulky shadow adjacent to the ulnar styloid process. In the absence of ulnar styloid erosion and uniform cartilage loss, two frequent changes in rheumatoid arthritis of the wrist, a specific diagnosis based solely on this soft tissue change is impossible. Any cause of synovial inflammation could result in an identical finding.

the pathologic changes associated with rheumatoid arthritis permits an educated guess as to what this water density mass might be.

Massive proliferation of the synovium is commonly seen in rheumatoid arthritis but is present in many other diseases as well. For example, fungal infections, tuberculosis, hemophilia and villonodular synovitis cause pathologic changes in the synovium. Hence, any of these diseases may result in localized swelling of synovium-lined bursae or joint capsules and secondary erosions of the underlying bones. Knowledge of the course and duration of the swelling, its pattern of distribution and its correlation with history and physical findings is essential to correctly diagnose the nonspecific radiographic finding of hypertrophied synovium.

Gout. Two types of localized increase in soft tissue occur in gouty arthritis: the first is an acute effusion or synovial proliferation within the joint capsule; the second is the formation of tophi in and around the joints.

Capsular distension from *any* inflammatory stimulus will result in periarticular soft tissue swelling. In gout, the inflammatory process is initiated by precipitated urate crystals resulting in an outpouring of fluid.

The fusiform swelling of the soft tissue surrounding the proximal interphalangeal joints of a patient with acute gout (Fig. 1–9) is much more extensive than that usually found in rheumatoid arthritis and involves swelling of the subcutaneous tissues as well as the capsule. This produces a change in the contour of the fingers. Since fluid distends the capsule uniformly, the distortion of the soft tissues is symmetrical on both sides of the finger.

Contrast this appearance with the soft

tissue changes at the distal interphalangeal joint of the middle finger. All of the periarticular swelling is on the radial side of the finger. This eccentricity indicates the presence of a subcutaneous tophus in this patient with gout.

SOFT TISSUE MASSES

Subcutaneous nodules are associated with rheumatoid arthritis and, less commonly, with other rheumatic diseases such as rheumatic fever, systemic lupus erythematosus and necrotizing arteritis. Soft tissue masses may accompany granulomatous diseases such as tuberculosis (cold abscess), sarcoidosis and leprosy. Gouty tophi, neurofibromas and mucoid cysts associated with primary osteoarthritis are three entities that must be considered when soft tissue masses are associated with bone and joint abnormalities. Tendon sheath xanthomas that accompany Type II hypercholesterolemia

and the histologically indistinguishable villonodular synovitis may appear as prominent periarticular masses and cause pressure erosions of the adjacent bone.

Tendon Sheath Xanthoma. The bulky soft tissue mass of a tendon sheath xanthoma (Fig. 1–10) distorts the normal silhouette of the finger. The underlying bone changes in the proximal phalanx attest to the chronicity of the mass. The destruction is caused by *pressure* from the juxtaposed xanthoma, with gradual resorption of the cortex forming a saucerlike defect.

Bony erosion produced by pressure from a long-standing overlying mass is a frequent occurrence and is not a diagnostic feature of a specific disease. It is commonly seen in assocation with gouty tophi. Destruction of bone is also characteristic of malignant soft tissue tumors that have invaded the adjacent bone.

Figure 1–9. Acute gout. Fusiform swelling of the proximal interphalangeal joints indicates massive capsular distension. The eccentric soft tissue mass adjacent to the distal interphalangeal joint of the middle finger (arrow) represents a tophaceous deposit. (Pure monosodium urate crystals are radiographically of water density). Marginal erosions alter the shape of the proximal phalanges. The flangelike projections of bone along the second and fourth proximal phalanges represent periosteal new bone, a radiographic finding occasionally seen in gout but more typical of the connective tissue disorders.

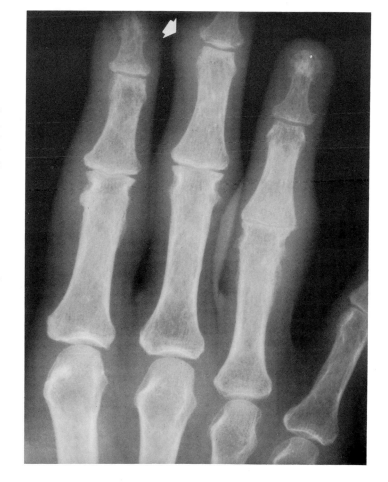

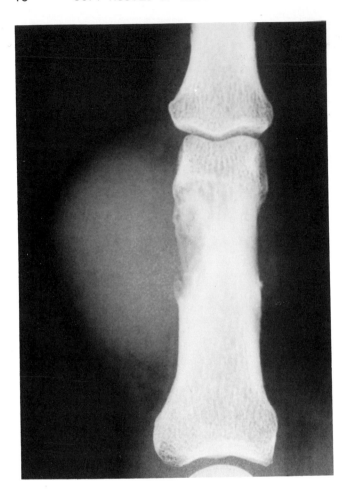

Figure 1–10. Tendon sheath xanthoma.

A localized soft tissue mass has produced a saucerlike pressure erosion of the adjacent bone. Any mass may cause a similar radiographic picture, and underlying bone erosion does not imply a malignant process.

Biopsy often may be the only definitive diagnostic procedure to distinguish among the vast spectrum of disease possibilities that range from benign to malignant and from local to systemic disorders.

Hypertrophic Osteoarthropathy. Clubbing of the fingers and symptoms of arthritis may accompany lung disease and, less commonly, gastrointestinal and liver abnormalities.

The bulbous configuration of the ends of the fingers is obvious in a patient with lung carcinoma (Fig. 1–11). Early bone changes accompany the soft tissue alterations and are typically seen in hypertrophic osteoarthropathy. The distal phalangeal tufts are beginning to resorb from the pressure of the proliferated soft tissue. This finding will be discussed in detail in Chapter 3.

Idiopathic Osteoarthropathy. A simi-lar increase in soft tissues is seen in the familial condition of idiopathic osteoarthropathy (pachydermoperiostosis). The elephant-like thickening of the skin is not limited to the distal portion of the finger but diffusely distorts the soft tissues of the entire digit (Fig. 1–12).

The shadows overlying the proximal interphalangeal joint bear further discussion. The redundant skin of the knuckle is frequently seen in films of normal hands if the soft tissue technique is excellent (see Figure 1–1) and must not be interpreted as a joint effusion. Exaggerated knuckle pads, as in Figure 1–12, may be the hallmark of a generalized infiltrative or proliferative condition such as pachydermoperiostosis or acromegaly. In addition, this condition is not infrequently associated with Dupuytren's contracture, and both findings may flag

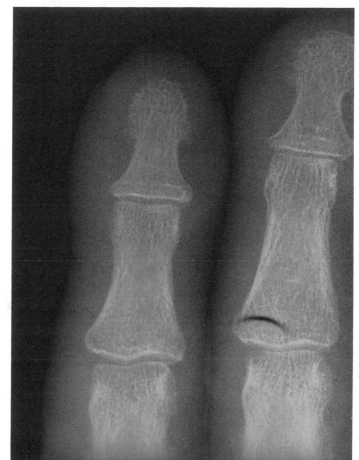

Figure 1–11. Hypertrophic osteoarthropathy.

Bulbous swelling of the tips of the fingers (clubbing) in a patient with an underlying lung tumor is easily detected on a film. Resorption of the terminal tufts seems to be related to the increased bulk of soft tissue and increased blood flow.

an unsuspected alcoholic. Exaggerated knuckle pads have been reported to accompany seizure disorders and a form of hereditary deafness. Although knuckle pad prominence may herald an underlying disease, it may also signify nothing more than an ex-marble champion.

SUBUNGUAL HYPERKERATOSIS

In addition to skin and subcutaneous abnormalities, nail changes may be captured on a radiograph. Subungual hyperkeratosis suggests a specific diagnosis in what might otherwise appear as a nonspecific arthritis: it is present in two disease conditions, psoriatic arthritis and Reiter's syndrome, and allows them to be differentiated from the frequently indistinguishable pattern of joint changes in rheumatoid arthritis. Radiographically, subungual hyperkeratosis is seen on a tangential projection of the nail as thickening and deformity of its base.

Psoriatic Arthritis. The thickened and deformed nails demonstrated in a patient with long-standing psoriatic arthritis (Fig. 1–13) represent the pathologic changes of onycholysis, onychophosis and subungual hyperkeratosis. Identical pathologic and radiographic changes of the nails are present in Reiter's syndrome, a condition which often has the clinical picture of psoriatic arthropathy. Even the skin lesions of Reiter's syndrome, keratodermia blenorrhagica, are often grossly and histologically indistinguishable from pustular psoriasis. Thus, although the presence of nail changes enables the radiologist and clinician to distinguish these two diseases from other arthritides, it provides no advantage in

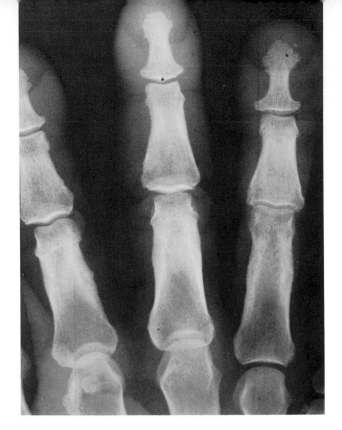

Figure 1–12. Idiopathic osteo-arthropathy.

Elephant-like thickening of the skin has caused clubbing of the distal fingers and exaggerated knuckle pads in addition to generalized increase in the bulk of soft tissue surrounding the phalangeal bones. Loss of the tufts accompanies the increase in overlying soft tissue.

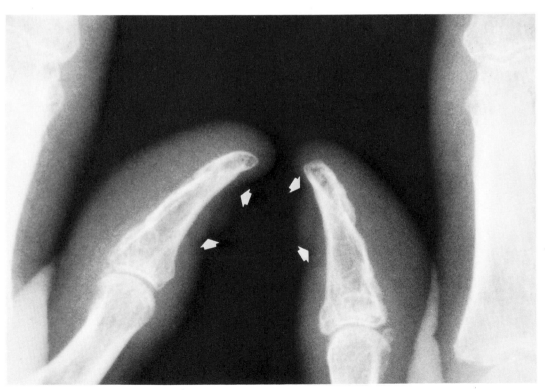

Figure 1–13. Psoriatic arthritis.

Subungual hyperkeratosis causes heaping up of the nail bed, as seen on both thumbs. Normally the nail casts a smooth, thin convex shadow over the tangentially viewed thumbs.

solving the diagnostic dilemma that frequently occurs between Reiter's syndrome and psoriatic arthritis.

LOCALIZED DECREASE IN SOFT TISSUE

Although localized soft tissue loss is most frequently associated with trauma, it may be seen in such rheumatic disorders as progressive systemic sclerosis

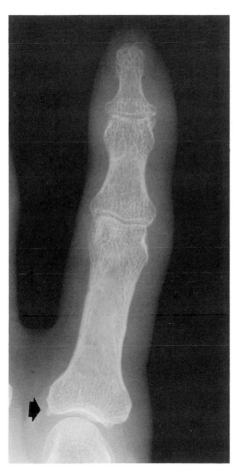

Figure 1–14. Progressive systemic sclerosis.

Tapering of the tip of the finger and concavity of the soft tissues adjacent to the middle phalanx indicate soft tissue atrophy. A fleck of amorphous calcium is seen at the metacarpophalangeal joint (arrow). Subcutaneous calcification should be searched for, as it is important substantiating evidence when a diagnosis of scleroderma is entertained.

(scleroderma), Raynaud's disease and accompanying resorptive arthropathies caused by such diverse entities as rheumatoid arthritis, psoriatic arthritis and neuropathic disorders.

Progressive Systemic Sclerosis. Atrophy and "tightening" of the skin are prominent features of progressive systemic sclerosis and can often be seen radiographically. The characteristic tapered appearance of the index finger of a patient with scleroderma is illustrated in Figure 1–14. Further evidence of the atrophic changes of sclerodactyly are manifested by loss of the normal redundant folds of the knuckle pads and a concave contour of the finger along the shaft of the middle phalanx.

SOFT TISSUE CALCIFIC DEPOSITS

In addition to quantitative changes in soft tissue, the presence, location and character of abnormal calcific deposits offer important information for diagnosing specific arthritides. Knowledge of normal anatomy permits localization of the calcium to the subcutaneous tissue, muscle, blood vessels, joint capsules, tendon sheaths or cartilage.

SUBCUTANEOUS TISSUE CALCIFICATION

Deposition of calcium in the subcutaneous tissues may indicate a systemic disorder such as progressive systemic sclerosis, hypervitaminosis D, hypoparathyroidism or pseudohypoparathyroidism; it also occurs in association with the abnormal elasticity of subcutaneous tissues in Ehlers-Danlos syndrome. The presence of soft tissue calcification may likewise signify local trauma, in areas of fat necrosis following frostbite or at sites of hemorrhage.

Progressive Systemic Sclerosis. Extensive amorphous calcific deposits are practically pathognomonic of progressive systemic sclerosis when they are located in the subcutaneous tissues, since the other disease conditions that are associated with this finding are so rare by contrast. In a patient with this disorder the bulky calcified mass that fills the ra-

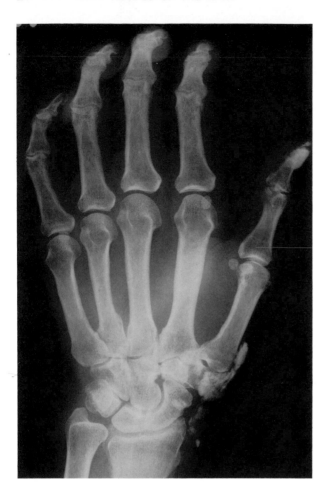

Figure 1–15. Progressive systemic sclerosis.

Amorphous deposits of calcium in the subcutaneous tissues are seen along the radial side of the wrist and have eroded the distal phalanx of the thumb. The fingers are flexed, reflecting the tightening of the skin. Extensive calcium deposits and flexion deformities, in association with normal joints, are characteristic of scleroderma.

dial side of the wrist and the amorphous calcified mass at the distal thumb that has eroded away half of the adjacent bone are large enough to be palpable clinically, but their calcium content must be detected by the radiograph (Fig. 1–15). Since the presence of subcutaneous calcification is substantiating evidence in the diagnosis of a clinically suspected case of scleroderma, the importance of a thorough inspection of the soft tissues is underlined. Referring back to the pre-

vious illustration of progressive systemic sclerosis (Fig. 1–14), one notes that a similar amorphous collection, almost hidden by the edge of the proximal phalanx, is present adjacent to the metacarpophalangeal joint. Such a calcium deposit reflects the pathologic change in the subcutaneous tissues; it may be present early in the disease and, if detected on a film, is a strong diagnostic sign of scleroderma.

Subcutaneous calcifications should not

Figure 1–16. CRST syndrome.

Three of the four components of the CRST syndrome are present in this hand, but only the soft tissue wasting of sclerodactyly and the extensive calcification within capsules and tendon sheaths are visualized on this reproduction. It is unusual to see such extensive deposition of calcium; this film offers an excellent opportunity to study the anatomy of the tendons and joint spaces of the hand.

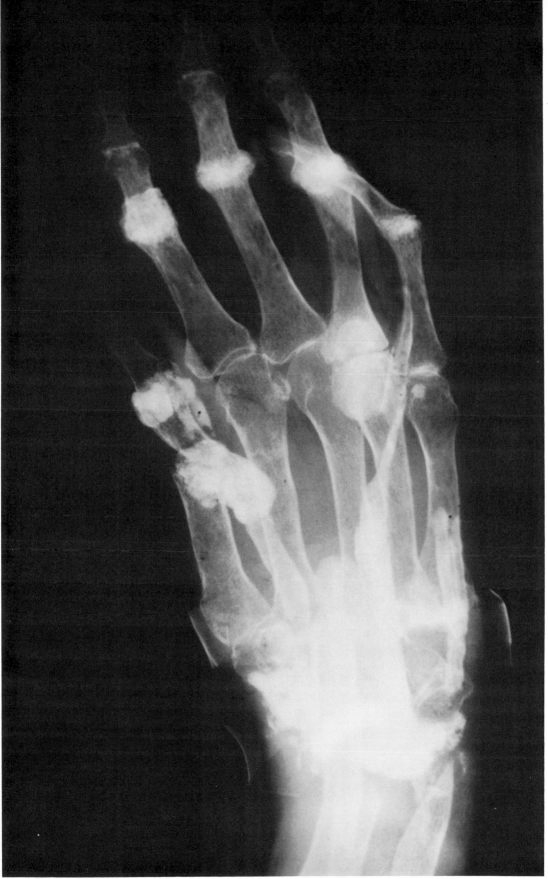

Figure 1–16. *See legend on opposite page.*

21

be confused with identical-appearing flecks of calcium at the periphery of joints. These dystrophic calcium deposits are indicative of degenerating cartilage with subsequent deposition of calcium. The importance of correctly pinpointing the position of a calcium deposit cannot be overemphasized, as it is often an important clue to a specific arthritis.

CAPSULAR CALCIFICATION

When calcium is present in the area of the capsule, it is important to distinguish free calcific deposits from calcified cartilage because the diagnostic possibilities are completely different. Small flecks of calcium within a joint capsule may indicate degenerative cartilage from any of several causes. Massive deposits of calcium are extracartilaginous and are most frequently associated with gout and renal failure. Occasionally extensive calcium deposits are seen in the joint capsules of patients with the CRST syndrome.

CRST Syndrome. The CRST syndrome is a variant of progressive systemic sclerosis that is characterized by the tetrad of calcinosis cutis; Raynaud's phenomenon, sclerodactyly and telangiectasia. Figure 1–16 illustrates the soft tissue wasting and calcinosis; in addition, Raynaud's phenomenon was clinically apparent in this hand.

The calcific deposits demarcate two anatomic compartments of the hand, the capsules and the tendons. Extensive deposits outline many of the metacarpophalangeal and interphalangeal joints as well as the radiocarpal and intercarpal joints of the wrist. The tubular calcification superimposed on the distal radius, the wrist and the metacarpal bones represents peritendinous deposits of calcium within the tendon sheath. Their extensive calcification offers an unusual opportunity to study the anatomic configuration and relation of tendons to the bones.

Gout. Large deposits of monosodium urate distort the soft tissues but cast no denser shadow than a collection of fluid (see Figure 1–9). Frequently, however, calcium is present in gouty tophi as calcium urate. Where this occurs, the nonspecific water density appearance of a soft tissue mass is converted to a readily recognizable sign suggestive of gout, as in Figure 1–17. The amorphous calcium deposits are intracapsular; they are thus easily distinguished from the subcutaneous calcification of scleroderma. In this patient (Fig. 1–17) they deform the capsules of the metacarpophalangeal joints asymmetrically. A gouty tophus may form in the subcutaneous tissues as well as in the capsule. When this occurs, the appearance of the tissues may resemble that in scleroderma; by the time calcification is present within a tophus, however, the clinical and radiographic evidence of gout is apparent and the two disease conditions are not likely to be confused.

Calcific Periarthritis. Rarely, a patient develops a red-hot joint, and when a film of the hand is obtained, calcium is revealed within the distended joint capsule. The condition is short-lived, the calcium disappears spontaneously, and there is no apparent renal or metabolic disorder to account for the deposition of calcium.

With the increasing use of renal dialysis, this entity, calcific periarthritis, is seen more frequently and has taken on a new importance. Its pattern of precipitation has characteristic features. *Clinically,* a patient experiences severe pain following dialysis. *Radiographically,* periarticular deposits of calcium appear. The sudden change in tissue pH following dialysis is great enough to cause precipitation of calcium in this relatively alkaline medium. Crys-

Figure 1–17. Chronic tophaceous gout.
Calcium deposited in tophi cast dense shadows within the capsules of the third, fourth and fifth metacarpophalangeal joints and adjacent to the distal phalanx of the thumb. The calcification is less dense than that deposited in the soft tissues of patients with progressive systemic sclerosis and can usually be distinguished easily on a radiograph.

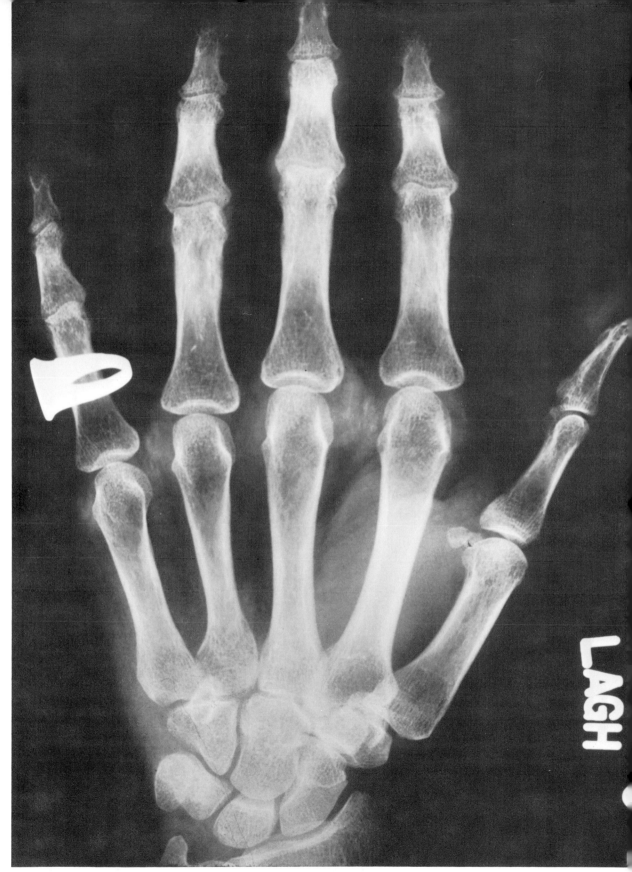

Figure 1–17. See legend on opposite page.

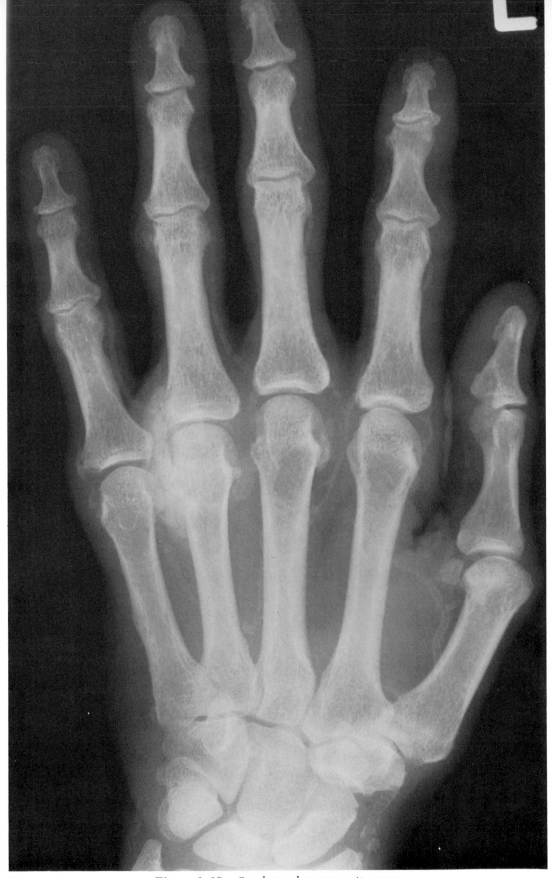

Figure 1-18. See legend on opposite page.

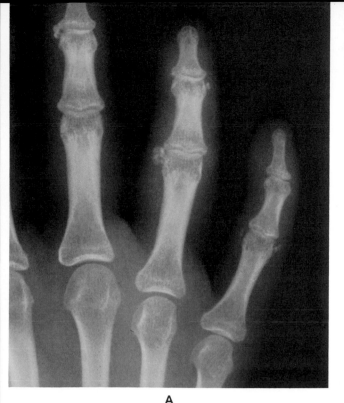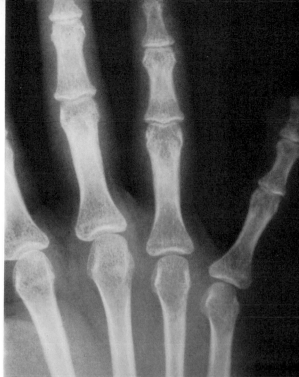

A   **B**

Figure 1–19. Calcific periarthritis.
  A. Calcific deposits and joint effusions are present in multiple joint capsules in a patient on chronic renal dialysis.
  B. Reversibility of the calcium deposits is documented by a film 10 months later and attests to the effectiveness of medical therapy.

tals initiate an outpouring of fluid in the synovium-lined capsule. A film of the affected joint will demonstrate the distention of the capsule from fluid as well as the increased density of calcium deposits.

Figure 1–18 demonstrates the similarity in appearance of these calcific deposits to that of the preceding example of gout. Large amorphous calcium collections distort the capsules of the fourth metacarpophalangeal joint and, less dramatically, the third metacarpophalangeal and fourth proximal interphalangeal joints. Aspiration is the only definitive procedure to distinguish the calcium hydroxyapatite crystals from tophaceous material; it is often made necessary by the fact that patients with renal failure frequently have elevated uric acid levels and a propensity to develop a gouty arthropathy. Since the treatment of these conditions differs, it is an important distinction to make.

Films of a second patient with calcific periarthritis demonstrate the reversi-

Figure 1–18. Calcific periarthritis.
  Although the distribution of inflammatory changes at the metacarpophalangeal and proximal interphalangeal joints is identical to the *pattern* of rheumatoid arthritis, the presence of calcium within the joint capsules excludes this diagnosis. Deposition of calcium occurs in hyperparathyroidism associated with renal failure and in chronic tophaceous gout. Only examination of the crystals differentiates these two conditions. Extensive vascular calcification is present in the radial and digital arteries.

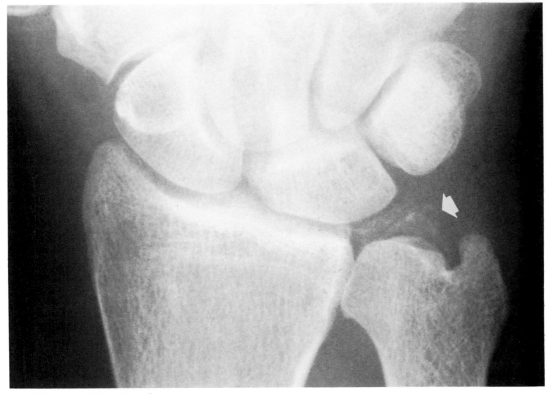

Figure 1–20. Pseudogout.
Calcified cartilage (chondrocalcinosis) in the absence of erosions and joint space narrowing is most frequently seen with pseudogout and hyperparathyroidism. In the wrist, the most common cartilage involved is the triangular fibrocartilage between the ulna and the proximal row of carpal bones (arrow).

bility of the calcific deposits with medical treatment and thus emphasize the importance of their early detection. The first film (Fig. 1–19A) reveals periarticular swelling and calcific deposits in multiple joints. A film taken 10 months later (Fig. 1–19B) is normal. The joint effusions are no longer present and the calcium has disappeared. Since calcium levels are often normal in patients with renal failure and phosphate levels are enormously elevated, resorption of the capsular deposits may be induced by decreasing the blood phosphate. Unfortunately, calcium deposited in the other areas of the body—the kidneys, arteries, lungs, heart and stomach wall—is irreversibly maintained.

CARTILAGE

The condition in which calcium is deposited in cartilage is called chondrocal-cinosis (*chondro*, "cartilage;" *calcinosis*, "calcium deposition"). This is a purely descriptive term and does not imply a specific disease process, although it is sometimes erroneously equated with pseudogout. The presence of chondrocalcinosis accompanies many arthritides. Most frequently it is seen in association with hyperparathyroidism, pseudogout and osteoarthritis. Less commonly it is present in patients with rheumatoid arthritis, gout, hemochromatosis and diabetes. It is always present in patients with ochronosis, but this is a rare disease and is not a diagnostic consideration in the usual patient with chondrocalcinosis.

Because chondrocalcinosis occurs in many arthritides, the finding of calcification in the cartilage is helpful in making a specific diagnosis only if the physician has noted the company it keeps. By following the method of approach of the ABC'S, significant clues to the diagnosis are not overlooked, and the presence of chondrocalcinosis becomes the keystone in diagnosis.

Pseudogout. As suggested by the name, the clinical manifestation of pseudogout mimics gout, joint pain and swelling being the prominent components. Although cystic changes occasionally are seen in the carpal bones and metacarpal heads in patients with pseudogout, generally the *isolated* finding of chondrocalcinosis signifies the presence of either pseudogout or hyperparathyroidism.

Figure 1–20, a film of the hand of a patient with pseudogout, illustrates the appearance of calcium deposited in cartilage. The faint shadow over the ulnar styloid process represents calcium within the fibrous triangular cartilage of the wrist (arrow). This is the most frequently calcified cartilage in the hand. Occasionally the hyaline cartilage between the first metacarpal and the greater multangular bone is also involved by this pathologic process.

SUGGESTED READINGS

Caner, J., and J. L. Decker. Recurrent acute (?gouty) arthritis in chronic renal failure treated with periodic hemodialysis. Amer. J. Med. *36*:571 (1964).

Caughey, D. E., and E. G. L. Bywaters. The arthritis of Whipple's syndrome. Ann. Rheum. Dis. *22*:327 (1963).

Dodds, N. J., and H. L. Steinbach. Gout associated with calcification of cartilage. New Eng. J. Med. *275*:745 (1966).

Dorfman, H. D., A Norman, and R. J. Smith. Bone erosion in relation to subcutaneous rheumatoid nodules. Arthritis Rheum. *13*:69 (1970).

Dymock, I. W., E. B. D. Hamilton, J. W. Laws, and R. Williams. Arthropathy of haemochromatosis: Clinical and radiological analysis of 63 patients with iron overload. Ann. Rheum. Dis. *29*:469 (1970).

Hayes, T. Lupus and calcinosis. Arch. Derm. (Chicago) *100*:17 (1969).

Hunder, G. G., T. F. Disney, and L. E. Ward. Polymyalgia rheumatica. Mayo Clin. Proc. *44*:849 (1969).

Johnson, C., C. B. Graham, and F. K. Curtis. Roentgenographic manifestations of chronic renal disease treated by periodic hemodialysis. Amer. J. Roentgen. *101*:915 (1957).

McCarty, D. J. On the crystal deposition diseases. Disease-A-Month (Chicago), March 1970.

Moskowitz, R. W., B. K. Harris, A. Schwartz, and G. Marshall. Chronic synovitis as a manifestation of calcium crystal deposition disease. Arthritis Rheum. *14*:109 (1971).

Moskowitz, R. W., and D. Katz. Chondrocalcinosis and chondrocalsynovitis. Amer. J. Med. *43*:322 (1967).

Swannell, A. J., F. A. Underwood, and A. St. J. Dixon. Periarticular calcific deposits mimicking acute arthritis. Ann. Rheum. Dis. *29*:380

Thompson, G. R., Y. Ming Ting, G. A. Riggs, M. E. Fenn, and R. M. Dennings. Calcific tendinitis and soft tissue calcification resembling gout. JAMA *203*:464 (1968).

Weston, W. J. De Quervain's disease—stenosing fibrous tendovaginitis at the radial styloid process. Brit. J. Radiol. *40*:446 (1967).

Williams, K. A., and J. T. Scott. Influence of trauma on the development of chronic inflammatory polyarthritis. Ann. Rheum. Dis. *26*:532 (1967).

Winterbauer, R. Multiple telangiectasia, Raynaud's phenomenon, sclerodactyly and subcutaneous calcinosis: A syndrome mimicking hereditary hemorrhagic telangiectasia. Bull. Johns Hopkins Hosp. *114*:361 (1964).

Chapter 2

ALIGNMENT ABNORMALITIES OF THE HAND

Abnormalities of joints may produce deviations in the spatial relationship of bones and can be detected by alterations in alignment. Standard projections of the hand are made in the prone, oblique and lateral views, and the fingers are carefully positioned by the technician. On viewing a film, it must be assumed that the part was correctly positioned. Hence, any deviation from the normal alignment of bone on a standard projection suggests limitation of motion or abnormal fixation of the joints.

Alteration in joint kinetics resulting in malalignment may be caused by disease of the cartilage, changes in the articulating ends of the bones, alterations in the joint capsule and ligaments or imbalance of the action of opposing muscles and tendons. Such deformities produce overlapping of bones or abnormal angulation, and additional projections to view the changes in three dimensions are often necessary to detect the precise abnormality.

Abnormalities of alignment can be grouped into four categories: flexion, hyperextension, deviation and subluxation. Characteristic patterns of change are associated with different arthritides: the importance of their detection is apparent.

FLEXION DEFORMITIES

Psoriatic Arthritis. Figure 2–1 illustrates obvious deformities of the fingers. At first glance, the question of an actual amputation of the index finger might be raised. However, by comparing the shadows of each of the four digits, the peculiar appearance of the index finger is explained. As each finger is positioned, a greater tendency toward an oblique projection occurs, becoming most exaggerated at the fifth finger. By virtue of this positioning phenomenon, the oblique projection of the fourth and fifth fingers unravels the peculiar shadows surrounding the distal second and third. The increased mass and *apparent loss* of the distal phalanges are in fact due to severe flexion deformities similar to those present in the fourth and fifth fingers. The "amputation" is only a visual distortion.

Dupuytren's Contracture. A more subtle example of flexion deformity is illustrated by a patient who developed Dupuytren's contracture (Fig. 2–2A). The dense shadow of the fifth finger is similar to those of the overlapping structures in the preceding examples. Its severity is evident from the disparity in height between this finger and the rest. Although the most dramatic radiographic finding is limited to the severe alignment abnormality of the fifth finger, the minor changes in the remaining fingers are important to recognize in order to establish the true *pattern* of the deformity. Although there may be many causes of an isolated flexion contracture, progressive deformity of the fingers with maximum flexion of the fifth finger is typical of the changes caused by Dupuytren's contrac-

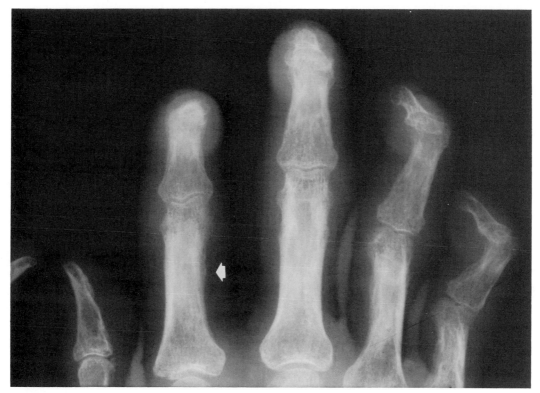

Figure 2–1. Psoriatic arthritis.

Foreshortening of the second and third fingers is due to severe flexion deformities rather than amputation as seen by the *increased soft tissue* density distally. The oblique projection of the fourth and fifth finger clearly defines the alignment abnormalities of all the fingers. Irregularity of the soft tissues over the fourth distal phalanx represents subungual hyperkeratosis with deformity of the nail. In addition to nail changes and flexion deformities, juxta-articular demineralization attests to inflammatory changes within the capsules. Thick periosteal new bone occasionally accompanies psoriatic arthritis (arrow).

ture. The evidence of flexion deformities is subtle. This patient appears to have lost the normal cartilage space that separates the articulating ends of the bones of the metacarpophalangeal joints. Closer scrutiny, however, demonstrates an overlap between the bases of the proximal phalanges and the heads of the metacarpals. A lateral view (Fig. 2–2B) graphically illustrates the flexion deformities of the metacarpophalangeal joints which have caused the fallacious appearance of cartilage loss and resulted in overlap of the ends of the bones. The fifth digit, which is most markedly affected by the contracture, cannot be straightened for the lateral projection and demonstrates

the severity of the flexion deformity at the proximal interphalangeal joint.

BOUTONNIÈRE DEFORMITY

The combination of flexion deformities of the proximal interphalangeal joints with hyperextension deformities of the distal interphalangeal joints results in a "boutonnière deformity." This is most commonly seen in rheumatoid arthritis but is also frequently associated with the deformities of systemic lupus erythematosus and Jaccoud's arthritis. The hand with a flexion deformity of the proximal interphalangeal joint and hyperextension of the distal interphalangeal joint is held as though one were securing a carnation in a lapel—hence the French term bou-

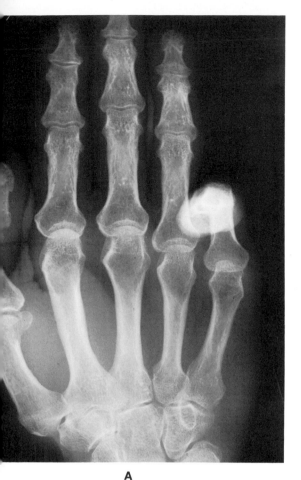

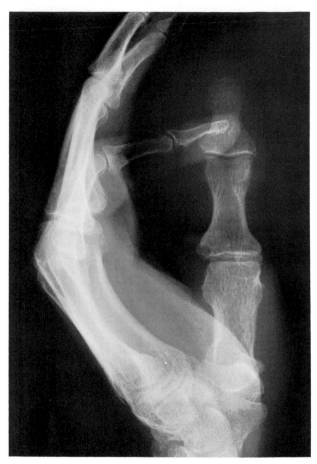

A   **B**

Figure 2–2.   Dupuytren's contracture.

A. Thickening and contracture of the palmar aponeurosis results in progressive foreshortening and flexion deformities of the fingers, most severely deforming the fifth finger. Overlap of the articulating ends of the bones indicates the flexion deformities in the other metacarpophalangeal joints.

B. Flexion deformities are more clearly delineated on the lateral view.

tonnière. The deformity is caused by detachment of the extensor tendon from the middle phalanx. As the tendon slips laterally, the knuckle projects through, and its *anatomic* appearance is that of a bone in a buttonhole. The laterally displaced tendon then acts as a flexor when the muscle contracts.

Systemic Lupus Erythematosus. Figure 2–3 demonstrates the typical boutonnière deformity in a patient with systemic lupus erythematosus. The presence of a flexion deformity at the proximal interphalangeal joint is evident. Although it is clinically apparent, radiographic visual-ization of the hyperextension of the distal interphalangeal joint requires additional views.

SWAN NECK DEFORMITY

A combination of flexion and hyperextension of the distal and proximal interphalangeal joints, respectively (in reverse order to that seen in the boutonnière deformity), results in a swan neck deformity. This occurs where the extensor tendon of the proximal phalanx is thickened and shortened or where the joint capsule of the distal interphalangeal joint is inflamed and distended so that the tendon slides over it. A tendon thus shortened or abnormally laterally positioned produces hyperextension of the proximal interphalangeal joint when it contracts. A compensatory flexion of the distal interphalangeal joint usually accompanies the hyperextension.

Systemic Lupus Erythematosus. The swan neck deformity is demonstrated in a patient with systemic lupus erythematosus (Fig. 2–4). Although the alignment deformities do not appear dramatic, their presence is significant because they indicate inflammation within the joints.

Malalignment in the *absence* of erosions of the joints is typical of patients with systemic lupus erythematosus. Figure 2–5*A* is a more dramatic example of the flexion and hyperextension deformities that are associated with this connective tissue disorder. There is flexion at the metacarpophalangeal joints, hyperextension of the proximal interphalangeal joints and flexion of the distal interphalangeal joints. The right angle configuration of the thumb is due to subluxation of the interphalangeal joint and is

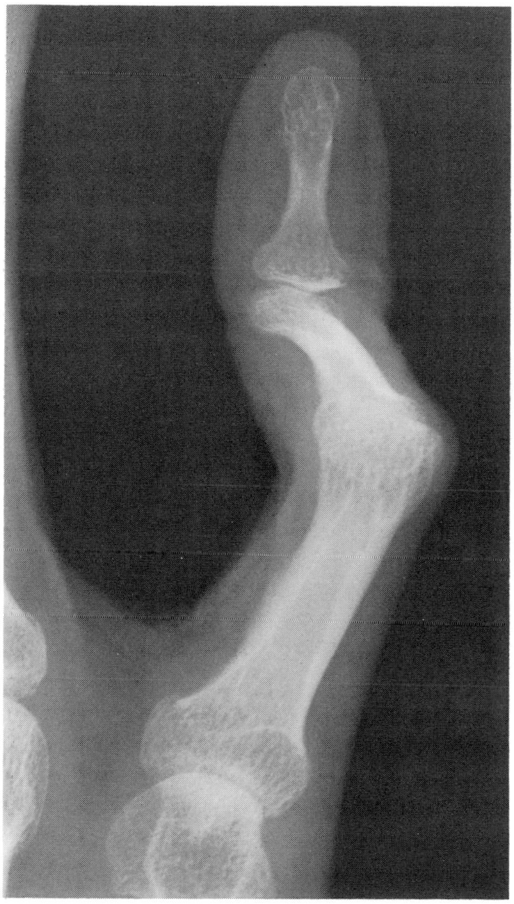

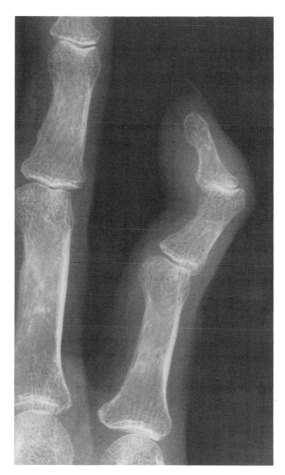

Figure 2–3. Systemic lupus erythematosus.

Flexion of the proximal interphalangeal joint and hyperextension of the distal interphalangeal joint result in a "boutonnière deformity." Alignment abnormalities in the absence of erosions reflect inflammatory changes in the joint with laxity of the capsule and ligaments. This most frequently occurs in systemic lupus erythematosus and Jaccoud's arthritis (post rheumatic fever).

Figure 2–4. Systemic lupus erythematosus.

The combination of hyperextension of the proximal interphalangeal joint and flexion of the distal interphalangeal joint results in a "swan neck deformity," the reverse of the "boutonnière." In addition to alignment abnormalities, diffuse osteoporosis is present.

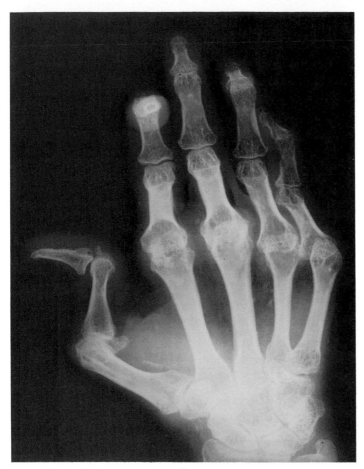

A

Figure 2–5. Systemic lupus erythematosus.

A. Overlap of the articular bones at the metacarpophalangeal joints indicates subluxation of the fingers. This frequently accompanies swan neck deformities of the digits, adding to their malfunction. Subluxation of the interphalangeal joint of the thumb is frequently seen in systemic lupus erythematosus, rheumatoid arthritis and Jaccoud's arthritis and renders a pinch impossible.

Illustration continued on opposite page.

frequently seen in systemic lupus erythematosus. The flexion and hyperextension abnormalities should be suggested by the overlapping bone shadows and the spurious loss of joint spaces on this view of the hand. However, the oblique view clearly and precisely reveals the abnormalities (Fig. 2–5B). A more classic wedge of swans is hard to find!

DEVIATION AND SUBLUXATION

Whereas flexion and extension deformities are best defined radiographically by the oblique view, other alignment abnormalities are better evaluated with the dorsovolar projection. These abnormal alignments may be classified according to two phenomena: deviation and subluxation. Normally, the axes of the bones of the hand form a straight line. Deviation from this straight line results in reduction of the normal 180 degree angle. Subluxation of two bones, by contrast, is present when the articulating surfaces of the bones are displaced. Hence the axes of the bones may remain parallel but are displaced or discontinuous.

It is somewhat hazardous to evaluate deviation deformity from a film, as positioning alone may cause a temporary deformity forever preserved on the radiograph. The X-ray technician may cause an ulnar deviation of the fingers by attempting to separate them. Generally, when the ulnar deviation is secondary to positioning of the fingers rather than to a pathologic process, the fifth finger shows the greatest amount of deviation. The opposite is true in pathologic conditions, where the fifth finger seems to act as a

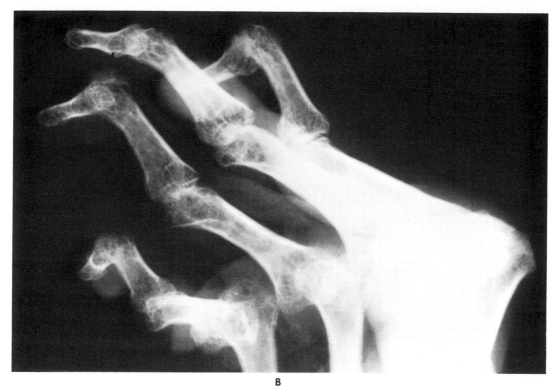

B

Figure 2–5. Continued. B. The oblique view of the hand defines far more clearly the alignment abnormalities.

buttress and demonstrates the least degree of deformity. This is not always true, though, and correlation with other evidence of a pathologic process is essential to prevent the erroneous interpretation of a pathologic condition in what is actually a normal hand.

REVERSIBLE SUBLUXATIONS

Not only may alignment abnormalities be spuriously produced, but a severely deformed hand may appear surprisingly normal on a film. As a matter of fact, it is extremely difficult to record the deformity of patients with systemic lupus erythematosus, since they characteristically have a reversible or "nonerosive arthritis." The mere pressure of the hand against the cassette straightens the deviated and subluxed fingers, and they return to a normal alignment. Since the least amount of pressure is exerted on the first and fifth digits when the palm is placed on the cassette, these may be the only areas that maintain their abnormal alignment. Hence, the rather subtle findings on a film of a hyperextended thumb and a swan neck deformity of the little finger may signify severe and extensive clinical abnormalities.

Systemic Lupus Erythematosus. The radiographic appearance of subluxation is illustrated in Figure 2–6. Instead of articulating with the metacarpal head, the base of the fifth phalanx has slipped laterally. Prior to her X-ray examination, all the fingers of this patient with systemic lupus erythematosus could be palpated between the metacarpal heads. Pressure of the hand against the cassette reduced all the subluxations except that of the fifth finger. Easy reversibility is typical of the deformities that are seen in the hands of patients with systemic lupus erythematosus.

Figure 2–7 shows a pathologic specimen of an interphalangeal joint illustrating volar flexion with preservation of the joint and only minimal loss of articular cartilage (arrows). Although it is unusual to see so little evidence of erosions of the cartilage and subchondral bone in rheumatoid arthritis, a subcutaneous rheumatoid nodule (double arrows) testifies to the origin of the arthritis. Osteoporosis is frequently seen in the connective tissue disorders and is evidenced in this example by the thin cortex and sparse trabeculae.

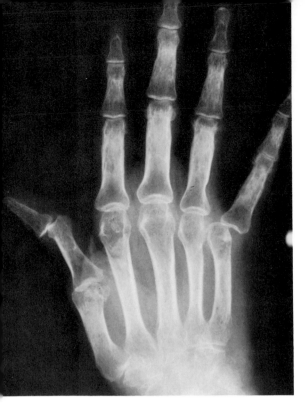

Figure 2–6. Systemic lupus erythematosus. Subluxation of the interphalangeal joint of the thumb and the fifth metacarpophalangeal joint are the sole *radiographic* remnants of the severe deformities affecting each finger. The slight pressure of the hand on the cassette was enough to reduce the other subluxations. Reversibility of the alignment abnormalities is characteristic of systemic lupus erythematosus because of the nonerosive nature of the arthritis. Juxta-articular demineralization accompanies the capsular laxity and both the subluxations and osteoporosis are secondary to inflammatory joint disease.

Figure 2–7. Rheumatoid arthritis.

Severe malalignment in the absence of joint destruction or pannus formation is most common in systemic lupus erythematosus but occasionally may occur in rheumatoid arthritis. The subcutaneous nodule on the extensor surface (double arrows) is typical of the location and histologic appearance of an excavated rheumatoid nodule. Marginal loss of cartilage (arrows) and early osteoporosis are also present. (Courtesy of The Arthritis Foundation.)

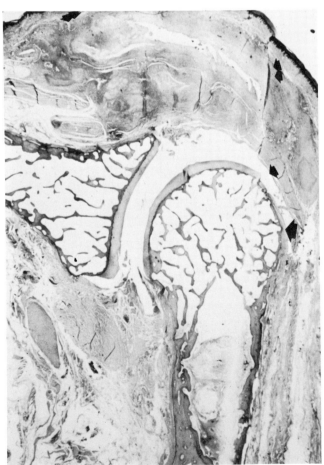

The reversibility of alignment abnormalities and the absence of erosions are typical of both systemic lupus erythematosus and Jaccoud's arthritis. Lack of pannus formation and minimal fibrous change during healing allow continued mobility of the involved joints.

Occasionally it is possible to capture severe subluxations on a film. If only minimal pressure is exerted by the hand on the cassette, reduction of the malalignment may be prevented. Figure 2–8A demonstrates deformities in a patient with systemic lupus erythematosus which were so extensive as to prevent her from using her hand. The ease with which the subluxations are reduced is evident in a second film of the same hand taken only moments later (Fig. 2–8B). Large erosions of the metacarpal heads are present, an unusual occurrence in this disease. However, these are related to pressure from the subluxed phalanges and have occurred from mechanical stresses and subsequent erosion rather than from inflammatory disease.

Hand films of these three patients with systemic lupus erythematosus (Figs. 2–5, 2–6 and 2–8) all have one finding in common: severe hyperextension of the thumb. This is so commonly seen in patients with this disease that its presence should strongly suggest the diagnosis. It is noteworthy that five of the six radiographs showing alignment deformities were of patients with systemic lupus erythematosus. Typically, in this connective tissue disease, of the four factors for evaluation of a joint film — soft tissue, alignment, bony mineralization and cartilage space — it is the *alignment* which is most severely affected.

Rheumatoid Arthritis. As evidenced by Figure 2–9, subluxation of the proximal phalanx and thick pannus (arrows) have resulted in total destruction of the metacarpophalangeal joint and pressure erosion of the distal metacarpal bone and the base of the phalanx in a patient with rheumatoid arthritis. The pathologic changes here are far more extensive than those shown in the radiographic illustrations of subluxation in patients with systemic lupus erythematosus; they underscore the irreversibility of the alignment abnormalities in this connective tissue disorder.

Figure 2–10 illustrates the alignment abnormality in a typical patient with rheumatoid arthritis. Subluxation and deviation of the fingers at the metacarpophalangeal joints are similar in their appearance to the findings in systemic lupus erythematosus. However, there are two important distinguishing features: the presence of *erosive changes* involving the articulating bones and the *irreversibility* of the subluxation. These differences reflect the more severe destructive changes within the joint capsules that are associated with rheumatoid arthritis.

Figure 2–11A demonstrates severe deformities seen in a patient with far-advanced rheumatoid arthritis. In addition to volar subluxation of the second and fifth fingers, the entire wrist is dislocated. Deformities of the interphalangeal joints and subluxation of the interphalangeal joint of the thumb complicate the radiographic picture and compound the inability of these fingers to function.

A film is essential if surgery to restore prehensile function of a severely subluxed thumb is contemplated. The presence of extensive erosions would make surgical fusion of the joint impossible.

The opposite hand of the same patient (Fig. 2–11B) illustrates the radiographic appearance of silastic prostheses restoring the function of the metacarpophalangeal joints. The wrist is subluxed and the overriding radius obscures the proximal row of carpal bones. The lateral view clarifies the change at the wrist, which can only be surmised from a single projection (Fig. 2–11C). A normal lateral wrist is included to illuminate the complex disarrangement (Fig. 2–12).

Juvenile Rheumatoid Arthritis. Two views of the hand of a patient with juvenile rheumatoid arthritis (Fig. 2–13) illustrate subluxations that are similar to the previous example of rheumatoid arthritis. In addition to the severe deformity of the wrist there are further alignment abnormalities of the first metacarpophalangeal joint and flexion of the interphalangeal joints. Such changes occur in patients who have had inadequate physiotherapy

Text continued on page 42.

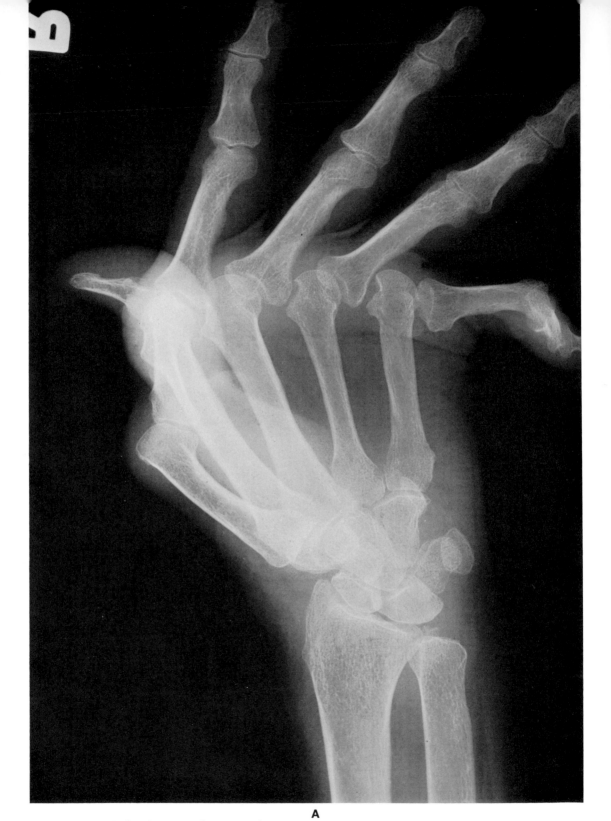

A

Figure 2–8. Systemic lupus erythematosus.

A. It is unusual to capture such severe deformities of lupus on a film since subluxations are usually easily reversed when the hand is flattened against the cassette. Large erosions on the radial side of the metacarpal heads are not generally associated with this connective tissue disorder and in this case appear to be related to pressure of the adjacent subluxed phalanges on the osteoporotic bones rather than to an underlying synovitis.

36

Illustration continued on opposite page.

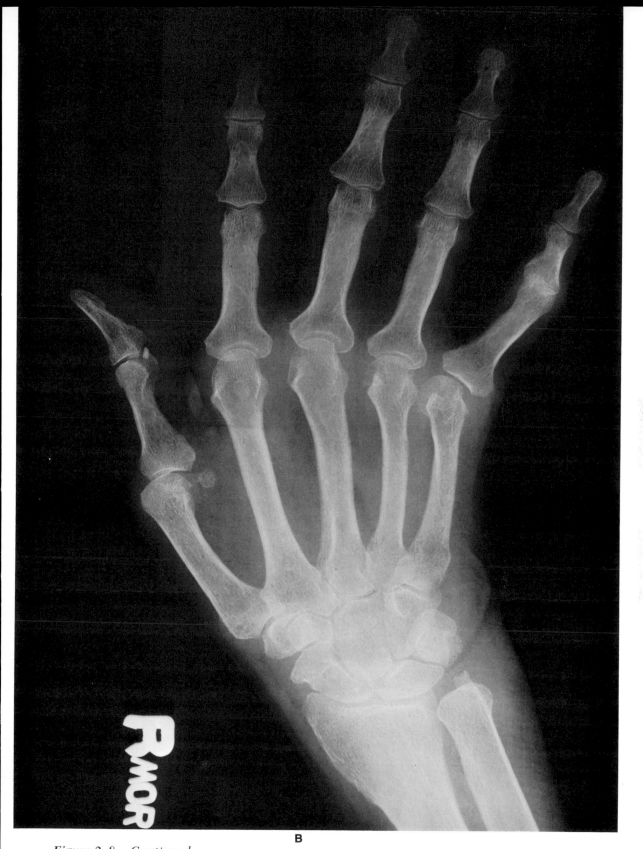

B

Figure 2–8. Continued.
 B. The easy reversibility of the deformities is documented on a film taken minutes after the first. Only slight ulnar deviation of the fingers and a boutonnière deformity persist as a testimonial to the ligament laxity in these joints.

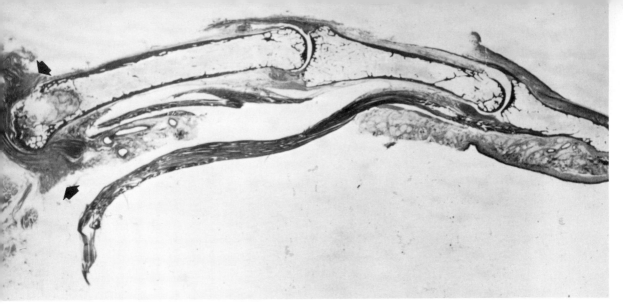

Figure 2–9. Rheumatoid arthritis.

Thick pannus formation (arrows) and volar subluxation of the proximal phalanx have contributed to total destruction of the joint and pressure erosions of the articulating ends of the bones. Osteoporosis is reflected in the pencil-thin cortex and sparse trabeculae of the cancellous bone. (Courtesy of The Arthritis Foundation.)

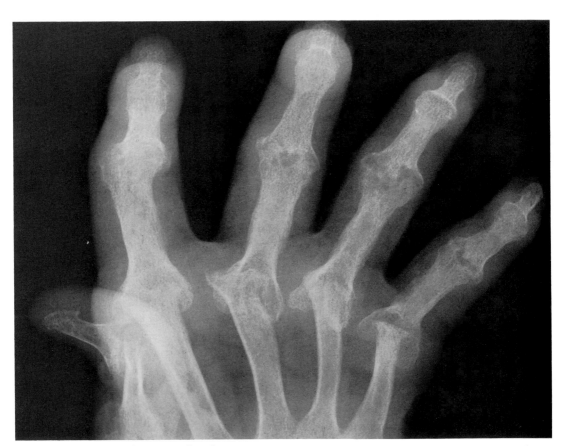

Figure 2–10. Rheumatoid arthritis.

When inflammation is extensive, as in rheumatoid arthritis, deposition of fibrous material and extensive erosions of the bones result in irreversible deviation or subluxation. The distribution is typical, involving the metacarpophalangeal and proximal interphalangeal joints. Flexion of the distal interphalangeal joints prevents evaluation of the joint spaces.

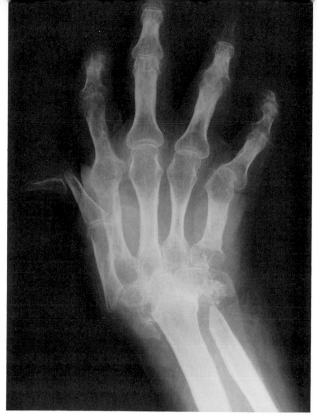

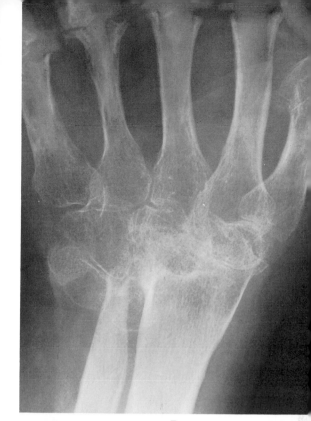

A

B

Figure 2–11. Rheumatoid arthritis.

A. Flexion of the fingers and subluxation of the interphalangeal joint of the thumb are less dramatic than the alignment abnormalities of the wrist. Volar displacement of the carpus obscures the proximal row of bones, and resorptive changes have whittled the distal ulna.

B. Similar changes are present in the opposite wrist.

C. The extent of the carpal dislocation is more apparent on the lateral view. Silastic implants have been introduced into the distal metacarpal bones to restore function of the fingers.

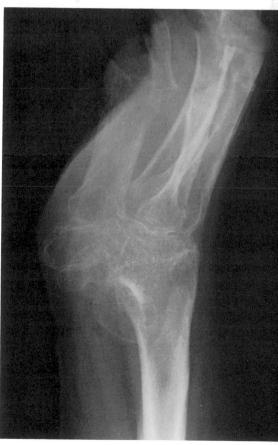

C

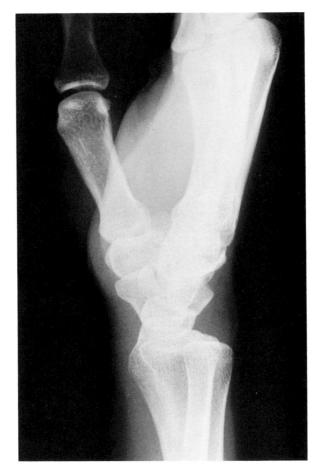

Figure 2-12. Normal lateral hand.
The normal relationship of the carpal bones to each other and to the radius and metacarpals is included for comparison.

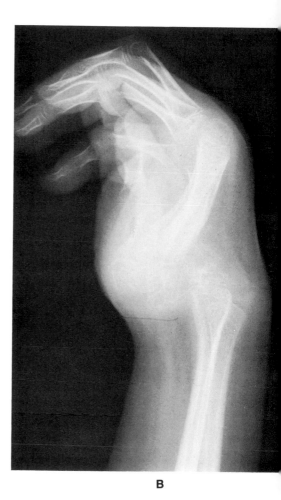

A

B

Figure 2–13. Juvenile rheumatoid arthritis.

A. Overgrowth of the metacarpal epiphyses, premature fusion, squaring of the proximal phalanges from apposition of periosteal new bone and diffuse osteoporosis are the hallmarks of the juvenile onset of rheumatoid arthritis. Erosions and alignment abnormalities are rare but debilitating sequelae of the inflammatory joint changes when they occur, as in this example.

B. The extreme carpal dislocation is only appreciated on the lateral view.

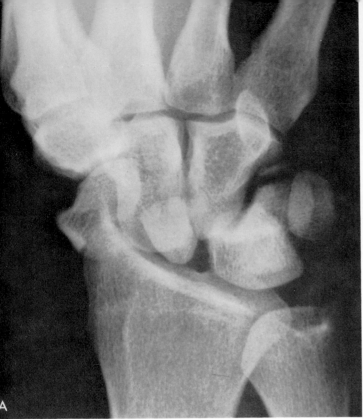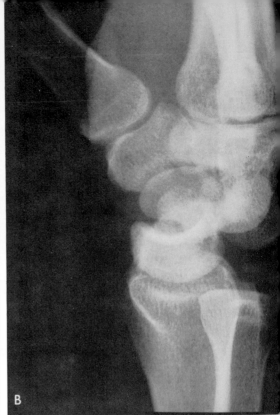

Figure 2–14. Perilunate dislocation.

An AP view of the wrist (A) frequently only hints at the dramatic disarray of carpal bones that may occur following trauma. Although fractures through the navicular, triquetrum and ulnar styloid testify to the magnitude of the force, the dorsal dislocation of the carpal bones is better appreciated on the lateral view (B). Only the lunate maintains its normal articulation, held in the hollow of the distal radius. Failure to recognize carpal dislocations results in a superimposed degenerative arthritis.

or have been unresponsive to it during the active phase of their disease. The residual deformity underlines the tragic consequences and permanent disability that may result from this inflammatory disorder.

Early fusion of the metacarpal epiphyses and a rectangular appearance of the proximal phalanges from periosteal new bone frequently accompany the pathologic changes of juvenile rheumatoid arthritis (see Chapter 3).

Traumatic Dislocation. In a perilunate dislocation, the lunate maintains a normal relationship with the distal radius, and the surrounding carpal bones dislocate dorsally. This disarray of carpal bones is seen in Figure 2–14A. Fractures are often associated, and are seen in this example in the ulnar styloid, the navicular bone and the triquetrum. The lateral view (Fig. 2–14B) clearly demonstrates the dislocated carpal bones which could easily be overlooked on a single projection. If such dislocation goes unrecognized, a severe osteoarthritis may ensue, with permanent limitation of motion.

SUGGESTED READINGS

Beausang, E., E. V. Barnett, and S. Goldstein. Jaccoud's arthritis: A case report. Ann. Rheum. Dis. 26:239 (1967).

Lubowitz, R., and H. R. Schumacher. Articular manifestations of systemic lupus erythematosus. Ann. Int. Med. 74:911 (1971).

Chapter 3

ABNORMALITIES OF BONY MINERALIZATION

Evaluation of bony mineralization must be approached in the same fashion as interpretation of soft tissues: is there too much or too little, and is this process generalized or is it limited to a localized area?

The problem of judging generalized alteration in bone density is even more hazardous than that of deciding whether there is an overall increase or decrease in soft tissue. Not only is there no base line on the same film by which to judge a change from normal, but to further complicate the decision, the bones may be altered in appearance from *technical factors* alone. Too much radiation (overpenetration) will blacken the film and appear to eradicate the trabeculae. Too little radiation will cause the bones to appear dense. How, then, can the pitfalls of overestimating pathologic involvement be avoided so that a patient is not condemned with a diagnosis of generalized osteoporosis when in truth it is only a heavy-handed technician?

Many elaborate techniques have been devised to establish a method for assessing mineral content of bone. One way is to include a standard with each film. This may be done by radiographing aluminum wedges of graded thickness or a series of lumbar vertebrae of different degrees of osteoporosis simultaneously with the hand. In this manner, a standard of known density is included on the film and will be affected by the same technical factors as the patient's bones. Since radiographic signs of osteoporosis always indicate far-advanced demineralization,

it has been hoped that by such methods osteoporosis may be detected with accuracy at an earlier time. In fact, these techniques are cumbersome and are not generally employed. Therefore, one is left with a single film upon which to base a decision. Not even an earlier comparative view will help, as variations in technical factors will affect the contrast between black and white and change the scale of grays. Fortunately, there are concrete clues which are reliable indicators of osteoporosis that can be used despite less than ideal films.

To use these clues it is first necessary to define a normal bone. A normal finger (Fig. 3–1) should have a sharp outline with no irregularity or jagged projections. The homogeneous dense cortex seen along both sides of the shaft encroaches on the spongiosa (medullary cavity). Its endosteal surface (the side toward the medullary cavity) is smooth and convex, with its greatest dimension at the level of the midshaft. The proximal and distal ends of each phalanx are demarcated by a sharp white continuous line of cortical bone. The periosteal side of the shaft (the outer margin) is smooth, and the entire frame of cortex is homogeneous and white. This contrasts with the spongiosa, which is gray at each end and progressively whitens as one approaches the midpoint of the shaft. At either end of the bone, in the epiphyseal and metaphyseal portions, individual trabeculae appear as thin white lines so numerous that they fill the ends of the bone. In the diaphyseal portion of the bone (the shaft), there

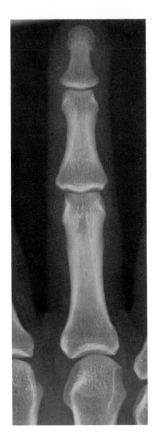

Figure 3–1. Normal bony mineralization.

The outline of the bones is smooth and unbroken, the cortex is homogeneous and encroaches on the spongiosa maximally at the midportion of the diaphysis. Trabeculae at the ends of the bones are delicate and numerous, and there is a gradual transition of the scale of grays from the end of the bone to the mid-diaphysis.

Figure 3–2. Normal distal interphalangeal joint.

The thick cortical bone and numerous trabeculae in the ends of the bones as well as the homogeneous shadow of the diaphysis are identical to the previous radiograph. The sharp continuous subchondral line that demarcates the articular margins of the bones is well-illustrated in this low-power photomicrograph. (Courtesy of The Arthritis Foundation.)

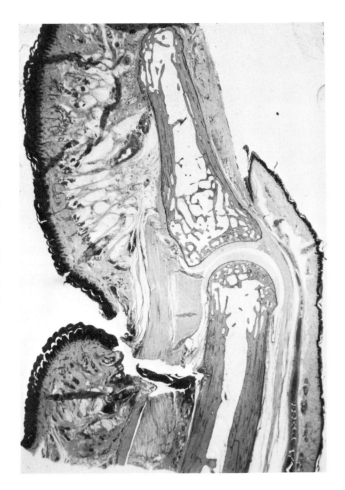

is a homogeneous ground-glass appearance, and individual trabeculae are not normally observed.

A sagittal section through a finger (Fig. 3–2) illustrates the normal appearance of cortical and cancellous bone in a 29 year old man and emphasizes the similarity between radiographic and microscopic appearance.

GENERALIZED OSTEOPOROSIS

The *width* of the *cortical* bone on film gives objective evidence of changes in the amount of bone. As bones become osteoporotic, the cortex begins to thin and the trabeculae of the spongiosa disappear. The trabeculae may likewise vanish if the dose of radiation is too great, but the width of the cortex cannot be altered by technical factors alone. Therefore, cortical thinning indicates loss of bone. In an osteoporotic bone, the central shaft will appear homogeneously gray from loss of trabeculae, and the cortex will stand out in sharp contrast, casting a distinct pencil-thin white image. This differs markedly from the normal wide frame which encroaches on the medullary portion of the normally mineralized bone.

Dermatomyositis. A film of a 26 year old woman with dermatomyositis who has been on high dosages of steroids manifests the classic changes of osteoporosis (Fig. 3–3). The outline of each individual bone of the hand is sharp and unbroken, but the cortex, instead of encroaching on the medullary cavity, is reduced to a thin white line. The entire center portion is homogeneous, giving a ground-glass appearance, and has lost the normal gradual change in density from epiphysis to midshaft. In addition, the trabeculae at the ends of the bones are markedly reduced in number from the normal.

JUXTA-ARTICULAR DEMINERALIZATION

In an inflammatory process involving the joint capsule, the ends of the bones that are enclosed by it often become de-

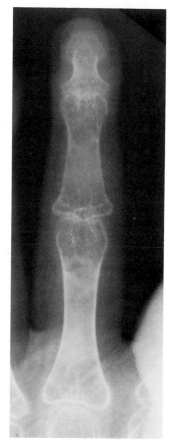

Figure 3–3. Osteoporosis.

In contrast to the normal finger, the cortex is reduced to a pencil-thin white line and the trabeculae are sparse. The sliding scale of grays that normally characterizes the spongiosa has been replaced by a homogeneous "ground glass" shadow. Osteoporosis in this patient with dermatomyositis is due to long-term steroid therapy.

mineralized; the shaft, however, is spared. The sliding scale of grays that is present in films of normal spongiosa is therefore lost, and the ends of the bones become black. The wide frame of cortical bone is unaltered by this process since it lies outside the capsule. Because this osteoporosis is localized to the ends of the bones, it is called *juxta-articular demineralization.*

Raynaud's Phenomenon. A hand film of a female patient with Raynaud's phenomenon (Fig. 3–4) illustrates the development of juxta-articular demineralization. The first film was taken when she noted the onset of cold sensitivity in her

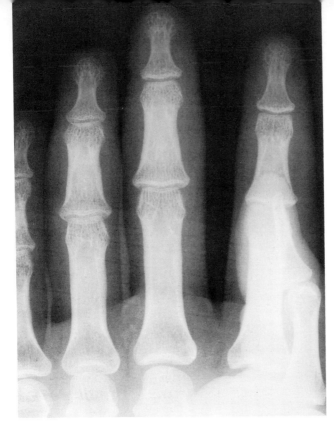

A

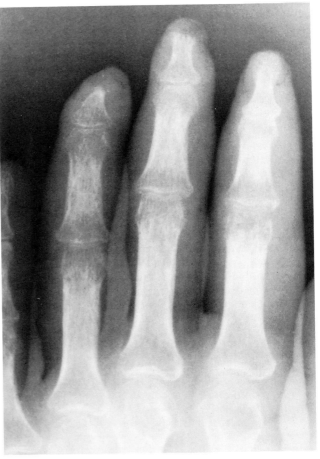

B

Figure 3–4. Juxta-articular de-mineralization.

A. Soft tissue swelling is the only abnormality seen at the onset of Raynaud's phenomenon in this patient with systemic lupus erythematosus.

B. Eighteen months later, the radiographic pattern of juxta-articular demineralization is apparent by the sharp transition between the gray ends of the phalanges and the white diaphyses. In addition, resorption of the distal phalanges has occurred in the third and fourth fingers, with associated loss of soft tissue.

Illustration continued on opposite page.

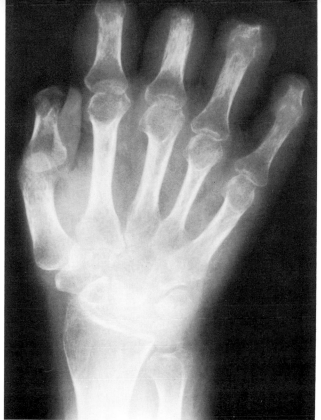

C

Figure 3–4. Continued.
C. This patient's opposite hand required surgical amputation because of the severe, unremitting vasculitis and gangrene.

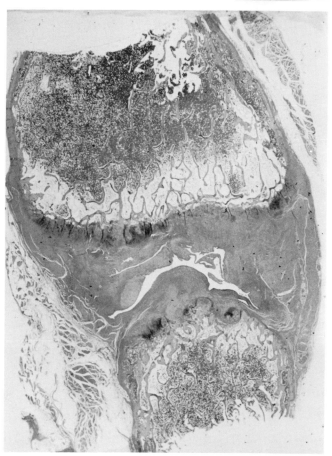

Figure 3–5. Juxta-articular demineralization.

The microscopic changes exactly duplicate the radiographic changes as seen by the sparse and thinned trabeculae at the ends of the articulating bones of a sternoclavicular joint. Pannus has completely replaced the normal intra-articular structures, destroying the fibrocartilage disc and the hyaline articulating cartilage of the bones. Irregularity of the margins of bone reflect the subchondral extension of the hypertrophied synovium. (Courtesy of Roger Terry, M.D.)

fingers (Fig. 3–4A). Diffuse soft tissue swelling of the fingers is the only abnormal finding on the initial examination. A film taken 18 months later (Fig. 3–4B) shows the radiographic manifestations of Raynaud's phenomenon secondary to scleroderma. The tips of the fingers are tapered, indicating soft tissue atrophy. There is resorption of the bone beneath. Juxta-articular demineralization is revealed by the sharp transition of *black* epiphysis to *white* shaft. Although the bones appear black on an overpenetrated film, technical factors cannot alter the transition of grays as one goes from epiphysis to midshaft. Hence, this *sudden* change in density is objective evidence of localized loss of mineral.

The condition of the patient's opposite hand necessitated surgical amputation to control unremitting gangrenous changes secondary to Raynaud's phenomenon (Fig. 3–4C).

The decreased density of articular bones is just as apparent on a microscopic section of a sternoclavicular joint as it is on a radiograph (Fig. 3–5). Inflammatory changes from rheumatoid arthritis have caused juxta-articular demineralization, with thin, sparse trabeculae. In addition, cartilage loss and subchondral erosions are evident.

SUBCHONDRAL DEMINERALIZATION

If the osteoporotic process is acute and rapid, as that which accompanies hyperemia or disuse, the bone is much less uniformly demineralized. The trabeculae immediately beneath the cortical margin disappear first, and the radiographic appearance is that of a black or radiolucent line paralleling the white cortical frame. The process is called *subchondral demineralization* because it occurs in the portions of bone covered by cartilage. In the hand it is seen in the carpal bones and the articulating ends of the long bones, where the trabeculae are normally well visualized and closely packed together.

Pyogenic Arthritis. A 30 year old man with staphylococcal arthritis presented with sudden swelling and redness of the wrist. A film corroborated the presence of an acute inflammatory arthritis (Fig. 3–6). The appearance of the carpal bones is fuzzy, as though their centers were out of focus, in contrast to their borders, which stand out more sharply than normal. The presence of soft tissue swelling and this peculiar fuzzy appearance of the bones are the radiographic hallmarks of an acute inflammatory process. The sharp white frame of cortical bone is exaggerated in its appearance because of the change just beneath it. Rapid demineralization has resulted in loss of trabeculae beneath the cortex and is evident as a parallel lucent line following its contour. In this example demineralization is particularly well demonstrated in the lesser multangular bone, the capitate bone and the ends of the second and third metacarpal bones.

The increased bone metabolism in an acute inflammatory or infectious process causes both osteoblastic and osteoclastic activity. Since it takes a hundred osteoblasts to replace the bone that one osteoclast can destroy, demineralization is the predominant finding early in an inflammatory process. Signs of the reparative phase are often subtle and must be searched for. Note in Figure 3–6, along the lateral aspect of the radius, a thin line of new bone paralleling the cortex; this is evidence of osteoblastic activity in the periosteum. The large lytic area in the radial epiphysis suggests that the infection has spread from the joint to involve the bone.

It is essential to recognize the significance of these minor radiographic changes. A suppurative arthritis rapidly destroys cartilage and bone, and the earlier appropriate antibiotic therapy is instituted, the more limited will be the permanent disability.

OSTEOMALACIA

It would be an oversimplification to suggest that the radiographic manifestations of osteoporosis and osteomalacia can always be easily differentiated. Osteomalacia results from insufficient mineral within the matrix of bone. It has among its causes inadequate absorption

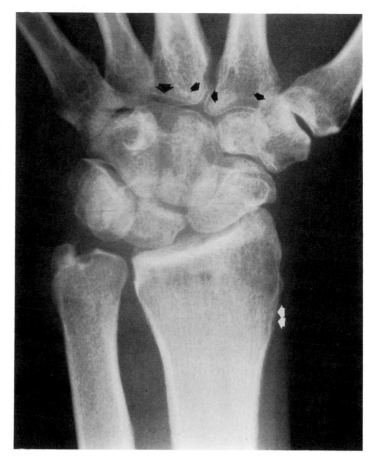

Figure 3–6. Subchondral demineralization.

Rapid loss of calcium is reflected radiographically as a fuzzy, out-of-focus appearance of the carpal bones and as an exaggerated white cortical margin owing to the parallel black line beneath it (arrows). Acute staphylococcal arthritis with its accompanying hyperemia has caused these changes. Secondary osteomyelitis of the radial styloid has occurred, with rarefaction of the end of the bone and an early line of periosteal new bone (double arrows).

of calcium, as in steatorrhea, and excessive loss of calcium, as occurs in renal tubular dysfunction. Although hyperparathyroidism results in both osteoporosis and osteomalacia, the predominent radiographic changes are those of osteomalacia. Radiographs of patients with this disorder offer an opportunity to contrast the findings in these two categories of bone disease.

Hyperparathyroidism. In osteomalacia, the cortical bone disappears in a very different manner from that in osteoporosis. Instead of an exaggerated pencil-thin white frame around a ground-glass matrix, the *opposite* phenomenon occurs. The distinction between the cortex and the medullary space is gradually lost. The once solid shadow cast by the cortex now blends subtly into the rest of the bone (Fig. 3–7A). In addition, extensive subperiosteal resorption of bone has given a shaggy appearance to the outer margin of the fingers. This is almost always more apparent on the radial side of the phalanges. The disease in this patient is far advanced: both sides of the fingers are irregular, the cortex is ill-defined and the loss of calcium has been so extensive in the distal phalanx that the soft tissues have collapsed on themselves, giving the appearance of clubbing. The vascular calcification paralleling the radial side of the finger is another complication of abnormal calcium metabolism.

The wrist of the same patient (Fig. 3–7B) demonstrates two more characteristic features of hyperparathyroidism: chondrocalcinosis involving the triangular cartilage above the ulna and at the base of the first metacarpal; and a cystic defect in the navicular bone, representing a brown tumor. Cystic lesions are not uncommon in *primary* hyperparathyroidism and histologically are indistinguishable from giant cell tumors.

The diagnosis of hyperparathyroidism

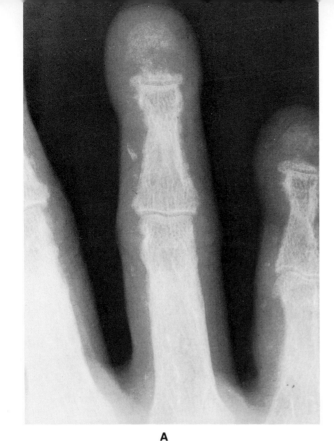

Figure 3–7. Hyperparathyroidism.

A. Vascular calcification of the digital arteries is seen, as well as the classic subperiosteal resorption of bone. The cortical and cancellous bone blend imperceptibly into each other. Loss of bone has been so extensive in the distal phalanges that collapse of the surrounding soft tissues mimics clubbing.

A

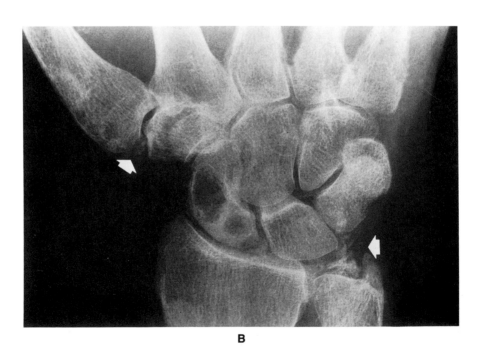

B

B. Two additional signs of hyperparathyroidism are seen in the wrist: calcification of the triangular cartilage and the articular cartilage between the greater multangular and first metacarpal bones (arrows), and a "brown tumor" that causes a radiolucency within the navicular bone.

50

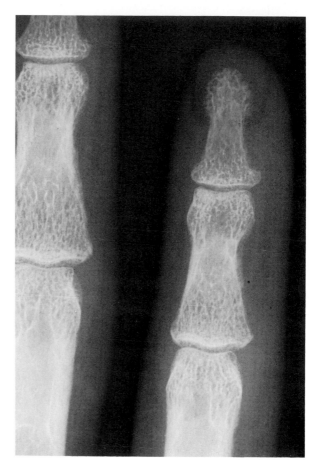

Figure 3–8. Hyperparathyroidism. Subperiosteal resorption causes an irregular contour, most advanced on the radial side of the middle phalanges. So much calcium has been resorbed that the cortex blends imperceptibly into the cancellous bone and the coarsened trabeculae give a lacelike texture to the bones.

is easy in this case. All of the radiographic findings associated with this disease are present on this single hand film: demineralization, subperiosteal resorption, vascular calcification, chondrocalcinosis and a brown tumor.

The finger of a second patient with this disease shows the changes of hyperparathyroidism at an earlier stage (Fig. 3–8). Coarsening of the pattern of trabeculae and a decrease in their total number are indicative of the presence of abnormal calcium metabolism. The few trabeculae that remain are thickened, giving a lacelike appearance to the cancellous bone. The cortical frame, which is normally sharp and homogeneous, is eroded and riddled with holes, indicating the extent of demineralization. In addition, the characteristic finding of subperiosteal bone resorption, although more subtle than that in the preceding example, is present in this case; this is the pathognomonic sign of hyperparathyroidism.

LOCALIZED RESORPTION OF BONE

When loss of bone is limited to one area, localized processes must be considered in the differential diagnosis. Identical erosions of bone occur with such dissimilar etiologies as granuloma, infection and tumor. The presence of a mass, no matter what the underlying histology may be, may cause increased osteoclastic activity; the result is a thinning of the bone around the mass. Therefore, because bone is limited in its manner of response to pathologic processes, localized rarefaction is not diagnostic of a specific disease. Further information must be sought from the film or from the

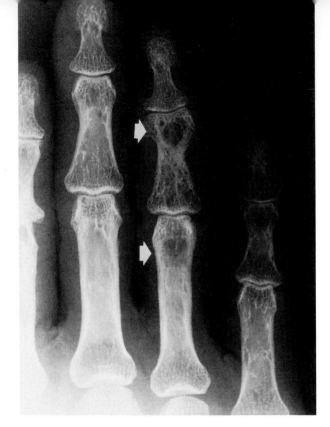

Figure 3-9. Sarcoidosis.
Coarsened, lacelike trabeculae and cystic lesions of the phalanges (arrows) indicate granulomatous involvement of the bone and are two of the osseous manifestations associated with sarcoidosis.

Figure 3-10. Sarcoidosis.
Diffuse soft tissue swelling is often the presenting finding in sarcoidosis and is seen here in the middle and ring fingers. Intraosseous granulomas cause smooth, punched-out lesions, as in the heads of the proximal phalanges. Rarely, resorptive changes and reactive endosteal new bone convert the phalanges to solid white, whittled cylinders (arrows). Subluxation of the distal interphalangeal joint of the middle finger has caused the confusing superimposition of shadows.

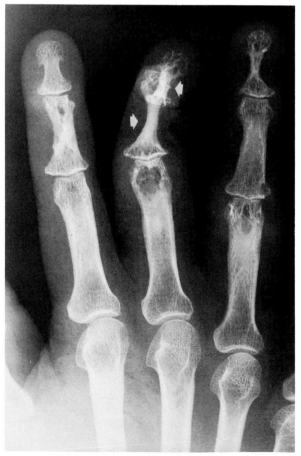

history and physical examination to establish a diagnosis. It may even be necessary to resort to biopsy for pathologic or bacteriologic confirmation.

Sarcoidosis. The bone changes of sarcoidosis (Fig. 3–9) are not unlike those of primary hyperparathyroidism. The texture of the bone is coarsened or lacelike, and the *endosteal* cortical surface loses its distinct margin. Note in Figure 3–9 two well-circumscribed holes in the proximal and middle phalanges; these indicate the presence of noncaseating granulomas. The solid mass of tissue causes pressure erosion of the overlying bone. Both the coarsened trabecular pattern and the cystic areas are indicative of abnormal tissue in the medullary space. If it were not for the subperiosteal resorption of bone in hyperparathyroidism, the radiographic findings of sarcoidosis could be easily confused with this entity.

Although joint pain is common in patients with sarcoidosis, actual bone changes are present in the phalanges in only about five per cent of patients. The most frequent type of alteration is illustrated by Figure 3–9. A much rarer finding is a resorptive arthropathy causing circumferential dissolution of the outer surfaces of the phalanges. This is seen in a far-advanced state in the middle and distal phalanges of the middle finger in Figure 3–10. Less severe changes are evident in the distal phalanx of the ring finger and the middle phalanx of the index finger.

Remarkably enough, patients with leprosy may manifest the same three radiographic patterns of change that are seen in sarcoidosis: lacelike coarsening, cystic punched-out lesions and resorptive pencilling of the phalanges. Biopsy of the cystic lesions in leprosy also demonstrates noncaseating granulomas indistinguishable from those of sarcoidosis. Only the presence of mycobacteria in the specimen conclusively indicates leprosy. The similarity of the radiographic and pathologic changes in these two diseases is startling. It lends credence to the long-discarded theory that sarcoidosis may be an infectious process from an atypical mycobacterium.

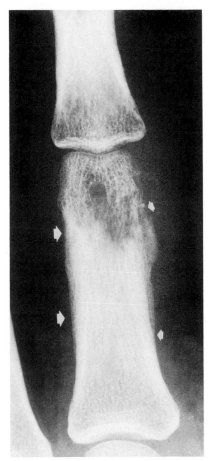

Figure 3–11. Coccidioidomycosis osteomyelitis.

Soft tissue swelling, ill-defined destruction of the phalanx and periosteal new bone (arrows) are typical of osteomyelitis.

Coccidioidomycosis. The pattern of destruction from coccidioidomycosis osteomyelitis, seen in Figure 3–11, illustrates the radiographic findings associated with a more rapidly destructive process of chronic granulomatous etiology. Three important findings on the film indicate the presence of a poorly contained infection: soft tissue swelling around the affected bone; absence of a sclerotic bony margin defining the area of destruction; and production of periosteal new bone (arrows).

Pyogenic Arthritis. Localized infection of the fifth metacarpophalangeal joint is illustrated in Figure 3–12. The pathogenesis of the two major radiographic signs of infection, localized soft

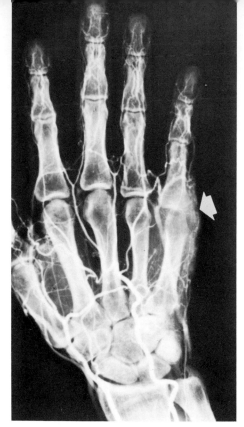

Figure 3–12. Infectious arthritis.

An arteriogram demonstrates the massive shunting of blood to an infected joint with increase in both the diameter of the digital artery and the number of small vessels in the periarticular soft tissues. Demineralization of the ends of the bones within the infected joint capsule reflect the hyperemia.

tissue swelling and bony demineralization, is demonstrated by this arteriogram. In examining the radiographic appearance of the vessels, one notes that not only is an abnormally large amount of blood being shunted to the infected area (seen in the increased diameter of the major feeding vessel) but numerous small vessels course through the swollen periarticular soft tissues.

Tuberculosis. The radiographic picture of tuberculous osteomyelitis (Fig. 3–13A) is similar to that of coccidioidomycosis. Extensive permeative destruction of the metaphysis and diaphysis and the solid layer of periosteal new bone along both sides of the shaft signal the presence of bone infection. The associated soft tissue swelling can only be seen on the lateral view of the hand and is characteristic of tuberculosis (Fig. 3–13B). The cold abscess that is as-

sociated with an underlying tuberculous osteomyelitis tends to be well defined, with distinct boundaries and preserved tissue planes, in contrast to the diffuse soft tissue swelling that occurs with a suppurative infection.

Metastatic Disease. Hematogenous spread of tumor to the distal extremities is rare. Bronchogenic carcinoma, however, is unique: since it is the only tumor not filtered through the lungs, it has a relatively greater statistical chance of being carried to the farthest parts of the body. Occasionally other tumors, such as breast carcinoma and neuroblastoma, metastasize to the hands and feet. Metastatic deposits arise in the same areas as hematogenous spread of infection: because of the sluggish circulation in the metaphysis, tumor emboli as well as bacteria tend to establish themselves at this point.

The similarity of findings in a patient with metastatic carcinoma of the lung (Fig. 3–14) to those in the foregoing cases of osteomyelitis emphasizes once more the limited manner in which bone can respond to a destructive focus. Only the rapidity of bone destruction and its reparative attempts (i.e., sclerotic new bone within the spongiosa or periosteal new bone) are captured by the film. These destructive changes from the deposit of carcinoma are evident. The entire shaft has a moth-eaten appearance, and the cortical margin is destroyed in several places. There is massive soft tissue swelling around the involved phalanx, and the entire picture could just as easily represent a rapidly destructive infection, as one might see with staphylococcus.

LOCALIZED DEPOSITION OF NEW BONE

Cortical new bone may be laid down along either the periosteal or endosteal surface. Its presence indicates a stimulation of osteoblastic activity by some underlying process and signifies an increase in metabolic activity. This may be a reflection of either a generalized increase in growth or a localized attempt at repairing or walling off a destructive

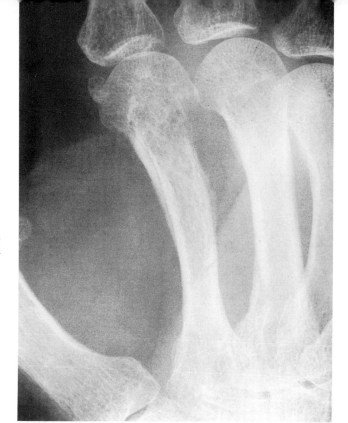

Figure 3–13. Tuberculosis.
A. Extensive permeative destruction of the second metacarpal bone is present, surrounded by a thick solid layer of periosteal new bone.

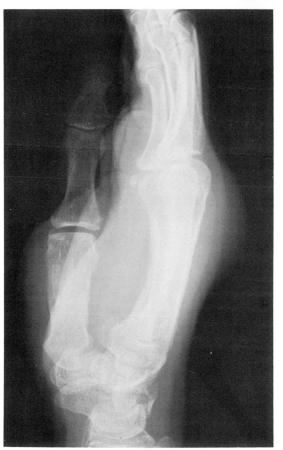

B. The localized soft tissue swelling (cold abscess) is best seen on the lateral view.

A

B

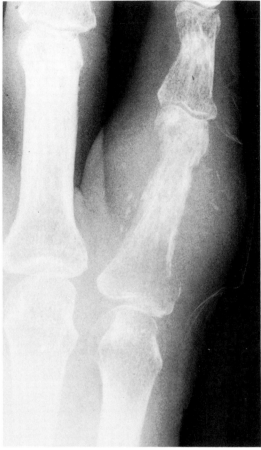

Figure 3-14. Metastatic tumor.
Occasionally metastases from a primary tumor will destroy a small bone of the hand. The radiographic picture is indistinguishable from osteomyelitis. Here, infiltration of the proximal phalanx and irregularity of the cortex are present, as well as a large extraosseous component of tumor distending the soft tissue, in a metastatic deposit from a primary bronchogenic cancer.

process. The latter mechanism has been demonstrated in preceding examples of osteomyelitis and metastatic tumor, where the primary process was local dissolution of bone and the secondary efforts at restoration were reflected in the periosteal new bone.

Periosteal New Bone

Cortical new bone may be associated with the inflammatory changes of rheumatoid arthritis, juvenile rheumatoid arthritis, Reiter's syndrome and, rarely, psoriatic arthritis. Of these four diseases, it is most commonly seen in juvenile rheumatoid arthritis and Reiter's syndrome; less than five per cent of patients with rheumatoid arthritis have periostitis. Characteristically, the periosteal new bone of juvenile rheumatoid arthritis and Reiter's syndrome is thick, whereas in rheumatoid arthritis the new bone appears in a thin layer that is easily overlooked.

Juvenile Rheumatoid Arthritis. The rectangular appearance of the proximal phalanges in a 10 year old child with juvenile rheumatoid arthritis (Fig. 3-15) is due to a thick layer of periosteal new bone that blends subtly with the cortex and fills the normal concavities of the bone. In addition, diffuse demineralization is present. Cupping of the epiphyses of the proximal phalanges, as seen in this example is not uncommon. It appears to be related to the pressure of the metacarpal head within an inflamed joint. Diffuse soft tissue swelling, a distinct feature of juvenile rheumatoid arthritis, is evident. The soft tissue abnormalities are not limited to distention of the joint capsules, as in the adult form of the disease. Absence of erosions in the presence of such severe changes is not uncommon in juvenile rheumatoid arthritis and is related to the thick protective layer of cartilage that caps the articular ends of the bones.

A section through the end of a phalanx illustrates the thickness of the articular cartilage in children (Fig. 3-16). Subchondral collections of lymphocytes indicate the presence of inflammation in this joint affected by juvenile rheumatoid arthritis. Destruction of bone and cartilage, however, has not occurred.

Reiter's Syndrome. Both synovitis (as reflected in juxta-articular demineralization) and periostitis are prominent findings in Reiter's syndrome (Fig. 3-17). The periosteal new bone along the proximal phalanges is thick and shaggy and is distinct from the underlying cortical bone. There is diffuse soft tissue swelling, causing *mild* flexion deformities at the interphalangeal joints. Severe deformities are not produced in the hands by Reiter's syndrome but are occasionally seen in the feet.

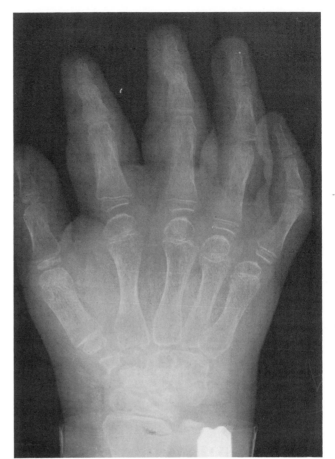

Figure 3–15. Juvenile rheumatoid arthritis.

Thick layers of periosteal new bone blend imperceptibly with the cortex, giving a rectangular configuration to the small bones of the hand. The diffuse soft tissue swelling and absence of erosions are characteristic, as well as the extensive osteoporosis.

Clinical differentiation between psoriatic arthritis and Reiter's syndrome is frequently difficult and sometimes impossible. Even the keratoderma blennorrhagica, the rash of Reiter's syndrome, is identical to pustular psoriasis. *Three* radiographic findings help to separate the two conditions. First, during an acute flare-up of Reiter's syndrome, bony demineralization is the most striking abnormality. In addition, although identical changes may be observed in psoriatic arthritis, the shaggy periosteal new bone is much more frequently seen and more pronounced in patients with Reiter's syndrome. Finally, it is rare for Reiter's syndrome to be associated with erosions in the hand, despite the fact that it may cause severe joint destruction in the foot; psoriatic arthritis, in contrast, is one of the most common causes of mutilating arthritis in the hand.

Rheumatoid Arthritis. Diseases associated with solid thick new bone, such as osteomyelitis, hypertrophic osteoarthritis, juvenile rheumatoid arthritis and Reiter's syndrome, must never be mistaken for rheumatoid arthritis. The periosteal new bone of the latter disease is never more than a thin single layer along the metaphysis, as seen in Figure 3–18.

At this point a word of caution in evaluating periostitis in the fingers is in order. In the standard prone projection of the hands, the thumb is always viewed laterally and the fourth and fifth fingers tend to assume an oblique position; this position brings into radiographic prominence a ridge of bone along the palmar surface of the phalanges. It is essential, therefore to take care not to interpret this normal ridge of bone as periosteal new bone.

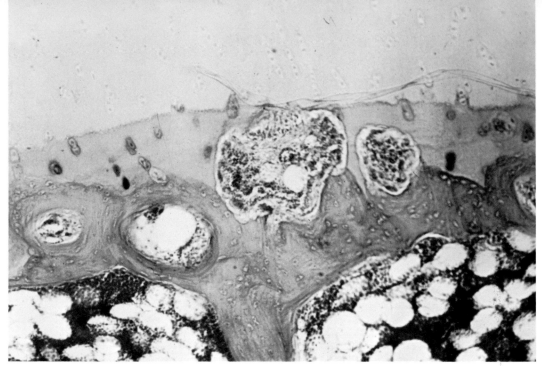

Figure 3–16. Juvenile rheumatoid arthritis.
A microscopic section illustrates the thick articular cartilage in a patient with juvenile rheumatoid arthritis. Although subchondral inflammatory cells are present, no destruction or erosions are evident. (Courtesy of Roger Terry, M.D.).

Hypertrophic Osteoarthropathy. The periosteal new bone in rheumatoid arthritis and Reiter's syndrome is frequently overshadowed by the more dramatic changes of capsular distention or juxta-articular demineralization. In contrast, periostitis is the *predominant* change in patients with hypertrophic osteoarthropathy, and the synovitis that accompanies this disease is less dramatic.

Even a brief glance at Figure 3–19, the hand of a woman with metastatic adenocarcinoma of the lung, reveals the extensive deposition of new bone surrounding every bony diaphysis. The normal ridge of bone on the volar surface of the thumb is in contrast with the prominent periosteal new bone on the opposite side. Periarticular soft tissue swelling of the fourth and fifth proximal interphalangeal joints indicates fluid within the capsular spaces.

Periostitis and synovitis are the primary manifestations of hypertrophic osteoarthropathy and may be present long before the lung disease becomes apparent. Although it is true that benign conditions of the lung, liver and gastrointestinal tract may occasionally be associated with hypertrophic osteoarthropathy, they are extremely uncommon. Any patient with periostitis as extensive as that seen in Figure 3–19 must be viewed as a tumor suspect; this amount of periosteal new bone is inconsistent with the pathologic changes in rheumatoid arthritis or Reiter's syndrome. All of these conditions may present with periarticular soft tissue swelling, juxta-articular demineralization and periostitis. A diagnosis must therefore be made on the pattern of radiographic changes, the findings in joint fluid and the clinical history.

Idiopathic Osteoarthropathy. Idiopathic osteoarthropathy, or pachydermoperiostosis, may be identical to hypertrophic osteoarthropathy in clubbing of the distal soft tissues, synovitis and infiltration of the skin and stomach wall. Despite the similarity of sites affected, the radiographic findings as well as the clinical information are distinctive enough that the two disease entities

Figure 3–17. Reiter's syndrome.

Juxta-articular demineralization and thick shaggy periosteal new bone are typical of the changes in Reiter's syndrome. Soft tissue swelling has caused flexion of the fingers. The absence of erosive changes within the joints is also characteristic of Reiter's syndrome when it affects the hands.

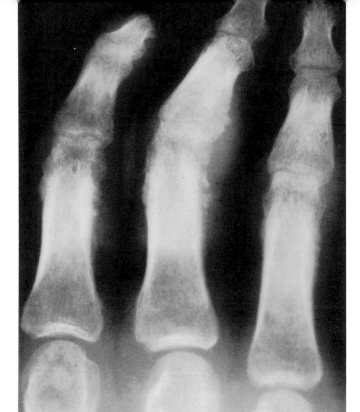

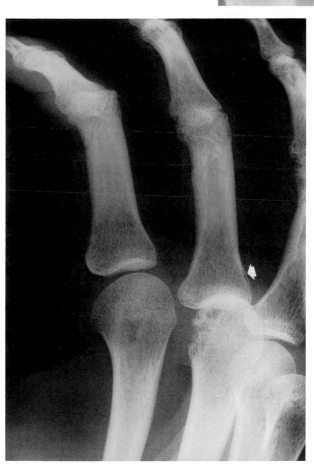

Figure 3–18. Rheumatoid arthritis.

The thin single layer of periosteal new bone at the base of the proximal phalanx is typical of the periostitis seen in rheumatoid arthritis (arrow). Simultaneous destruction of cartilage and articular bone occurs at the metacarpophalangeal joints and is indicated radiographically by joint space narrowing and irregularity of the radial surface of the metacarpal head.

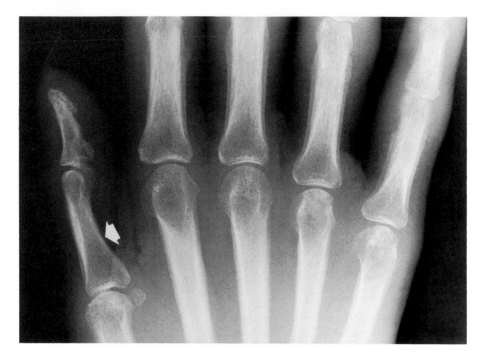

Figure 3–19. Hypertrophic osteoarthropathy.

When periosteal new bone is the most *prominent* radiographic finding, hypertrophic osteoarthropathy should be the first diagnosis. Less obvious but just as important is the presence of synovitis, as reflected by the juxta-articular demineralization and joint effusions. The normal volar ridge of bone along the first proximal phalanx (arrow) has a distinctly different appearance from the periostitis on the opposite side of the bone.

should not be confused. The onset of idiopathic osteoarthropathy, which only rarely occurs in women, is in adolescence. The skin changes are more extensive than those in hypertrophic osteoarthropathy and are not limited to the tips of the fingers. Although patients complain of joint pain, synovitis is not a prominent feature of idiopathic osteoarthropathy, and little or no capsular swelling is present. The appearance of periosteal new bone is more subtle than in hypertrophic osteoarthropathy. In the idiopathic form it is not seen as a separate layer of bone: most frequently it blends into the cortex, altering the *contour* of the diaphysis, as in juvenile rheumatoid arthritis, by filling in the normal concavity. The contribution to the widened cortex may be from the endosteal as well as the periosteal side and is apparent because the medullary space becomes narrowed.

Figure 3–20A demonstrates these findings in an 18 year old boy. Admittedly the manifestations are subtle, and without a strong clinical suspicion they most certainly would be overlooked. Soft tissue clubbing at the ends of the fingers (Fig. 3–20B) is frequently associated with resorption of the terminal tufts, as seen in this patient. This substantive piece of evidence may confirm the suspicion aroused by minor changes in the cortical bone; however, young patients may normally have *no* tufts, and so this finding alone is therefore not significant.

Acromegaly. In contrast to the diffuse layering of periosteal new bone seen in the previously mentioned arthritides, localized production of new bone in acromegaly occurs at very characteristic points in the fingers. Accelerated osteoblastic activity occurs at the sites of attachment of tendons and capsules, causing projections or spikes of new bone along the smooth outer contour (see Figure 3–21). In the distal phalanx, this results in a proximal exaggeration of the

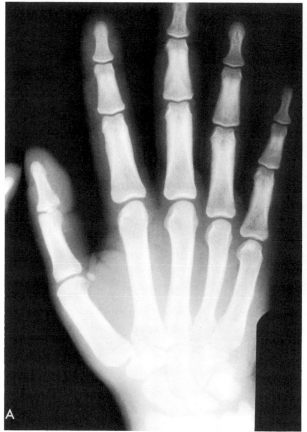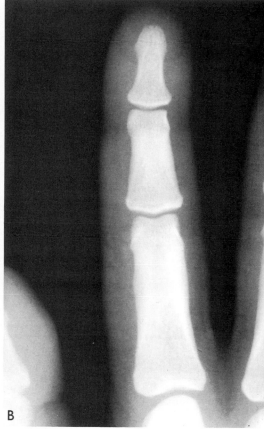

Figure 3-20. Idiopathic osteoarthropathy.

A. Diffuse increase in soft tissue may be most apparent at the tips of the fingers (clubbing), and loss of the terminal tufts accompanies this change. A slight decrease in the concavity of the diaphysis of the small bones of the hand indicates the subtle addition of periosteal new bone, which typically fuses imperceptibly to the underlying cortex.

B. A detailed view of the index finger illustrates the squared appearance of the proximal and middle phalanges.

size of the terminal tuft as well as overgrowth of the base of the phalanx such that the bony projections tend to grow towards each other.

Since patients with idiopathic osteoarthropathy frequently have spade-shaped hands from the infiltrated skin, they are often initially suspected of having acromegaly. Films are essential in distinguishing the two diseases. The *exaggerated* tufts of acromegalics stand in striking contrast to the *absence* of tufts in patients with pachydermoperiostosis. In addition, the changes in bone mineralization further distinguish the two diseases. Acromegaly is associated with os-

teoporosis. Thinning of the cortical margin and loss of trabeculae are apparent in the acromegalic hand illustrated in Figure 3–21 and in the microscopic specimen shown in Figure 4–2. Radiographic examination of pachydermoperiostosis, however, reveals the opposite: a widened bony cortex and a narrowed medullary space.

Osteophytes

Osteoarthritis. Any discussion of local production of new bone would be incomplete without mention of os-

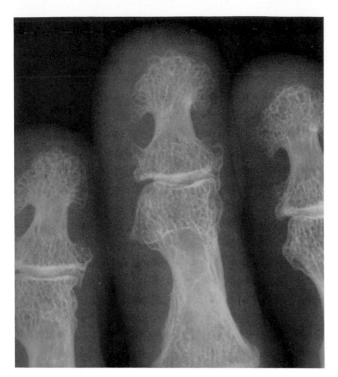

Figure 3–21. Acromegaly.

Overgrowth of bone at the sites of capsular and tendinous attachment is a late finding in acromegaly. Irregularity of the tuft and exaggeration of its projections, as well as overgrowth of the base of the distal phalanx, are more evident than the slight increase in soft tissues in this example. Marginal narrowing of the distal interphalangeal joint is present; and thinning of the cortex of the phalanges and loss of trabeculae—indicate degenerative arthritis and osteoporosis, two additional findings in acromegaly.

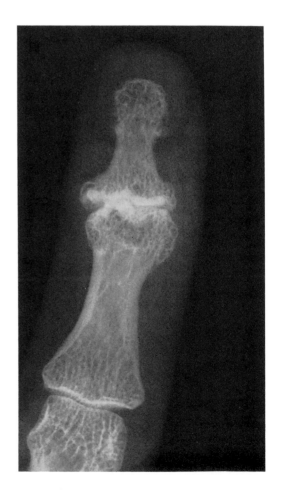

Figure 3–22. Osteoarthritis.

The smooth overgrowth of the base of the distal phalanx is typical of the osteophytes produced secondarily to degeneration of articular cartilage. They are distinguished from the more flamboyant projections of acromegaly by their horizontal axis. Eburnation or sclerosis of the unprotected articular edge of bone commonly accompanies loss of cartilage as seen in this example.

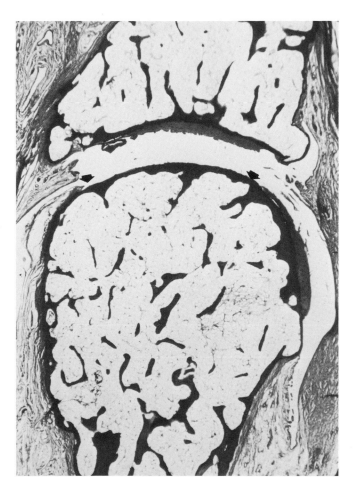

Figure 3–23. Osteoarthritis. Irregular loss of cartilage along both articulating surfaces is accompanied by a thickened subchondral margin of bone (arrows). Narrowing of the joint is not apparent, but a small osteophyte at the base of the distal phalanx deforms the normal contour. (Courtesy of The Arthritis Foundation.)

teoarthritis. In the hands, the distal interphalangeal joints and the first carpalmetacarpal joint are most frequently involved. The proximal interphalangeal joints are affected less frequently. New bone is formed around degenerating cartilage, and since cartilage is most poorly nourished at its periphery, narrowing and osseous outgrowth are found at the margins of a joint space. As the protective cushion of cartilage is destroyed, trauma to the bare articulating ends of the bones stimulates osteoblastic activity, and sclerosis or eburnation ensues. Such changes are evident in Figure 3–22.

The radiographic findings of irregular loss of cartilage and osteophytes along the margin of the joint are similar in appearance to the findings on microscopic section (Fig. 3–23). The abnormal thickness of the subchondral bone (due to eburnation) is more manifest upon comparison with the microscopic section of a normal joint. (Fig. 3–2).

Terminal Phalangeal Sclerosis

The counterpart of periosteal new bone is endosteal new bone, which widens the cortical frame from the inside rather than from without (Fig. 3–24A). The diameter of the bone remains unchanged, but the medullary cavity is reduced. This deviation is most commonly seen in conditions resulting in abnormal bone marrow, such as marrow fibrosis and adult sickle cell disease, and is most striking in the hereditary abnormality of osteopetrosis. A local form of endosteal new bone, when limited to the distal phalanges, occasionally is seen in patients with connective tissue disorders. Because it occurs only in the distal phalanges, this condition is called terminal phalangeal sclerosis.

The presence of terminal phalangeal sclerosis is diagnostically significant when it affects *all* the fingers of *each* hand: this finding is most commonly associated with rheumatoid arthritis. The widened cortex may completely fill the spongiosa and be seen as a solid cylinder of white bone. The fifth finger is usually most dramatically involved; the remaining distal phalanges, because of their greater diameter, may not be completely filled in with cortical new bone. When the process involves only one finger or appears radiographically as localized plaques of new bone in several fingers, the diagnostic possibilities are increased.

Besides rheumatoid arthritis, terminal phalangeal sclerosis has been associated with progressive systemic sclerosis, dermatomyositis, disseminated lupus erythematosus and psoriatic arthritis. Although this condition is most often found in patients with connective tissue disorders, examples of the diffuse form have

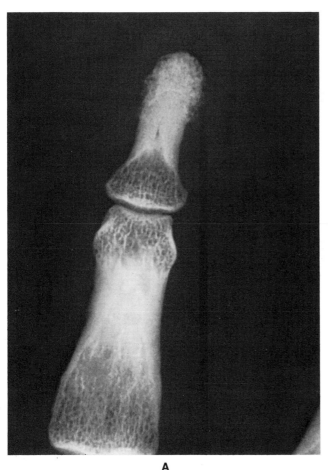

A

Figure 3–24. Rheumatoid Arthritis.

A. The dramatic white distal phalanx is due to endosteal bone obliterating the medullary space.

Figure 3–24. B. When terminal phalangeal sclerosis is seen in all the distal phalanges it is most commonly associated with rheumatoid arthritis. The white bones contrast with the juxta-articular demineralization.

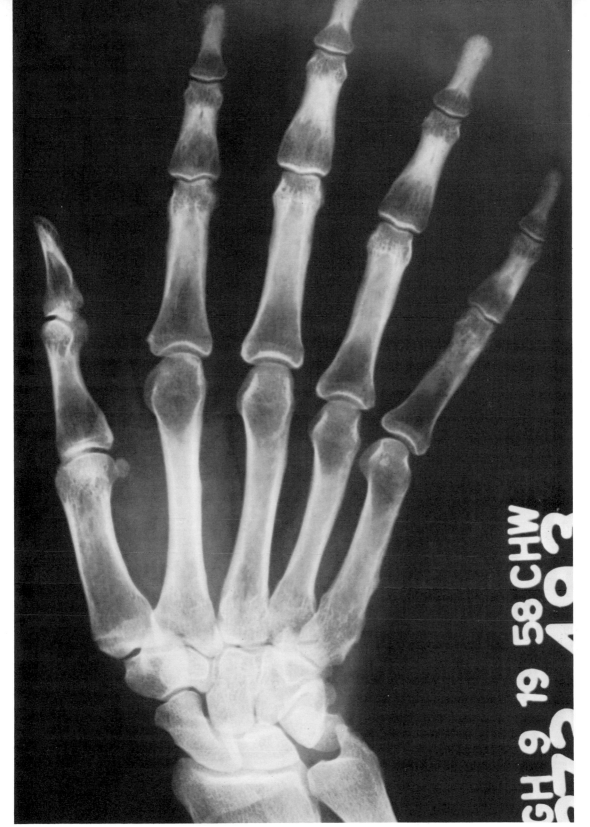

B *Figure 3–24. See legend on opposite page.*   65

Illustration continued on following page.

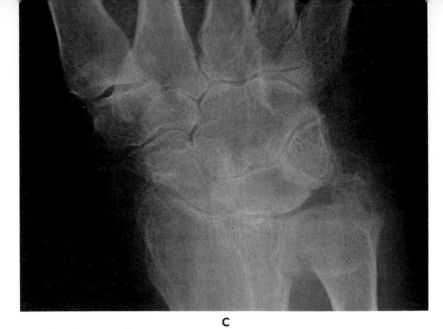

C

Figure 3-24. *Continued.*
C. Eleven years later the characteristic changes of rheumatoid arthritis are present, and uniform cartilage loss with joint space narrowing in the wrist is seen.

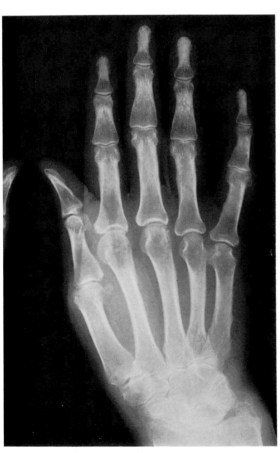

D. In addition to inflammatory changes of the wrist, diffuse demineralization is present, but the terminal phalangeal sclerosis remains unchanged.

D

been seen in chronic active hepatitis and sarcoidosis. In normal patients, although an occasional plaque of sclerotic bone may be present, *diffuse* sclerosis is *never* seen.

The pathogenesis of terminal phalangeal sclerosis is unknown, but the condition is unrelated to clinical signs of vasculitis or the use of steroids. When it occurs, it is evident on the earliest films and remains unchanged in appearance despite progression of the disease. Amazingly enough, despite its dramatic appearance, it is never noticed unless the observer is aware of the entity.

In patients with rheumatoid arthritis, terminal phalangeal sclerosis occurs more frequently than periostitis and is therefore a useful diagnostic sign. As an example, the hand of a patient with clinical complaints of joint pain was completely normal on initial examination, with one striking exception. All of the terminal phalanges were solid white (Fig. 3–24B). Eleven years later, the classical changes of rheumatoid arthritis became apparent. There were narrowing of the cartilage space of the wrist and erosions of the carpal bones (Fig. 3–24C, D); interestingly enough, the sclerotic signs in the distal phalanges had remained unchanged over this long period of time.

SUGGESTED READINGS

Bywaters, E., A. Dixon, and J. Scott. Joint lesions of hyperparathyroidism. Ann. Rheum. Dis. 22:171 (1963).

Calenoff, L. Angiography of the hand: Guidelines for interpretation. Radiology 102:331 (1972).

Engleman, E. P., and H. M. Weber. Reiter's syndrome. Clin. Orthop. 57:19 (1968).

Feist, J. H. The biologic basis of radiologic findings in bone disease. Radiol. Clin. N. Amer. 8:183 (1970).

Greenfield, G. B., H. A. Schorsch, and A. Shkolnik. The various roentgen appearances of pulmonary hypertrophic osteoarthropathy. Amer. J. Roentgen. 101:927 (1967).

Gumpel, J. M., C. J. Johns, and L. E. Shulman. The joint disease of sarcoidosis. Ann. Rheum. Dis. 26:194 (1967).

Harbison, J. B., and C. M. Nice. Familial pachydermoperiostosis presenting as an acromegaly-like syndrome. Amer. J. Roentgen. 112:532 (1971).

Kelly, P. J., W. J. Martin and M. B. Coventry. Bacterial (suppurative) arthritis in the adult. J. Bone Joint Surg. Amer. 52A:1595 (1970).

Laws, J. W., R. A. E. Sallab, and J. T. Scott. An arteriographic and histologic study of digital arteries. Brit. J. Radiol. 40:740 (1967).

Lynn, R. B., R. E. Steiner, and F. A. K. Van Wyk. The digital arteries of the hands in Raynaud's disease. Lancet 1:471 (1955).

Marshall, T. R., D. Neustadt, W. F. Chumley, and M. L. Kasdan. Hand arteriography. Radiology 86:299 (1966).

Murray, R. D. Steroids and the skeleton. Radiology 77:729 (1961).

Rimoin, D. L. Pachydermoperiostosis (idiopathic clubbing and periostosis): Genetic and physiologic considerations. New End. J. Med. 272:923 (1965).

Scanlon, G. T., and A. R. Clemett. Thyroid acropachy. Radiology 83:1039 (1964).

Scharer, L., and D. W. Smith. Resorption of the terminal phalanges in scleroderma. Arthritis Rheum. 12:51 (1969).

Scott, J. T., R. A. E. Sallab, and J. W. Laws. The digital artery design in rheumatoid arthritis—further observations. Brit. J. Radiol. 40:748 (1967).

Sherman, R. S. General principles of the radiologic diagnosis of bone disorders. Radiol. Clin. N. Amer. 8:173 (1970).

Siltzbach, L. E., and J. L. Duberstein. Arthritis in sarcoid. Clin. Orthop. 57:31 (1968).

Soila, P. Roentgen manifestations of adult rheumatoid arthritis with special regard to the early changes. Acta Rheum. Scand. Suppl. 1, 1958.

Stenseth, J. H., O. T. Clagett, and L. B. Woolner. Hypertrophic osteoarthropathy. Dis. Chest 52:62 (1967).

Whalen, J. P., P. Winchester, L. Krok, R. Desihe, and E. Nunez. Mechanisms of bone resorption in human metaphyseal remodeling. Amer. J. Roentgen. 112:526 (1971).

Chapter 4

ABNORMALITIES OF THE CARTILAGE SPACE

The cartilage space frequently offers the definitive diagnostic evidence to differentiate one arthritis from another. Despite its prominent participation in a disease process, this area must be analyzed last to avoid overlooking important peripheral information.

The normal diarthrodial joint (Fig. 4–1) has a uniform crescent of cartilage covering the articular ends of the bones. The synovium is a thin layer of cells lining the capsule of the joint (arrow). Synovial fluid lubricates the joint and separates the articular cartilages. The bony margins of the ends of the bones are defined by a continuous sharp line (black on the microscopic section, white on a radiograph).

Inflammatory processes that involve the joint capsule initiate a series of changes that affect the synovium, the cartilage and the articulating ends of the bones. Excessive fluid is often the first sign of a joint abnormality; examples of this radiographic finding were given in Chapter 1. Progressive destruction of the cartilage narrows the joint space, and proliferation of synovium results in erosions and irregularities of the margins of the bones.

Different arthritides characteristically affect certain joints in the hand preferentially, and the distribution of the pathologic involvement may be diagnostic. Furthermore, the configuration of the erosion and the character of its margin offers additional evidence of the specific underlying arthritis. For example, the poorly marginated erosion of rheumatoid arthritis is in many cases sufficiently distinct from the sharply defined lesion of gout with its overhanging edges to suggest from the film alone a most probable diagnosis. Similarly, the location of joint changes at the proximal interphalangeal and distal interphalangeal areas and the presence of osteophytes at the margins are typical of osteoarthritis. Rheumatoid arthritis, in contrast, affects the metacarpophalangeal and proximal interphalangeal joints and is made noteworthy by the *absence* of osteophytes, sclerotic margins and overhanging edges.

As will become evident, most arthritides that cause destructive changes in the joint capsule initiate a progressive series of events beginning with *narrowing* and *erosions* that may eventually lead to total obliteration of the joint if the process is not interrupted.

Occasionally, the cartilage space is not narrowed but is widened. This deviation is so uncommon that its presence is always a significant clue in unraveling a puzzling diagnostic problem.

WIDENED CARTILAGE SPACE

The joint space may be widened by four mechanisms: increase in the actual size of the cartilage, interposition of fluid between the cartilage surfaces, deposition of fibrous material between the articular ends of the bones at the end stage

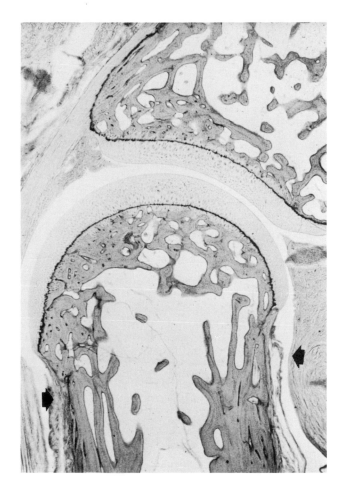

Figure 4-1. Normal diarthrodial joint.

A sagittal section illustrates the extent of the joint capsule, the appearance of the articular hyaline cartilage, and the microscopic appearance of normal cortex and spongiosa. The appearance of the sharp continuous subchondral line of bone is identical to that on a radiograph. (Courtesy of The Arthritis Foundation.)

of a destructive process and resorption of the ends of the bones.

CARTILAGE OVERGROWTH

Acromegaly. Widening of the joint space is one of the hallmarks of acromegaly, and its occurrence in all the joints shown on a hand film should suggest the possibility of that diagnosis, hopefully before the patient has changed glove size three times. Initially, the cartilage increases in bulk just as the soft tissues enlarge.

A midsagittal section through an interphalangeal joint (Fig. 4–2) demonstrates the microscopic changes of cartilage overgrowth. It has caused separation of the articulating ends of the bones and a concave configuration of the base of the distal phalanx. Additional hallmarks of acromegaly are also evident: diffuse osteoporosis and proliferation of bone at

the point of capsular attachment (arrow). These findings are particularly striking when compared with the microscopic section of a normal joint.

Following overgrowth of cartilage from acromegaly, premature degeneration causes joint narrowing and the characteristic changes of osteoarthritis.

Figure 4–3 demonstrates the radiographic appearance of widened spaces between the metacarpophalangeal joints. Proliferation of cartilage at the second metacarpophalangeal joint has resulted in an exaggerated concavity of the base of the proximal phalanx similar to that seen in microscopic section. Even at this stage of the disease, early degenerative changes are present. Calcification at the periphery of the distal interphalangeal joints and early osteophytes developing at the bases of the middle phalanges sig-

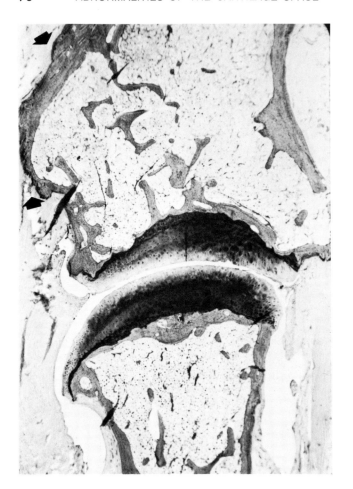

Figure 4–2. Acromegaly. Overgrowth of the articular cartilage has widened the joint and caused a cuplike configuration of the base of the phalanx by pressure from the increased cartilage. Thinning of the trabeculae and cortex reflects the osteoporosis that is seen in acromegaly. A projection of new bone deforms the contours of the phalanx (arrows) and is typical of the spurs that develop in response to stress from capsular and ligamentous attachments. (Courtesy of The Arthritis Foundation.)

nal the senescent changes in the cartilage.

EFFUSION

Rheumatoid Arthritis. A massive effusion in the acute inflammatory stage of an arthritis may occasionally force the bones apart, as in the following example of a patient with rheumatoid arthritis (Fig. 4–4*A*). The widened joint space (arrow) is an isolated phenomenon, in contrast to the uniform involvement in acromegaly. The film shows an increased soft tissue density outlining the distended joint capsule, and an abnormally wide separation between the metacarpal head and its proximal phalanx as well as the adjacent metacarpal head. A later film (Fig. 4–4*B*) illustrates the transient nature of the periarticular swelling and bone separation. Residual irregularities of the articular surfaces of the bones in-

dicate the erosive nature of the disease. Progressive changes of the third and fourth metacarpophalangeal joints are also apparent and are characteristic of rheumatoid arthritis.

FIBROUS DEPOSITION

Acute effusions and cartilage overgrowth may widen the joint space early in the series of pathologic changes. Fibrous deposition, on the other hand, widens a joint as an end-stage event. This occurs most commonly in psoriatic arthritis and Reiter's syndrome. Radiographic and historical evidence differentiate an early arthritis from a chronic condition.

BONE RESORPTION

Bone resorption may occasionally be excessive, resulting in a whittled appearance of the phalanges and a widening of the joint spaces from actual shortening of the bones. Most commonly, resorptive

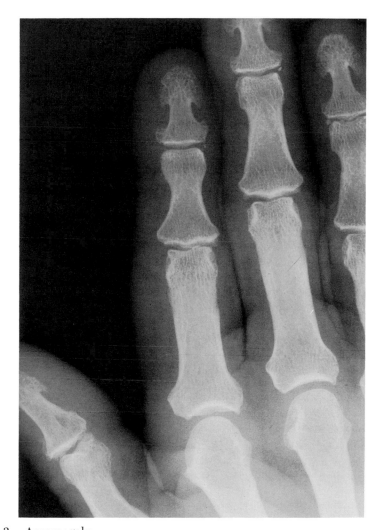

Figure 4–3. Acromegaly.

The widened joint spaces reflect overgrowth of the articular cartilage, and the concavity of the base of the phalanx is similar to that seen in the preceding microscopic section. Calcification at the periphery of the distal interphalangeal joints indicates early senescence of the cartilage and superimposed degenerative joint disease.

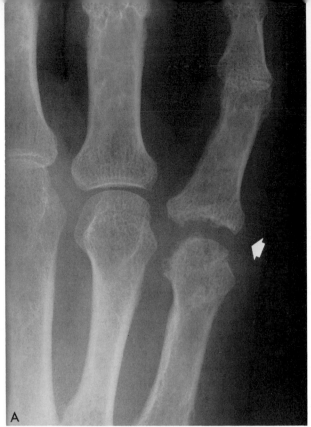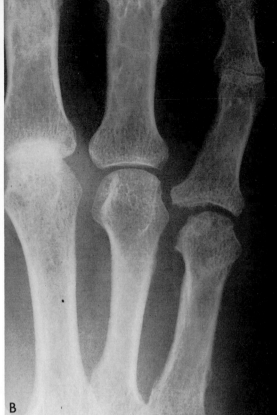

Figure 4–4. Rheumatoid arthritis.

A. Acute widening of a joint may be due to a capsular effusion, as seen here in the fifth metacarpophalangeal joint (arrow).

B. Subsidence of the acute inflammation has resulted in a more normal approximation of the articular bones, but irregularities of the subchondral bone indicate inflammatory destruction. The third and fourth metacarpophalangeal joints are uniformly narrowed.

arthropathies are associated with rheumatoid arthritis and psoriatic arthritis when they occur in the hand, but identical deformities may result from neuropathic conditions in the hand, as in leprosy and syringomyelia.

JOINT DESTRUCTION

The series of events that leads to destruction of a joint in rheumatoid arthritis is initiated by the changes in the synovium. The combination of effusion, synovial proliferation and hyperemia causes changes in the underlying bone that are visible radiographically very early in the disease. A group of patients, all with rheumatoid arthritis, have been selected to demonstrate the radiographic manifestations of inflammatory joint destruction.

DEMINERALIZATION

The earliest finding that may confirm a clinical suspicion of inflammatory arthritis is loss of the sharp cortical margin of the metacarpal head, indicating demineralization. Because the ulnar side is often faceted it is more difficult to evaluate. Therefore, although the entire surface of bone is involved, early evidence of demineralization is only valid when it is observed on the radial side (arrow), as it is in Figure 4–5*A*, a patient with rheumatoid arthritis. Additional evidence of demineralization is indicated by a decrease in the number of trabeculae in the metacarpal head—in this example, best seen in the fourth finger. An erosion on the ulnar side of the fourth metacarpal reflects the extent of synovial proliferation.

A later film of the same joints (Fig. 4–5*B*) attests to the significance of these minimal findings and confirms their importance as early signs of an inflammatory process. Extensive marginal erosions

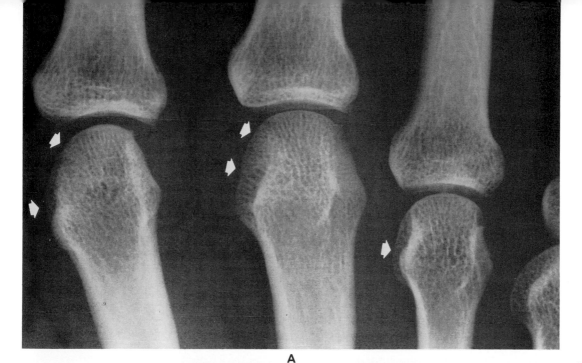

A

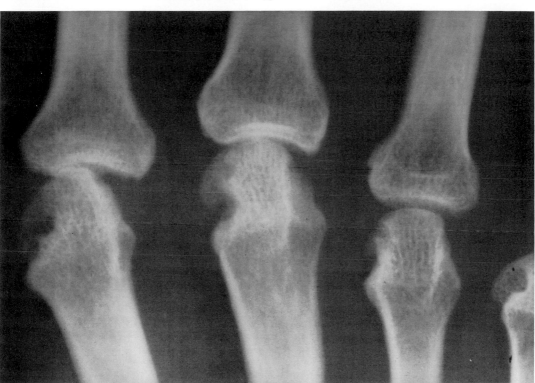

B

Figure 4–5. Rheumatoid arthritis.

A. Interruption of the continuous white subchondral line (arrows) reflects proliferation of synovium and subsequent erosions of adjacent bone. Thus, although this is a seemingly minor radiographic finding, it indicates extensive destructive changes within the joint space.

B. A later film reveals the typical marginal erosions, verifying the significance of the earlier abnormality. *Simultaneous* narrowing of the joint spaces is typical of the pattern of changes that occur in rheumatoid arthritis involving the metacarpophalangeal joints.

deform the heads of the metacarpal bones. This is a common site for erosions, since the bone is particularly vulnerable at the point where the articular cartilage ends. Uniform destruction of cartilage in the second and third metacarpophalangeal joints has resulted in marked narrowing of the entire cartilage space.

The earliest evidence of joint inflammation that is reflected in the bone is an interruption of the continuous sharp white subchondral line. When occurring in several places, this gives what is referred to as the "dot-dash" appearance. Again, it is most readily detected on the radial side of the metacarpal head. Pathologically it represents fingers of proliferated synovium eroding into the bone. The configuration is most easily understood when a microscopic section of an inflamed joint (Fig. 4–6) is compared to

the normal (Fig. 4–1). Interruption of the continuous subchondral line of bone has occurred along both the articular edges in the areas where synovium has proliferated and destroyed the cartilage. The process is most advanced along the margins, and contiguous "rat-bite" erosions of the subchondral bone are also present (arrows). In addition to the hypertrophied synovium (pannus) growing over the articular cartilage, fibrous ankylosis is beginning to restrict the mobility of this interphalangeal joint.

Interruption of the subchondral bone is illustrated radiographically in Figure 4–7. Comparing the appearance of the joints in this patient, one can see that the cortical margin of the middle finger has more dot than dash, suggesting very little intact cortex. Although this radiographic finding seems insignificant, it represents severe inflammatory joint involvement.

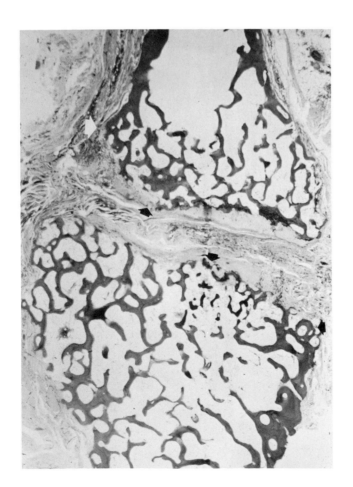

Figure 4–6. Rheumatoid arthritis.

Severe inflammatory changes of an interphalangeal joint are evident from the pannus formation covering the articular ends of the bones. Almost complete loss of cartilage has occurred, and obliteration of the subchondral lines is similar to the preceding radiograph. Poorly circumscribed marginal erosions in areas of excessive synovial proliferation are characteristic of the type of articular destruction in rheumatoid arthritis (arrows). (Courtesy of The Arthritis Foundation.)

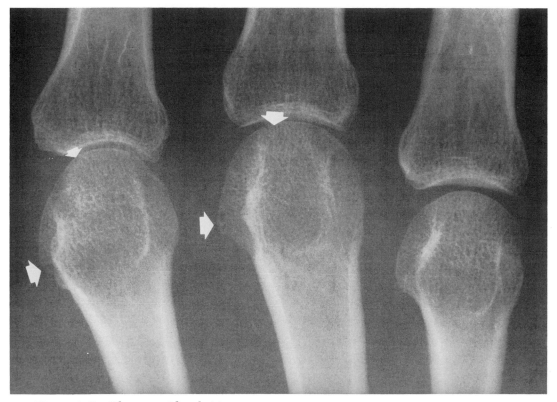

Figure 4–7. Rheumatoid arthritis.
· The dot-dash configuration of the subchondral line (arrows) and simultaneous narrowing of the joint space indicate inflammatory involvement of the third and fourth metacarpophalangeal joints. The pattern of changes is typical of the manner in which rheumatoid arthritis affects the joints.

In this patient, the third and fourth metacarpophalangeal joint spaces are markedly narrowed, indicating extensive cartilage destruction. The extent of the narrowing is evident when the involved joints are compared to the normal fifth metacarpophalangeal joint. It is very common in rheumatoid arthritis to see the "dot-dash" changes in the bone accompanied simultaneously by uniform loss of cartilage at the *metacarpophalangeal joints.*

CARTILAGE LOSS

The articular cartilage is destroyed in a uniform manner in rheumatoid arthritis. Hence, the joint space narrows symmetrically. This distinguishes rheumatoid arthritis from such arthritides as tuberculosis, gout and chronic low-grade infection. The latter diseases tend to at-

tack the margins of the joint first where the protective cap of cartilage ends and the synovium originates and, thus, destroy the cartilage and the underlying bone in an irregular manner. Similarly, osteoarthritis is easily distinguished from rheumatoid arthritis by its peripheral joint space narrowing. Unlike the inflammatory arthritides, however, the cartilage destruction is related to the relatively poor nutrition peripherally rather than to the location of the synovium.

The preceding examples have demonstrated the classical pattern of change associated with rheumatoid arthritis. *Simultaneous* narrowing of the joint space and erosion of the subchondral bone occurs at the *metacarpophalangeal joints.* The *proximal interphalangeal joints,* on the other hand, are usually affected to a *lesser* extent than the metacarpophalangeal joints in rheumatoid arthritis, and the narrowing is seen *before* erosions are visible on a film. This is probably due to the difficulty in detecting small cortical defects on such nonspherical surfaces as the ends of the phalanges.

Figure 4–8 illustrates both patterns of joint destruction as well as the typical distribution of rheumatoid arthritis as it affects the fingers. Joint destruction of the metacarpophalangeal joint is far advanced as compared with the changes at the proximal interphalangeal joint. There is capsular distention, indicated by the periarticular soft tissue swelling at the metacarpophalangeal joint, and subluxation, viewed as an overlap of the ends of the bones. Erosions deform the radial and ulnar sides of the metacarpal head. Only the uniform loss of cartilage at the

proximal interphalangeal joint attests to the severity of the disease in this area. The articular ends of the bones are unaltered. Juxta-articular demineralization coexists with the joint space changes and substantiates the presence of inflammatory joint disease. The fine line of periosteal new bone, barely visible at the base of the proximal phalanx (arrow), is an additional sign of the inflammatory process of rheumatoid arthritis. It is better projected on the oblique view of this hand shown in the previous chapter (see Figure 3–18).

Juvenile Rheumatoid Arthritis. The pattern of distribution and the type of erosions are identical in rheumatoid arthritis and juvenile rheumatoid arthritis, and often only the age of onset will distinguish the two. Because of the initiation of an inflammatory process during

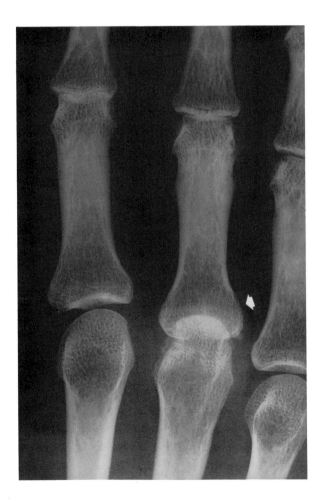

Figure 4–8. Rheumatoid arthritis. Frequently, monarticular involvement of the second or third metacarpophalangeal joint occurs in rheumatoid arthritis and destructive changes there are out of proportion to the remaining joints. Capsular distention and erosions are present at the third metacarpophalangeal joint, in addition to joint narrowing and flexion. The proximal interphalangeal joints in rheumatoid arthritis generally are affected less severely than the metacarpophalangeal joints, and narrowing precedes detectable signs of erosion, as illustrated in this example. The fine line of periosteal new bone (arrow) is an additional sign of rheumatoid arthritis.

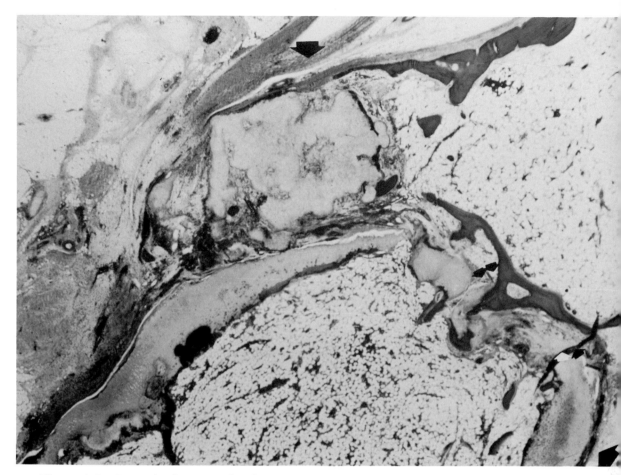

Figure 4-9. Juvenile rheumatoid arthritis.
Severe destructive changes are far less common when rheumatoid arthritis has a juvenile onset. A sagittal section through a metacarpophalangeal joint illustrates the thick articular cartilage and its propensity to proliferate (arrows). Despite these protective attributes, complete destruction of cartilage in the center of this joint and bridging bony trabeculae illustrate the beginnings of bony ankylosis (double arrows). (Courtesy of The Arthritis Foundation.)

the active growth phase of a bone, superimposed alterations in maturation, growth and fusion of the epiphyses may occur and differentiate the juvenile onset variety from adult rheumatoid arthritis.

The important role of the thick articular cartilage in protecting the underlying bones is illustrated in a microscopic section from a patient with juvenile rheumatoid arthritis (Fig. 4–9). Proliferation of cartilage (arrows) occurs readily in young patients and protects the adjacent articular bones from the destructive changes of pannus formation. Despite this protective capacity, there is loss of cartilage centrally, and bony spicules are beginning to bridge the gap between the two bones in this example (double arrows).

Figure 4–10 shows the hand of a 14 year old child with juvenile rheumatoid arthritis and illustrates the type of joint destruction and bony erosions that may occur in this disease. The metacarpophalangeal joints are uniformly narrowed, and erosions are extensively seen in the metacarpal heads. The phalangeal epiphyses, however, are unaffected by the inflammatory arthritis. Similar joint narrowing and erosions are present in the

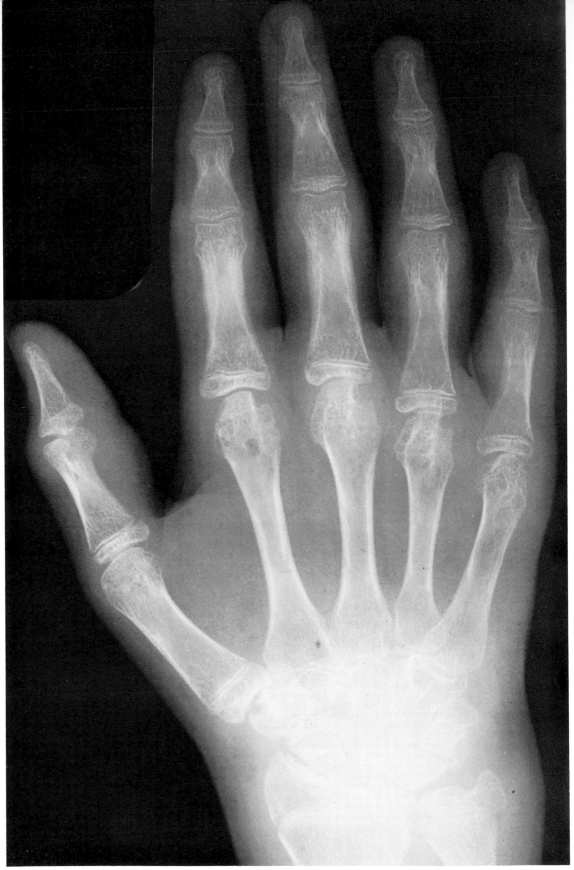

Figure 4–10. *See legend on opposite page.*

78

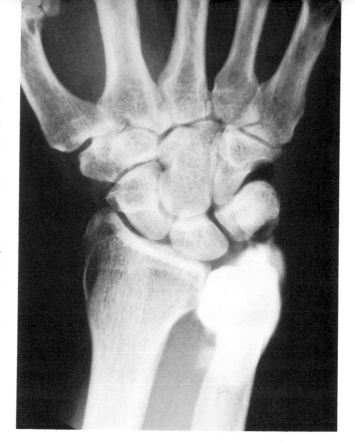

Figure 4–11. Normal wrist arthrogram.

The three joint spaces of the wrist are documented by an arthrogram. The radioulnar joint is outlined by Hypaque and the intercarpal joint by gas, which has diffused irregularly between the carpal bones and the metacarpals, obstructed in many areas by the intercarpal ligaments, so that a uniform black outline of the cartilage space is not obtained. Absence of gas and Hypaque in the radiocarpal joint verifies the distinct boundaries of the three joints in a normal wrist. All three joints are frequently involved in rheumatoid arthritis, communication between them resulting.

carpal bones as well. The rectangular appearance of the proximal phalanges results from apposition of periosteal new bone along the diaphyses. Generalized osteoporosis is also present and is so common in juvenile rheumatoid arthritis that its occurrence in combination with erosions and periostitis should always suggest this diagnosis.

CYST FORMATION

Although cysts may be seen in the metacarpal bones and phalanges, as was demonstrated by the preceding example of juvenile rheumatoid arthritis, it is more common to see *shallow erosions* of the articular bones of the *fingers* and cysts in the carpal bones. This occurs for two reasons. Because of the blocklike shape of the carpal bones, erosions in the wrist are as likely to be viewed en face as tangentially. Thus they will *appear* as cysts within the bone rather than interruptions of the cortical margin. However, true intraosseous cysts, completely surrounded by bone, may also form and are most commonly seen in rheumatoid arthritis and gout. These cysts are produced by invagination of synovium or deposition of tophaceous material within the bone itself. Where cysts occur in rheumatoid arthritis they are generally in patients who work with their hands, e.g., laborers: their occurrence may be related to intermittent bursts of increased pressure within the joint capsule of the wrist, enhancing the ability of the synovium to implode into the subchondral bone.

There are three separate joint spaces of the wrist: the radioulnar, the radiocarpal and the intercarpal. Figure 4–11 outlines two of them and emphasizes their separate anatomic compartments in a normal patient. Contrast material was injected into the radioulnar joint, and although

Figure 4–10. Juvenile rheumatoid arthritis.

Joint narrowing and erosions of the metacarpal heads are seen, as well as diffuse osteoporosis. The rectangular appearance of the proximal phalanges is due to periosteal new bone. The carpal joint is similarly involved, with loss of cartilage uniformly between the bones and multiple erosions.

there was extravasation superiorly, there was no flow of the material between the radius and carpal bones. Gas was introduced between two of the carpal bones and immediately diffused around all of them (seen as a slight increase in the *blackness* between the bones); it, too, failed to enter the radiocarpal joint.

A film of a male patient with rheumatoid arthritis demonstrates the appearance of cysts (Fig. 4–12) in the bones of all three joint compartments. The cysts are most prominent along the margins of the radial epiphysis and the radial side of the radioulnar joint. However, they are also evident in the base of the first metacarpal and in the greater multangular and navicular bones.

That the radiograph is, in effect, the gross specimen becomes obvious when the microscopic appearance of a rheumatoid cyst is compared to its radiographic image (Fig. 4–13). The articular cartilage is locally destroyed, and the expanding subchondral cyst erodes the bone but causes no proliferative response; the margins are thus sharp but not sclerotic.

Identical bone changes have been seen in patients with gout. For this reason it would be an oversimplification to suggest that this picture (Fig. 4–12) is pathognomonic of rheumatoid arthritis. The uniform narrowing of the cartilage between the radius and proximal row of carpal bones, however, is *more typical* of the changes in rheumatoid arthritis. Thus the pattern of involvement of the entire wrist as well as the character of the erosive changes are helpful in differentiating the two confusing entities.

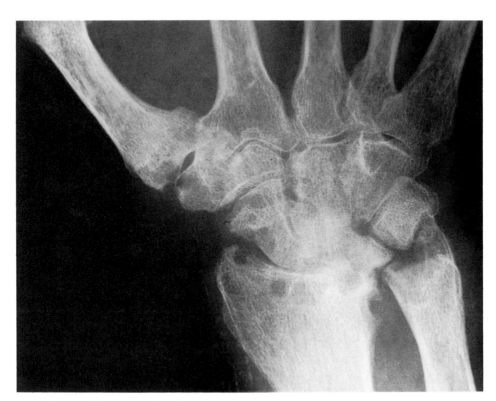

Figure 4–12. Rheumatoid arthritis.
Uniform narrowing of the radiocarpal joint space is a frequent finding in rheumatoid arthritis. Erosions of the carpal bones and ulnar side of the radial epiphysis implicate inflammatory involvement of these two additional joint spaces. Subchondral cysts and sharply defined punched-out lesions are more frequently seen in patients who work with their hands and may be related to intermittent bursts of increased intra-articular pressure.

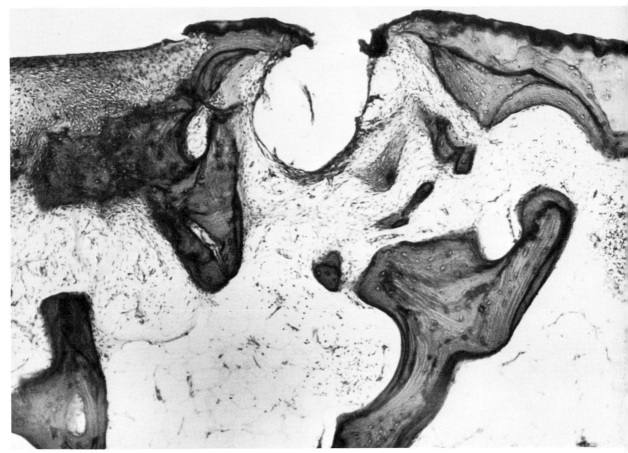

Figure 4–13. Rheumatoid arthritis.

A subchondral cyst is sharply demarcated, extending from the articular surface into the subchondral bone. It does not have the thick sclerotic margin of bone that is seen in gout. (Courtesy of The Arthritis Foundation.)

THE "RAT-BITE" EROSION OF RHEUMATOID ARTHRITIS

Rheumatoid arthritis characteristically does not stimulate the production of new bone. Therefore, the erosions have poorly defined edges, as though the bone had been nibbled away. This was well demonstrated in the microscopic section of a joint affected by rheumatoid arthritis (Fig. 4–6).

Massive synovial proliferation and extensive erosive changes of the bones of the wrist (Fig. 4–14) are an exaggeration of the findings that were present in the previous patient with rheumatoid arthritis. These changes have most severely af-fected the radioulnar and radiocarpal joints. Every projection catches the erosions tangentially, and their contiguity with the cartilaginous space is evident. They do not resemble intraosseous cysts at this advanced stage. The scalloped appearance of the distal ulna demonstrates the "rat-bite" erosion of rheumatoid arthritis.

The Carpal Tunnel Syndrome. Since erosions occur with pannus formation, the bone changes are accompanied by adjacent soft tissue masses. Both synovial hypertrophy and deposition of fibrous tissue alter the joint space. Occasionally in patients with rheumatoid arthritis, these

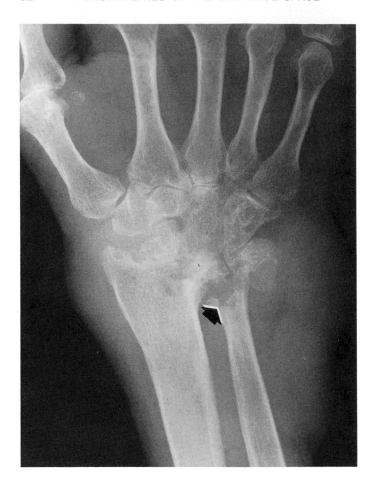

Figure 4–14. Rheumatoid arthritis.

Massive synovial proliferation deforms the soft tissue of the wrist. Destruction of cartilage and erosions most severely involve the articular bone of the radiocarpal joint. A large, poorly marginated "rat-bite" erosion has hollowed the distal ulna (arrow).

changes are sufficiently extensive in the wrist to cause entrapment of the median nerve, the "carpal tunnel" syndrome.

Visualization of the volar soft tissues of the wrist can be obtained only by projecting them away from the bones. This is done by placing the wrist on the cassette and pulling the fingers back to get them out of the beam of radiation. This view of the carpal tunnel is obtained on a patient with rheumatoid arthritis (Fig. 4–15), where extensive erosions of the carpal bones can be seen. Since nerve entrapment is secondary to soft tissue abnormalities, and the radiograph evaluates only abnormalities of the bones, the film is helpful only in providing a *clue* to the etiology of the nerve entrapment syndrome but does not delineate the pathology involving the median nerve itself.

Most frequently, the carpal tunnel syndrome is due to such primary soft tissue problems as deposition of amyloid or distention of the soft tissues from chronic swelling, as occurs in myxedema or pregnancy. In such conditions, the radiograph is normal. Occasionally it is caused by an occult fracture of the hook of the hamate bone. The carpal tunnel projection is the view of choice to discover this abnormality.

A normal carpal tunnel view is included for comparison (Fig. 4–16).

THE OVERHANGING EDGE OF GOUT

The *configuration* of the erosion as well as its *location* may be helpful in distinguishing one arthritis from another. As the previous examples have illustrated, the erosions of rheumatoid arthritis look as though a bite was taken out of the bone. The absence of any new bone results in a poorly marginated lesion with ill-defined edges. Gout characteristically stimulates new bone formation, and the

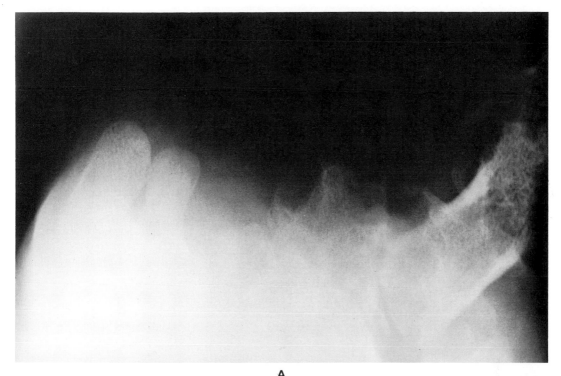

A

B

Figure 4–15. Carpal tunnel syndrome.

A. Occasionally synovial proliferation in rheumatoid arthritis causes entrapment of the median nerve. Although the soft tissue abnormality cannot be visualized, the erosions of the carpal bones are apparent on this carpal tunnel view, indicating the extensive inflammatory involvement of the joint.

B. A view of the wrist demonstrates the degree of arthritis that has led to synovial proliferation and the carpal tunnel syndrome.

83

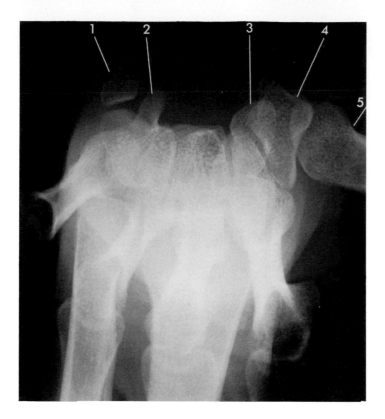

Figure 4–16. Normal carpal tunnel view.

The carpal tunnel view is obtained by placing the wrist on the cassette and pulling the fingers back to get them out of the line of the X-ray beam. The tube is angled cephalad 30 degrees. The normal appearance of the soft tissue and bones is in marked contrast to the previous example.

1, pisiform; *2,* hamulus; *3,* navicular; *4,* multangular; *5,* first metacarpal.

erosions are *well-defined,* often with a *sclerotic margin.* They are frequently associated with tophi, so that the soft tissue mass is localized, in contradistinction with the diffuse periarticular swelling of rheumatoid arthritis.

In addition, at the periphery of the erosion of gout, growth of a shell of new bone may partially encompass the tophus. This splayed rim or overhanging edge, like the sclerotic margin of the erosion, is new bone stimulated by the presence of the tophus. It is not seen in rheumatoid arthritis. That this is new bone, and not the margin of a scooped-out erosion, is demonstrated by a series of films where the *development* of the *overhanging edge* can be followed. The initial film shows a localized tophus (Fig. 4–17A, arrow) adjacent to the middle phalanx. Later, a projection of new bone is produced that begins to encompass the lower margin of the soft tissue deposit (Fig. 4–17B). Finally, a typical erosion within the proliferated wedge of new bone is seen (Fig. 4–17C). Progressive destruction of the metacarpal heads and the large cuplike deformity of the base of the third proximal phalanx have occurred during a two year interval. Although the bony erosions persist in the fingers, many

of the tophi have disappeared with medical therapy.

Although Figure 4–18A is a section through the sternoclavicular joint, the pathologic changes from multiple tophi found here are equally pertinent in understanding the changes in the peripheral joints of the body. Because this specimen was fixed in absolute alcohol, the urate crystals are preserved and are seen as the dark staining material in the cartilage, subchondral bones and synovial membrane. The tophi are sharply defined by a sclerotic margin of new bone (arrows), the solid white margin that is present on the radiograph. A closeup of a subchondral tophus (Fig. 4–18B) illustrates the sharp punched-out character of the erosion and its edge of new bone.

The erosions of gout are often distinctive enough that they should not be confused with the punched-out lytic lesions that occur in rheumatoid arthritis. Referring back to Figure 4–12, note that a rheumatoid erosion along the margin of the radial styloid process is not unlike the smaller erosions of gout in the previous illustration. Unlike gout, the edges are neither lifted up nor splayed, and there is no associated mass. The erosion of the radius at the radioulnar articulation, by

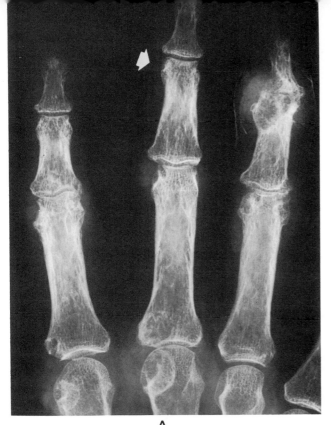

A

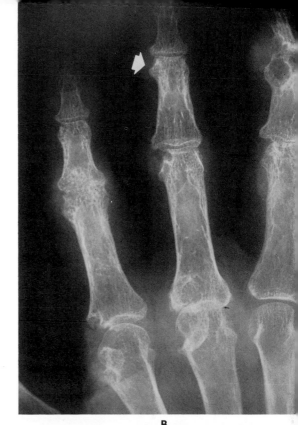

B

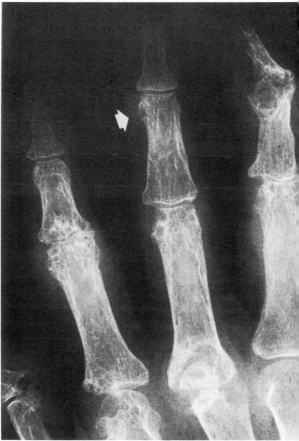

C

Figure 4–17. Gout.

A. Multiple soft tissue tophi are visualized because of their calcium content. A faint mass is present adjacent to the middle phalanx of the long finger (arrow).

B. One year later, a wedge-shaped shelf of bone has been produced (arrow) adjacent to the soft tissue tophus.

C. The following year, an erosion of the edge of the bony spur has occurred, with an overhanging edge (arrow). The tendency to stimulate growth of new bone is also observed as a well-defined sclerotic margin with a splayed edge of bone surrounding the large tophus in the distal fourth finger. Progressive destruction of the metacarpophalangeal joint and a cuplike invagination of the proximal phalanx are identical to the changes so frequently seen in rheumatoid arthritis.

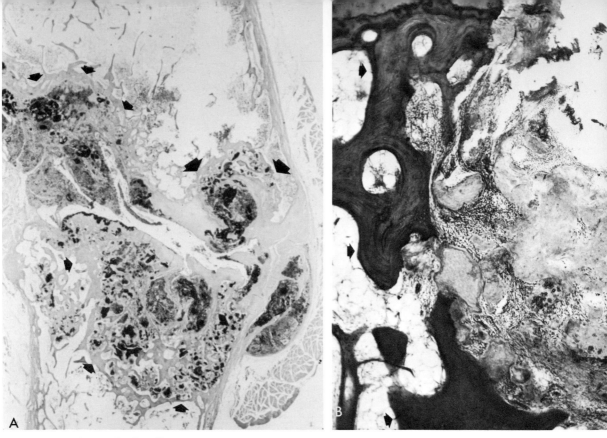

Figure 4–18. Gout.

    A. A sagittal section through the sternoclavicular joint of a patient with chronic tophaceous gout illustrates three characteristic pathologic findings: a soft tissue tophus, adjacent articular erosions and a condensation of cortical bone at the base of the erosion (arrows) giving the sclerotic margin to the radiographic image.

    B. A close-up view of a marginal erosion shows destruction of the bone and extension into the articular cartilage. Thick bony trabeculae give the erosion a well-defined edge (arrows) identical to the sclerotic border seen on the radiograph (Courtesy of The Arthritis Foundation.)

contrast, mimics the changes of a gouty erosion and suggests a word of caution. Although the overhanging edge is typical of gout, it occasionally may be seen in rheumatoid arthritis, and the distinction between the two entities must be made from all the radiographic and clinical information.

FIBROUS AND BONY ANKYLOSIS

    Obliteration of the cartilage in an inflammatory arthritis may be followed by fibrous or bony ankylosis of the joint. Since fibrous tissue is of water density, the extreme limitation of motion caused by such tissue is only appreciated clinically. The radiologist continues to see space between the articulating ends of the bones and may not appreciate the degree of joint destruction. With bony ankylosis, on the other hand, the reason for immobility is evident on the film. Trabeculae bridge the joint space and form a continuum of bone.

    Rheumatoid Arthritis. Rheumatoid arthritis may cause bony ankylosis of the carpal bones of the hand and the tarsal bones of the feet. This is practically never seen in the interphalangeal joints, no matter how severe or advanced the destructive process may be. The characteristic distribution is seen in Figure 4–19. The carpal bones are fused together and to the base of the metacarpal bones.

    Psoriatic Arthritis. Patients with psoriatic arthritis can be divided into three categories, depending on the distribution of their disease. One-third will

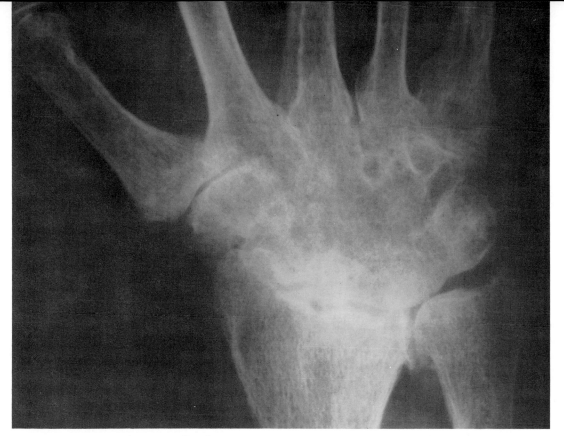

Figure 4-19. Rheumatoid arthritis.

Bony ankylosis of the carpal bones and the carpal-metacarpal joints occurs in rheumatoid arthritis. No matter how advanced the disease, bony ankylosis is rarely seen in the interphalangeal joints, an important distinguishing characteristic from psoriatic arthritis.

have a distribution indistinguishable from rheumatoid arthritis, with involvement of the wrist, the metacarpophalangeal joints and the proximal interphalangeal joints. One-third will have destructive changes limited to the distal interphalangeal joints. A final third will have a combination of the two patterns. Whenever the distal interphalangeal joints are involved in a patient who otherwise appears to have rheumatoid arthritis, psoriatic arthritis should be considered. Since the arthritis may herald the skin condition, this diagnostic possibility may not have been a clinical consideration. Psoriasis should be even more strongly considered when the distal joints are *more extensively* involved than the proximal joints and when proliferative new bone is present, as this pattern is very unusual in rheumatoid arthritis.

Even when the *pattern* of distribution is identical to that in rheumatoid arthritis there are distinguishing features that im-

plicate psoriatic arthritis as the underlying disease. A patient with a 35 year history of arthritis demonstrates all five of the radiographic findings peculiar to psoriatic arthritis (Fig. 4–20*A*).

1. Despite the chronicity of the disease, the mineralization of the bones is normal—a rare occurrence in rheumatoid arthritis, but occasionally seen in psoriatic arthritis.

2. Bony ankylosis occurs in the fingers in psoriatic arthritis, but when seen in the hands of patients with rheumatoid arthritis it is limited to the wrist. It is present in this patient (Fig. 4–20*A*) in the interphalangeal joint of the thumb, where it appears as a continuous solid shaft of bone.

The opposite hand of the same patient is more extensively involved and demonstrates three additional signs of psoriatic arthritis (Fig. 4–20*B*).

3. Diffuse soft tissue swelling (the "cocktail sausage digit") and fluffy peri-

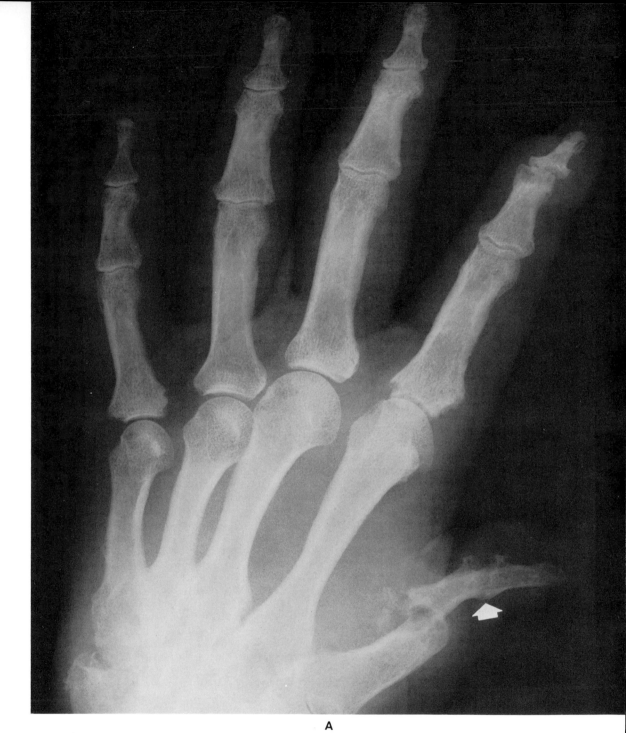

A

Figure 4–20. Psoriatic arthritis.

A. Bony ankylosis of the interphalangeal joint of the thumb (arrow) and prominent erosions of the base of the proximal phalanges are typical of the changes in psoriatic arthritis. Despite the chronicity of the disease, the bone mineralization is normal.

B. The opposite hand shows more advanced destructive changes. Bony ankylosis of the third proximal interphalangeal joint is associated with resorption of the adjacent bone. The foreshortened bones have caused a redundancy of the soft tissue and the picture of "main en lorgnette," or opera-glass hand. Excessive deposition of fibrous tissue has widened the joint spaces of the fourth and fifth proximal interphalangeal joints. Extensive deformity of the distal interphalangeal joints is seen. Shaggy periosteal new bone (along the ulnar side of the fifth metacarpal bone; arrow) is occasionally seen in psoriatic arthritis.

88

Illustration continued on opposite page.

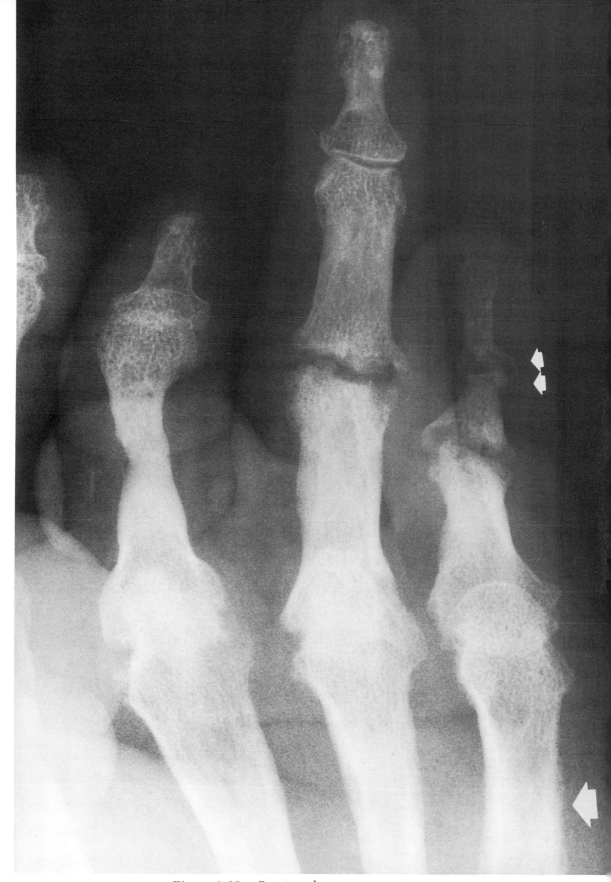

Figure 4–20.   Continued.   **B**

ostitis occasionally occur in psoriatic arthritis and are seen at this patient's fifth metacarpal bone (Fig. 4–20B, arrow). Identical changes occur more frequently in Reiter's syndrome and thus serve merely to distinguish these two rheumatoid variants from rheumatoid arthritis.

4. Severe involvement of the distal interphalangeal joints commonly accompanies similar changes in the more proximal joints in psoriatic arthritis (double arrows). Although the distal interphalangeal joints may be narrowed and eroded in *rheumatoid arthritis*, this is extremely rare, and when it occurs, it is less extensive than the destruction at the more proximal joints.

5. Extensive deposition of fibrous material within the joint space may result in separation of the articular ends of bones (seen in the proximal interphalangeal joint of the fourth finger). This *widened* joint space in the absence of resorptive whittling of the articular bones is diagnostic of psoriatic arthritis. Although fibrous deposition and widened joints occur in Reiter's syndrome, severe destructive changes may be found in the feet but are very rare in the hand. An acute effusion may widen a joint space also, but this is an early occurrence. By the time destructive changes have eroded the ends of the bones, a widened joint space is mute evidence of the end stage of psoriatic arthritis.

The microscopic appearance of fibrous ankylosis is seen in Figure 4–21. The articular cartilage has been totally destroyed and the ends of the bones are eroded. Proliferative new bone widens the base of the more distal phalanx. Diffuse osteoporosis is also present. The cor-

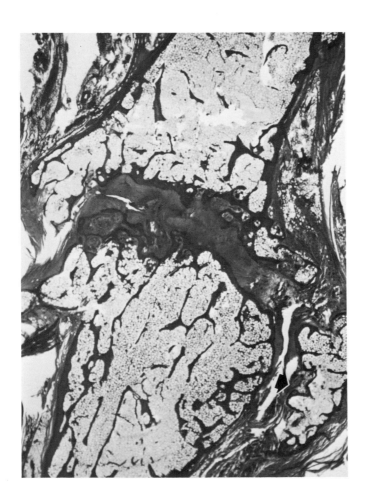

Figure 4–21. Fibrous ankylosis.

Excessive fibrous deposition and irregular erosions of the articular surfaces of the bone may be the end stage of an inflammatory arthritis. Accompanying the joint changes are diffuse osteoporosis and erosion of the sesamoid bone (arrow). (Courtesy of The Arthritis Foundation.)

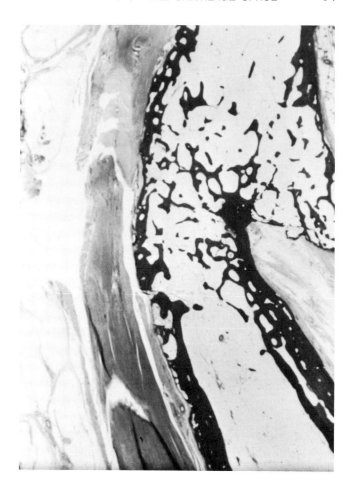

Figure 4-22. Bony ankylosis. A sagittal section of an interphalangeal joint shows total destruction of the joint and continuous lines of bone connecting the two articulating surfaces. (Courtesy of The Arthritis Foundation.)

tical bone is a pencil-thin line, and the trabeculae are markedly decreased in number.

Bony ankylosis, on the other hand, obliterates the joint space by continuous lines of trabeculae and cortical bone. As seen in Figure 4–22, concentric resorption of bone has narrowed the proximal phalanx. No evidence of inflammation is present, and at this stage the patient is left with a painless but rigid finger.

A second pattern of distribution of psoriatic arthritis is illustrated by Figure 4–23A. The arthritis is limited to the distal interphalangeal joints; the rest of the hand is normal. Inability to see a joint space may be due either to flexion deformities with overlap of the ends of the bones or to loss of the articular cartilage and actual joint narrowing. Oblique views are often necessary to make the distinction, as in this example. When joint narrowing is due to flexion, the cortical margins are superimposed on each other, whereas cartilage loss results in apposition of their edges. The oblique projection (Fig. 4–23B) verifies the joint space destruction and demonstrates bony ankylosis which has united the middle and distal phalanges. The ring finger appears only partly fused. This degree of demineralization is unusual in psoriatic arthritis and is undoubtedly attributable to the postmenopausal condition of this 67 year old woman.

Since osteoarthritis characteristically affects the distal interphalangeal joints, it must be differentiated from distal involvement by psoriatic arthritis. Although the two conditions may be indistinguishable, certain findings are helpful. Bony ankylosis is rare in osteoarthritis.

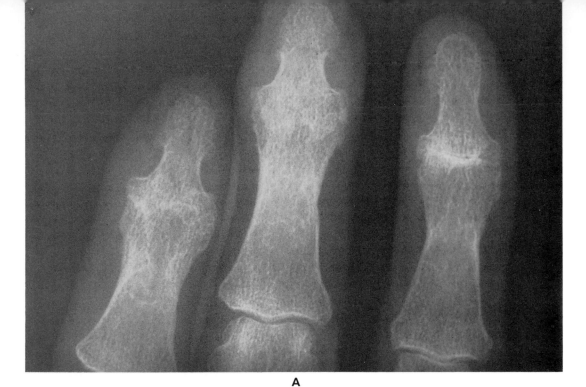

A

B

Figure 4–23. Psoriatic arthritis.

A. Obliteration of the distal interphalangeal joint spaces with bony ankylosis occurs most commonly in psoriatic arthritis. Occasionally it occurs in osteoarthritis, but the two diseases can be diagnosed by the presence of Heberden's nodes in the latter and nail changes in the former.

B. The oblique view verifies the ankylosis, as continuous arcs of trabeculae are seen crossing the narrowed joint space.

Both diseases may produce irregular joint narrowing and erosions, but proliferative changes in the form of marginal osteophytes are seen in osteoarthritis. Resorption of bone and widening of the joint space is not seen in osteoarthritis. In addition, distal interphalangeal involvement in psoriatic arthritis accompanies psoriasis of the overlying nail, and examination of the patient distinguishes the two diseases.

ARTHRITIS MUTILANS OR "MAIN-EN-LORGNETTE" DEFORMITY

A glance at Figure 4–24 explains the origin of the French term for the deformity called "opera-glass hand." The soft tissues telescope on each other as the underlying struts of bone are resorbed, resembling a collapsed opera glass.

The specific pathologic process leading to a resorptive arthropathy is unknown. Alteration in the *control* of the rich glomus network of capillaries that surrounds each joint has been suggested as the mechanism by which the dissolution of bone is initiated.

Whatever the stimulus to concentric resorption of bone may be, Figure 4–25 illustrates its histologic appearance. A closeup of the cortical margin of the phalanx from a patient with psoriatic arthropathy demonstrates the increased osteoclastic activity along the periosteal surface. The osteoclasts have "bitten off" chunks of bone along the margin leaving holes (arrows). Continuation of this process will result in concentric loss of the bony cortex of the phalanx.

A contributing factor in the production of an opera-glass hand may relate to mechanical factors. Continued pull of the muscles in areas of cartilage destruction may cause progressive resorption of the ends of the bones from pressure of the articular ends against their unprotected surfaces.

The ends of the bones may be widely separated as resorption takes place, or they may fuse by fibrous and bony ankylosis, as seen in a pathologic specimen from an opera-glass hand (Fig. 4–26). In this example, the phalanges are short and tapered, and complete obliteration of the distal interphalangeal joint with bony ankylosis is present. Fibrous tissue has replaced the articular cartilage in the proximal interphalangeal joint, and reactive sclerosis of the ends of the bones casts a dense black shadow adjacent to the fibrous tissue. These microscopic changes will be seen in the following example of juvenile rheumatoid arthritis.

Whenever a picture of arthritis mutilans or resorptive arthropathy is seen in the hand, four disease conditions must be considered: rheumatoid arthritis, psoriatic arthritis, juvenile rheumatoid arthritis and neuropathic diseases. Very rarely progressive systemic sclerosis will cause a similar resorptive phenomenon. Lipoid dermatoarthritis may produce a classic opera-glass hand, but this entity is so rare that it is not a practical consideration.

Juvenile Rheumatoid Arthritis. Rarely, resorptive changes will occur to such an extent in a patient with juvenile rheumatoid arthritis that the final picture is that of an opera-glass hand with redundant soft tissues and whittled bones (Fig. 4–27). The metacarpophalangeal joints are subluxed and destruction and reactive sclerosis similar to that in the preceding pathologic specimen are seen in the proximal interphalangeal joints. Severe osteoporosis and bony ankylosis of the entire wrist are additional tragic residua of juvenile rheumatoid arthritis.

Cupping of the base of the phalanges is commonly seen in resorptive arthropathies. The microscopic section of a joint from a patient with rheumatoid arthritis suggests that this may be due in part to deposition of fibrous material and subsequent erosion (Fig. 4–28). The fact that it affects the distal side of the joint rather than the proximal may be related to the forces within the joint from continued muscle pull.

JOINT CHANGES ASSOCIATED WITH NEW BONE FORMATION

Osteoarthritis. Both primary generalized osteoarthritis and erosive osteoarthritis are specific disease entities that warrant distinction from the general

Text continued on page 97.

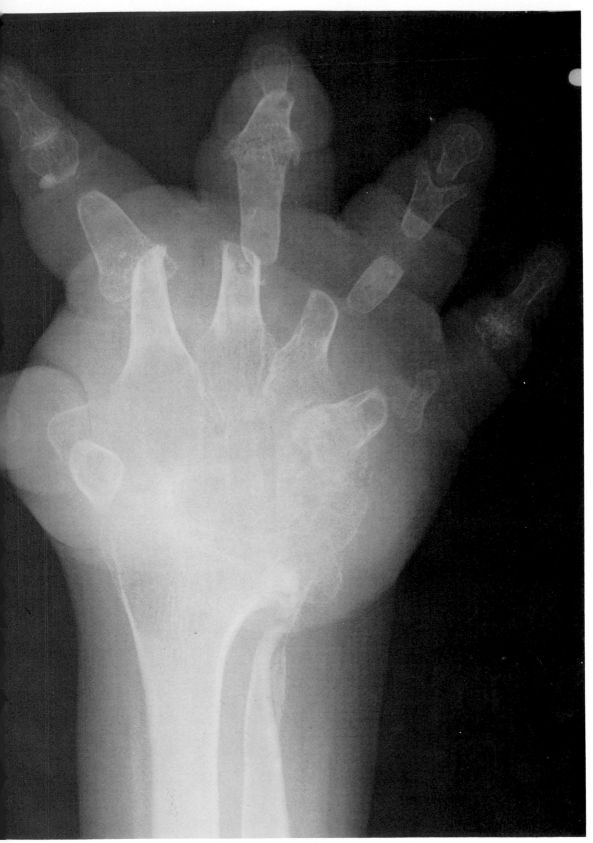

Figure 4–24.   See legend on opposite page.

Figure 4-25. Resorptive arthropathy.

A photomicrograph offers a close look at the periosteal surface of a phalangeal bone from a patient with hand changes similar to those seen in the preceding radiograph (Fig. 4–24). Large "bites" of bone are being removed by the active osteoclasts, leaving white holes along the margin and decreasing the width of the bone (arrows). Continuation of this resorption will result in a whittled or pencilled appearance of the bone. (Courtesy of The Arthritis Foundation.)

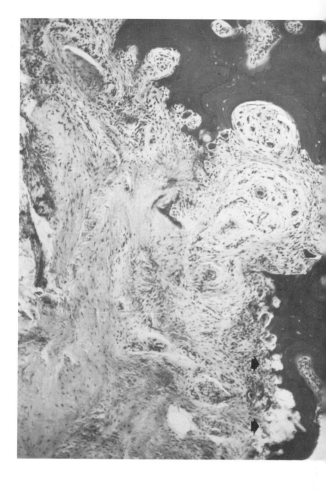

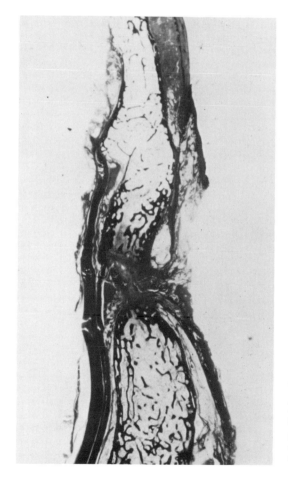

Figure 4-26. The "opera-glass" deformity.

Joint destruction and resorption of the ends of the articular bones causes shortening of the strut of bone and redundancy of the overlying soft tissues. Although the soft tissues are not seen in this preparation, the whittled bones, the fibrous ankylosis of the proximal interphalangeal joint and the bony fusion of the distal interphalangeal joint are typical of the end stages of psoriatic arthritis, a frequent culprit in this rare mutilation of the hand. (Courtesy of The Arthritis Foundation.)

Figure 4-24. The "opera-glass" hand in rheumatoid arthritis.

The hand is aptly named. The telescoped skinfolds result from resorption of the articular ends of the bones and subsequent destruction of the joints and foreshortening of the fingers. Concentric resorption, beginning at the periosteal surface of the cortex, causes a pencilled effect, as seen at the third, fourth and fifth metacarpophalangeal joints. When the proximal bone is affected more extensively, continuous pull of the tendons across a destroyed joint space results in invagination and a pencil-in-cup deformity, as seen in the second metacarpophalangeal joint. Resorption of the distal ulna often accompanies the changes in the digits.

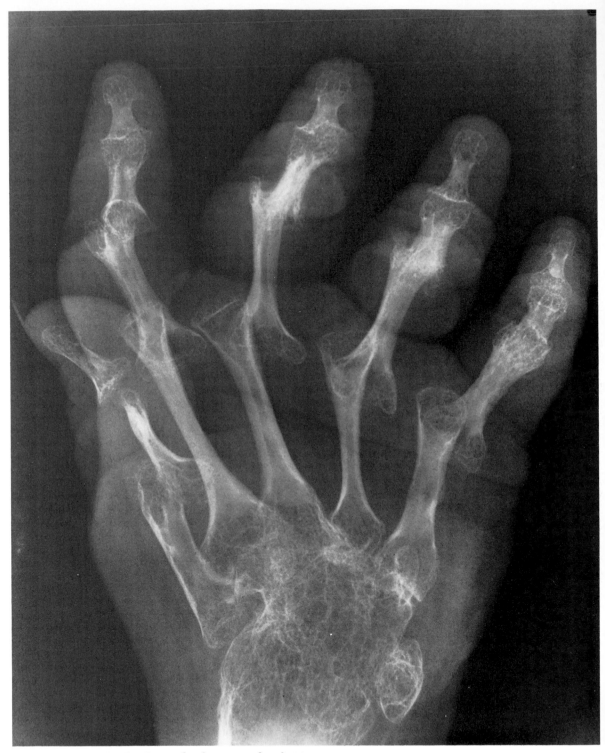

Figure 4-27. Juvenile rheumatoid arthritis.

Resorptive arthropathies may rarely be seen in juvenile rheumatoid arthritis, causing a typical "main en lorgnette" or "opera-glass" hand deformity. The redundant soft tissues have folded on each other over the shortened phalangeal bones. Subluxation of the fingers and bony ankylosis of the wrist add to the deformity. The generalized, severe osteoporosis is typical of juvenile rheumatoid arthritis.

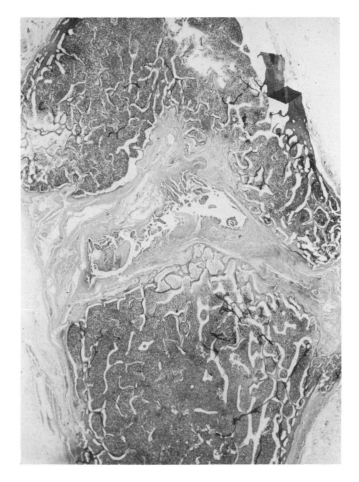

Figure 4-28. Rheumatoid arthritis.

Cupping of the base of a phalanx is commonly seen in resorptive arthropathies. Excessive deposition of fibrous material, as in this example, coupled with continuous tendinous pull across the damaged joint may account for the radiographic changes. (Courtesy of The Arthritis Foundation.)

term of degenerative arthritis. Primary generalized osteoarthritis was originally described by Kellgren and is frequently referred to as Kellgren's arthritis. It occurs in postmenopausal women and affects the distal and proximal interphalangeal joints and the first carpometacarpal joint of the wrist. Occasionally the metacarpophalangeal joints are involved, but this involvement is minor as compared with that of distal joints.

When erosions of the articulating surfaces of bone form a major component of the pathologic picture, a distinction is made between Kellgren's arthritis and erosive osteoarthritis. It is important to be aware of the latter entity and its potential confusion with rheumatoid arthritis. Although the histology of the synovium during the acute phase of erosive osteoarthritis is similar to that in rheumatoid arthritis, its occurrence in the *prox-*

imal and *distal* interphalangeal joints with sparing of the metacarpophalangeal joints and the absence of systemic symptoms should suggest the correct diagnosis. Unlike rheumatoid arthritis, erosive osteoarthritis is a self-limited disease, and although it leaves permanent deforming sequelae, it does not have the more ominous complications of rheumatoid arthritis.

Changes in both Kellgren's arthritis and erosive osteoarthritis are characterized by non-uniform narrowing of the joint space and development of new bone at the margins (osteophytes) and are indistinguishable from those in degenerative joint disease. However, degenerative changes imply trauma, and the occurrence of primary generalized osteoarthritis and erosive osteoarthritis appears to be spontaneous. In both conditions, the large weight-bearing joints of the body may be affected. As in the hand, the changes are those of irregular joint narrowing with associated osteophytes.

The hand of a woman with typical primary generalized osteoarthritis shows the classical configuration and distribution of this disease (Fig. 4–29A). There is a wavy appearance to the contour of the fingers which is as obvious clinically as it is radiographically. It is quite typical of osteoarthritis and is due to two factors: the lateral subluxation of one phalanx on the other and the presence of osteophytes which exaggerate the offset of the joint margins and distort the overlying soft tissue. This proliferative new bone is palpable and is called a "Heberden's node" when it occurs at the distal interphalangeal joint (Fig. 4–29B). Frequently the node is much more prominent clinically than it is on the radiograph; this is due to cartilage which caps the osteophyte but casts only a water density shadow.

Typically, in both types of osteoarthritis the distal interphalangeal joints are affected first, and their involvement is out of proportion to the changes in the proximal interphalangeal joints. Figure 4–29A shows early manifestations of the disease in the second and fourth proximal interphalangeal joints. Narrowing occurs at the periphery of the joint, where the cartilage degenerates earliest. The metacarpophalangeal joints are spared in both primary and erosive osteoarthritis, with the exception of the articulation of the base of the first metacarpal with the carpal bone (the trapeziometacarpal joint). This third area of the hand is affected in this patient.

In this example, the classical pattern of distribution for osteoarthritis is present: the distal interphalangeal joints, the proximal interphalangeal joints and the first carpal-metacarpal articulation. The

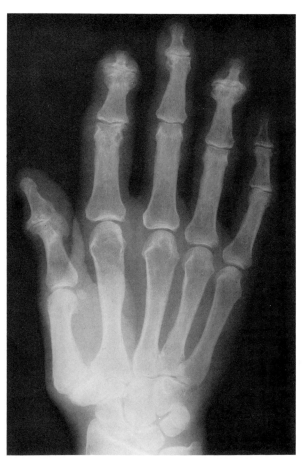

A

Figure 4–29. Primary generalized osteoarthritis.

A. The pattern of joint involvement often suggests a specific disease, as in this hand. Osteoarthritis affects the distal interphalangeal and proximal interphalangeal joints as well as the first carpal-metacarpal articulation and spares the metacarpophalangeal joints and the rest of the wrist.

Illustration continued on opposite page.

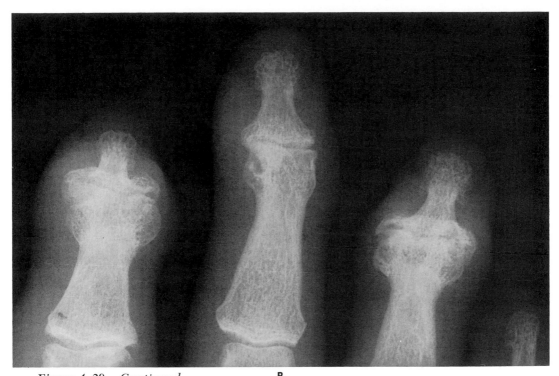

Figure 4–29. Continued. **B**

B. A close-up of the distal interphalangeal joints illustrates the typical radiographic changes: irregular cartilage loss; osteophytes, adding to the dimension of the articulating ends of the distal phalanges; and lateral subluxation of the bones, causing a wavy appearance to the finger and a classical Heberden's node.

pattern of distribution excludes a connective tissue disease as does the presence of new bone or osteophytes.

Mucoid cysts of the soft tissues are occasionally seen in patients with erosive osteoarthritis and should not be confused with rheumatoid nodules. They appear and disappear spontaneously and are clinically insignificant. The periarticular mass seen in Figure 4–30 is out of proportion to the early developing osteophytes and cannot be considered a Heberden's node. This is the typical appearance of a mucoid cyst in a patient with osteoarthritis.

When lateral subluxation and osteophytes develop at the *proximal* interphalangeal joints they are called "Bouchard's nodes." These are seen in Figure 4–31.

Acromegaly. Osteophytes are formed in response to the degeneration of cartilage and develop at the periphery of joints along the margins of the bones. They must not be confused with the pro-

liferative new bone that accompanies acromegaly. The latter develops as part of a general tendency in acromegaly for all tissues to proliferate and is seen at points of maximal stress on the underlying bone. Osteoblastic stimulation tends to produce spicules of bone where capsules and tendons insert.

Figure 4–32 demonstrates typical widening of the cartilage spaces at the metacarpophalangeal joints. The prominent knuckle pads reflect the soft tissue hypertrophy. The proximal interphalangeal joints and distal interphalangeal joints are beginning to show the degenerative changes that signify early senescence of the overdeveloped cartilage. The narrowing of the lateral aspects of the joint spaces is the radiographic sign of loss of cartilage.

Neuropathic Arthropathy. Ectopic or soft tissue deposition of bone is rare in the hand although it is a common accompaniment of neuropathic changes in other regions of the body. A female pa-

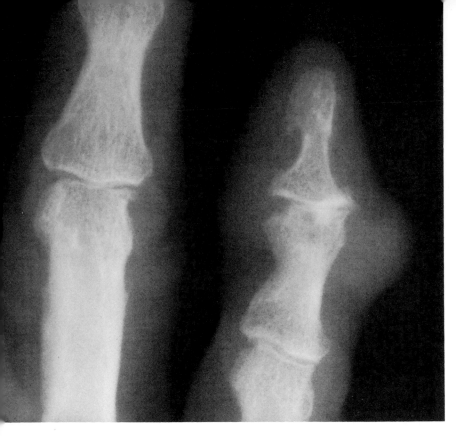

Figure 4–30. Osteoarthritis with a mucoid cyst.

Joint narrowing, eburnation and osteophytes characterize the changes of osteoarthritis. A prominent soft tissue mass, a mucoid cyst, is a frequent finding in postmenopausal women with this condition.

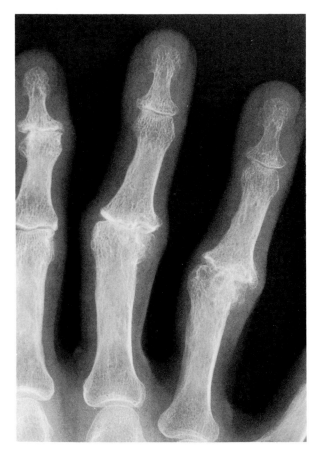

Figure 4–31. Erosive osteoarthritis.

Lateral subluxation with osteophytes at the proximal interphalangeal joints constitutes a Bouchard's node. The irregular erosions of the articular surfaces reflect the active synovitis and differentiate the radiographic picture from primary generalized osteoarthritis.

Figure 4–32. Acromegaly.

Cartilage overgrowth at the metacarpophalangeal joints is striking and contrasts with the peripheral joint narrowing present in the interphalangeal joints. This seeming contradiction is clarified when one recalls that the enlarged cartilage is vulnerable to early degenerative changes and a superimposed osteoarthritis. Bony proliferation has expanded the tufts and the base of the distal phalanges and has caused jagged projections of bone along the metaphyses and diaphyses of the proximal phalanges and metacarpal bones.

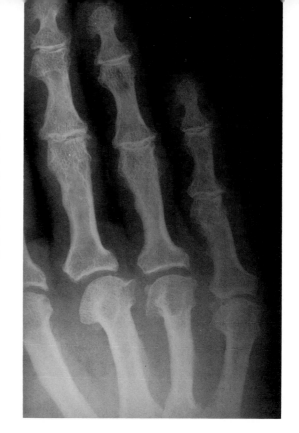

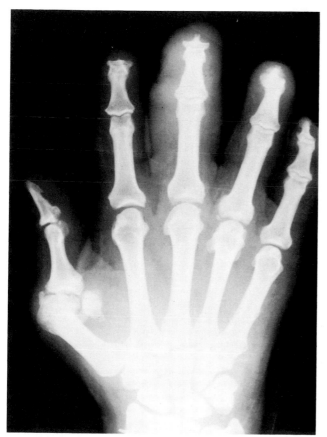

Figure 4–33. Syringomyelia.

Chronic soft tissue swelling and loss of the tips of the fingers from repeated episodes of trauma have altered the appearance of the hand since an earlier film (see Figure 1–3). Degenerative changes of the first metacarpophalangeal joint are characteristic of neuropathic arthropathies, with excessive ectopic bone in the soft tissues adjacent to a disorganized joint.

101

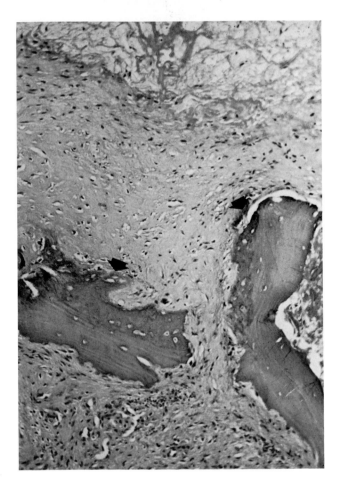

Figure 4–34. Neuropathic arthropathy.

A photomicrograph illustrates the mechanism of the enlarging bone fragments within soft tissues. Fragments of dead bone (with empty lacunae) are being enlarged by apposition of new bone along the edges (arrows). Although disorganization of the joints typifies a neurotrophic condition, the prominent periarticular new bone cannot be accounted for by fragmentation of the articular ends of the bones alone. (Courtesy of The Arthritis Foundation.)

tient with syringomyelia has developed this characteristic formation of new bone adjacent to the base of the thumb (Fig. 4–33). This patient had a long history of chronic massive effusion with distortion of the soft tissue; a film of this same hand early in the course of her disease showed this finding (see Figure 1–3). With loss of sensation, recurrent unrecognized trauma is most frequently inflicted on the tips of the fingers, and underlying damage to these bones occurs. In addition to the ectopic new bone, marked resorptive changes can be seen involving the distal phalanges of the second, third and fourth fingers, corresponding to areas of old burns and lacerations that had accrued over the seven year interval.

It is apparent that the amount of bone adjacent to the base of the thumb is more than could be accounted for by fragmentation of the adjacent articular bones. It is

characteristic of neuropathic arthropathies to develop new bone in the soft tissues. A biopsy specimen from a neuropathic joint (Fig. 4–34) illustrates the possible mechanism. Fragments of dead bone with empty lacunae are in the process of being enlarged as appositional new bone is formed around them.

SUGGESTED READINGS

Avila, R., D. G. Pugh, C. H. Slocumb, and R. K. Winkelmann. Psoriatic arthritis: A roentgenologic study. Radiology 75:691 (1960).

Grahame, R., and J. T. Scott. Clinical survey of 354 patients with gout. Ann. Rheum. Dis. 29:461 (1970).

Green, F. A. Distal interphalangeal joint disease and nail abnormalities. Ann. Rheum. Dis. 27:55 (1968).

Harrison, M. O., R. H. Freiberger, and C. S. Ranawat. Arthrography of the rheumatoid wrist joint. Amer. J. Roentgen. 112:480 (1971).

International Congress Series #61. Radiologic

Aspects of Rheumatoid Arthritis. Excerpta Medica Foundation.

Jayson, M. I. V., D. Rubenstein, and A. St. J. Dixon. Intra-articular pressure and rheumatoid geodes (bone cysts). Ann. Rheum. Dis. 29:496 (1970).

Marshall, T. R. Radiographic changes in rheumatoid arthritis in the digits. Radiology 90:121 (1968).

Martel, W. The overhanging margin of bone: A roentgenologic manifestation of gout. Radiology 91:755 (1968).

Martel, W. The pattern of rheumatoid arthritis in the hand and wrist. Rad. Clin. N. Amer. Aug. 1964, p. 221.

Martel, W., Murray, R. A., and I. F. Duff. Cervical spine involvement in lipoid dermatoarthritis. Radiology 77:613 (1961).

Martel, W., Holt, J. F., and J. T. Cassidy. Roentgenologic manifestations of juvenile rheumatoid arthritis. Amer. J. Roentgen. 88:400 (1962).

McAfee, J. G., and M. W. Donner. Differential diagnosis of radiographic changes in the hands. Amer. J. Med. Sci. 245:592 (1963).

McClain, E. J., and J. H. Boyes. Missed fractures of the greater multangular. J. Bone Joint Surg. (Amer.) 48A:1525 (1966).

O'Hara, L. J., and M. Levin. Carpal tunnel syndrome and gout. Arch. Int. Med. 120:180 (1967).

Peter, J. B., C. M. Pearson and L. Marmar. Erosive osteoarthritis of the hands. Arthritis Rheum. 9:365 (1966).

Phillips, R. S. Carpal tunnel syndrome as a manifestation of systemic disease. Ann. Rhem. Dis. 26:59 (1967).

Rodnan, G. P. The nature of joint involvement in progressive systemic sclerosis (diffuse scleroderma): Clinical study and pathologic examination of synovium in twenty-nine patients. Ann. Int. Med. 56:422 (1962).

Sholkoff, S. D., M. G. Glickman, and H. Steinbach. Roentgenology of Reiter's syndrome. Radiology 97:497 (1970).

Silbiger, M. L., and C. C. Peterson, Jr. Sjogren's syndrome: Its roentgenographic features. Amer. J. Roentgen. 100:554 (1967).

Silver, M., and O. Steinbrocker. Resorptive osteopathy in inflammatory arthritis. "Absorptive arthritis;" "Opera glass hand." Bull. Hosp. Joint Dis. 15:211 (1954).

Templeton, A. W., and I. D. Zim. The carpal tunnel view. Missouri Med. 61:443 (1964).

Vainio, K. Rheumatoid changes in the metacarpophalangeal region as a cause of Bunnell's sign. Ann. Rheum. Dis. 26:328 (1967).

Weinstein, J. D., H. M. Dick, and S. A. Grantham. Pseudogout, hyperparathyroidism and carpal-tunnel syndrome. J. Bone Joint Surg. (Amer.) 50A:1669 (1968).

EXERCISES

INTRODUCTION

The following Exercises, which round out the preceding four chapters on the hand, and the Exercises following each subsequent chapter, are presented for several reasons. We have included some because they summarize the classic radiographic manifestations of an arthritis in a single picture. Some offer an opportunity to see non-bony manifestations of an arthritis. Many provide an opportunity to underscore important diagnostic clues that we have found helpful in distinguishing one arthritis from another. And finally, we have included some films simply because they have been particularly exciting to decipher.

Without benefit of history or physical examination, a methodical search of the film alone often provides the information necessary to establish a diagnosis. At times, however, it is impossible without knowledge of the distribution of the arthritis in the patient or without laboratory data to suggest anything more conclusive than a list of possibilities. Nevertheless, it is equally important to realize the extent of reliability of a film alone as it represents the gross pathologic specimen, and to understand its limitations because of nonspecific findings. For this reason, no clinical information is provided before the Answer to each Exercise.

The discussion that follows the unknown illustration or illustrations reveals the diagnosis, and additional radiographs may be included if pertinent. For the most part, the Exercises are on the left-hand page and the Answers are on the right, but occasionally the answer may be directly under the picture to save space, and care must be taken to avoid inadvertently observing the answer.

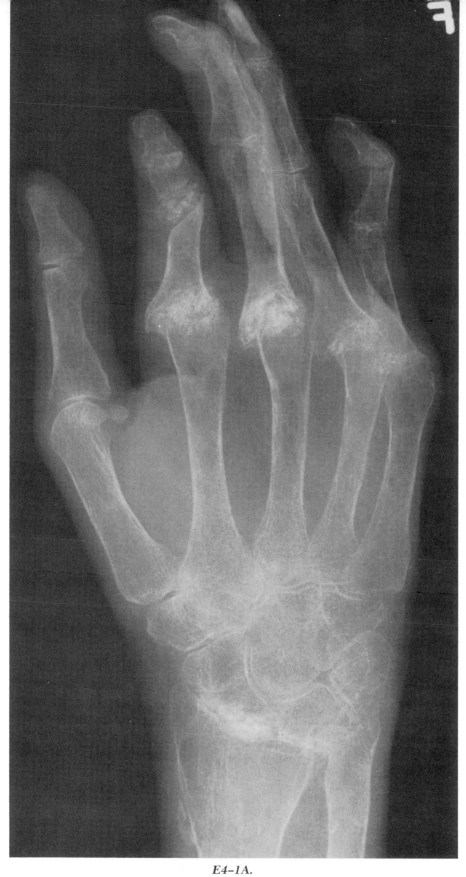

E4–1A.

Exercise continued on following pages.

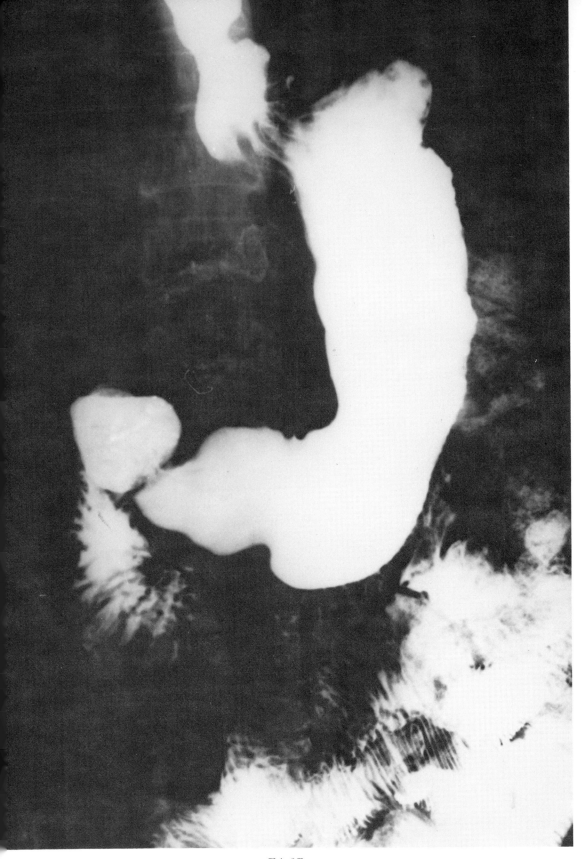

E4–1B.

E4–1. This first Exercise exemplifies the "ABC'S" approach since each category contains an abnormality. Even though this is an extreme example of the *CRST syndrome*, the spectrum of radiographic findings leads one to the appropriate diagnosis.

SOFT TISSUE. The soft tissues are wasted, as is best seen adjacent to the fifth metacarpal bone and its proximal phalanx. Loss of the tip of the second finger and decrease in the bulk of soft tissues around the terminal tufts reflect gangrene accompanying Raynaud's phenomenon. Subcutaneous calcifications abut the distal radius and fill the radiocarpal joint, the second and third metacarpophalangeal joints and the proximal interphalangeal joint of the index finger.

ALIGNMENT. There is volar subluxation of the fingers at the metacarpophalangeal joints and a swan neck deformity of the fifth finger, reflecting a mild inflammatory arthritis with laxity of the joints.

BONY MINERALIZATION. Although it may indicate nothing more than a postmenopausal state, severe generalized osteoporosis should always suggest a possibility of systemic adrenocorticosteroid medication. In stark contrast to the washed-out appearance of the bones, a wedge of solid cortical bone whitens the distal phalanx of the fourth finger. Even when generalized to all the distal phalanges, terminal phalangeal sclerosis is far from pathognomonic of a connective tissue disorder. Its patchy presence in the ring finger of this patient with progressive systemic sclerosis only increases the curiosity as to its pathogenesis.

CARTILAGE SPACE. The abnormality of intra-articular deposition of calcium is apparent in multiple joints. Erosion of the juxta-articular bones, a rare finding in scleroderma, relates to the adjacent calcium deposits rather than an inflammatory erosive arthritis. The proximal interphalangeal joint of the second finger is actually widened by the extensive pressure erosion from the large amorphous collection of calcium.

The barium study of this patient illustrates the changes in the upper gastrointestinal tract when it is involved in the changes of progressive systemic sclerosis. Normally the esophagus empties its contents immediately. This film shows the last swallow of barium still residing in the distal esophagus, despite the fact that enough time has passed to outline the entire jejunum.

Foreshortening of the esophagus is common when the gastrointestinal tract is involved in the changes of scleroderma. Not infrequently, small hiatal hernias evolve and further complicate esophageal emptying as peptic esophagitis supervenes to narrow the distal portion as in this example.

Delayed emptying of the stomach and duodenal sweep and dilatation of the jejunum indicate extensive gastrointestinal tract involvement. The appearance of sharply defined, thin valvulae distinguishes this condition from dilatation of the small bowel by mechanical obstruction, which widens and effaces the valvulae. Small bowel thickening and dilatation may be so extensive and passage of its contents so sluggish that a malabsorption *syndrome* may develop. The radiographic picture of a malabsorption *pattern*, however, never occurs.

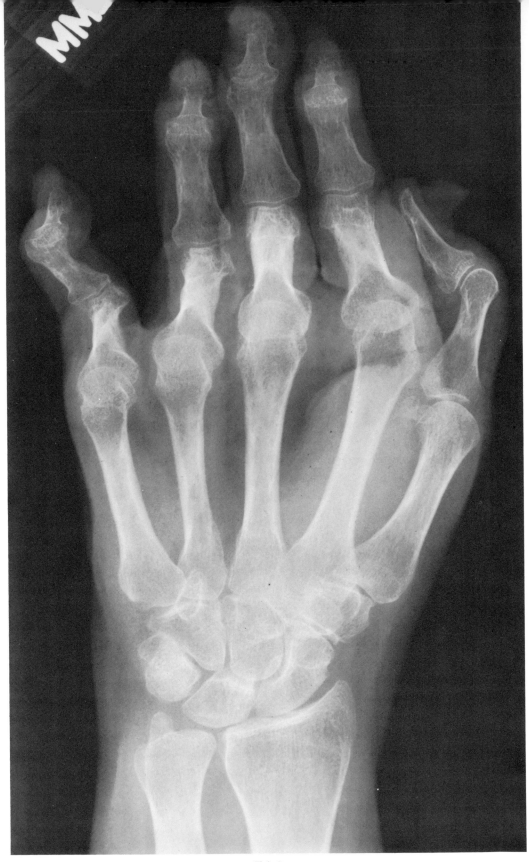

E4-2.

E4–2. The soft tissue findings give this hand away. The grotesque distortion of the nails is from subungual hyperkeratosis. Swan neck deformities without associated erosions are more commonly seen in systemic lupus erythematosus and Jaccoud's arthritis and, although present in this example, are an uncommon occurrence in *psoriatic arthritis*.

Even more fascinating than the radiographic evidence of joint laxity was the distribution of arthritis in this woman: the right knee, the right foot and the right elbow were involved in addition to the right hand. All the joints on this patient's left side were symptom-free and radiographically normal. Unilateral arthritis always suggests a past incident that has resulted in disuse and hence protection of the joints from destruction, such as poliomyelitis or stroke. This woman had had neither, and her unilateral arthritis remains a mystery.

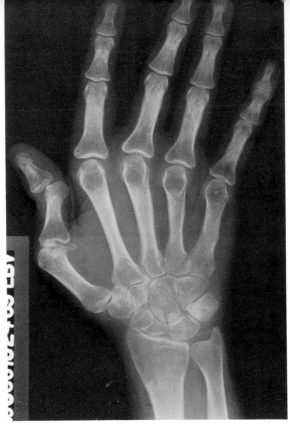

E4–3.

E4–3. Despite the easily overlooked abnormalities, the presence of subtle and seemingly insignificant changes in alignment and bony mineralization signify a severe illness. Ulnar deviation at the metacarpophalangeal joints, subluxation of the interphalangeal joint of the thumb and juxta-articular demineralization are often the only radiographic findings in *systemic lupus erythematosus.* In fact, these minor changes in a patient with chronic arthritis and signs of a systemic disease should always suggest the possibility of this connective tissue disorder, as they are so frequently seen in the hands of patients where arthritis is a major complaint.

E4–4. To obtain an admission of drug abuse is difficult and often the film offers the first clue of such a history by revealing one of the frequent complications of injections.

When this patient was admitted to the hospital complaining of exquisite pain in her hand, a routine chest film offered more information than anticipated. Even as sterile an abstraction as a radiograph can portray the agony of addiction. No ad-

mission of drug abuse was necessary after seeing the telltale syringes and spoon in the pocket of her blouse (E4–4A).

Her initial hand film (E4–4B) was not normal either. There were signs of early juxta-articular demineralization and soft tissue tapering of the end of her index finger, the radiographic signs of vasculitis or Raynaud's phenomenon. Accidental injection of Seconal into the artery several days earlier had brought this girl to the hospital with severe arterial spasm. The changes are similar to the vasculitis of a connective tissue disorder, but the sequence of events in *vasculitis from drug abuse* is measured in days and weeks rather than months and years. In the past, this occurred as an accidental mishap of anesthesia. Today it is being seen more and more frequently in emergency rooms and private offices, and if not recognized, irreversible destruction from the ensuing vasculitis follows. In this case, even heroic measures failed, and surgical amputation of the second and third fingers was necessary (E4–4C). Juxta-articular demineralization of the hand remains as evidence of this self-induced vasculitis.

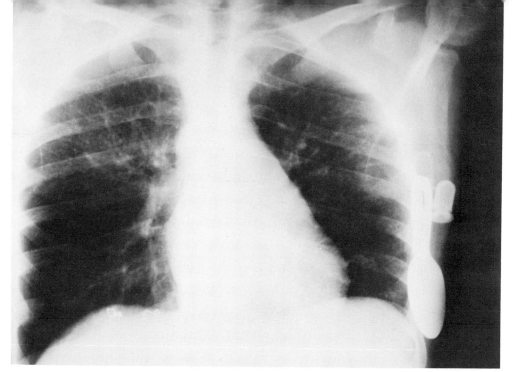

E4-4A.

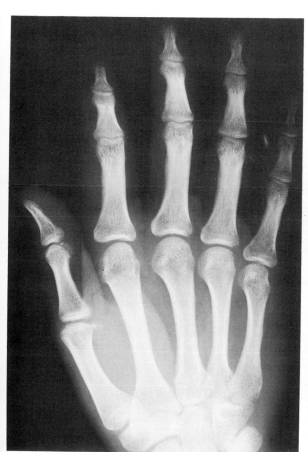

E4-4B.

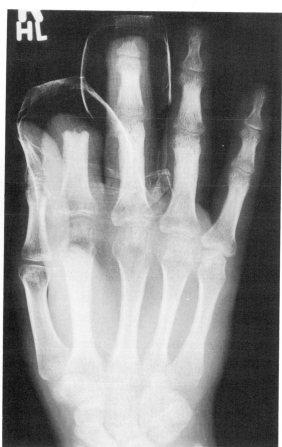

E4-4C.   Three weeks later.

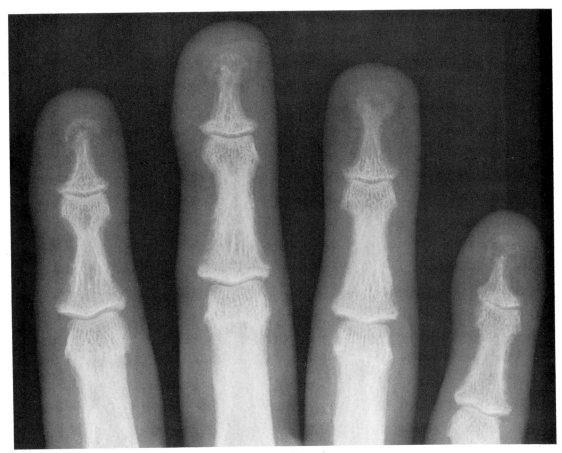

E4–5A.

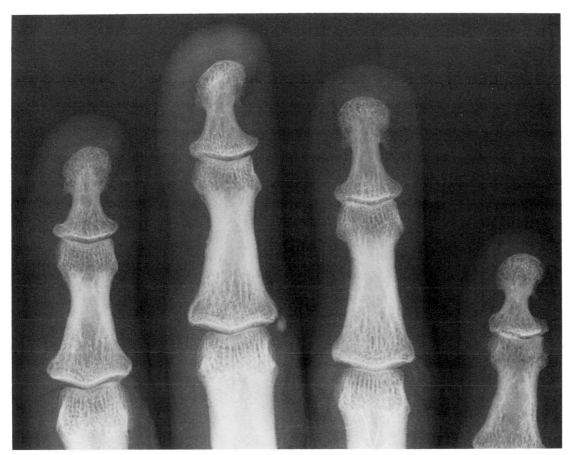

E4–5B.

E4–5. Few signs are pathognomonic in medicine. Subperiosteal resorption is. Such extensive cortical loss as is seen in these middle and distal phalanges could only mean one disease—*hyperparathy-* *roidism.* The parathyroid adenoma was removed, and the bony mineralization returned to normal, as documented by a film taken several years later (E4–5*B*).

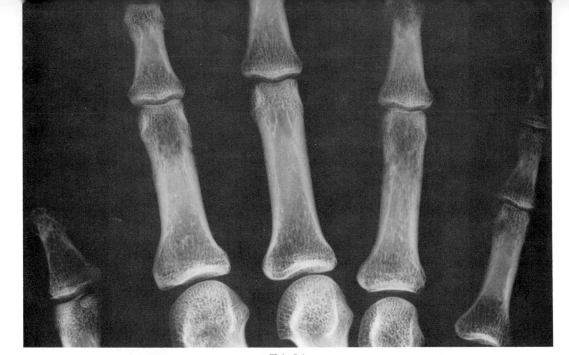

E4-6A.

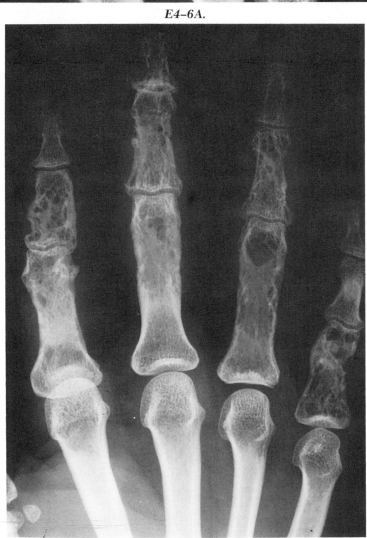

E4-6B. Several years later.

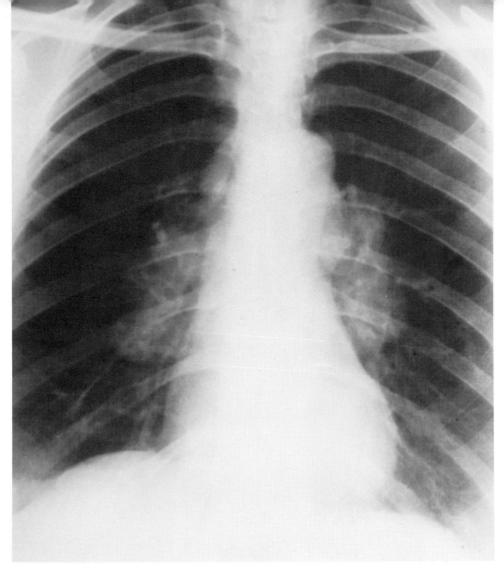

E4–6C.

E4–6. "Faith loves to lean on time's destroying arm"* — and diagnosis does too.

The passage of time converts the non-descript finding of localized trabecular thinning (of the distal ends of the second and fourth proximal phalanges) into the well-defined coarse, lacelike destruction suggestive of diffuse granulomatous involvement of the medullary cavities. Both leprosy and sarcoidosis may occasionally affect the small bones of the hand so extensively. The chest film illustrates the classical triangular nodal involvement of sarcoid: there is a potato-like configuration of the hilar nodes and an enlarged azygos node forming the apex of the triangle and filling in the arm of the right main bronchus and distal trachea.

With the advent of adrenocorticosteroid therapy for *sarcoidosis* it is rare to see the classical small, punched-out lesions of the hands, much less the far-advanced granulomatous involvement of the marrow cavity that deforms this woman's hands.

_____

*Oliver Wendell Holmes

115

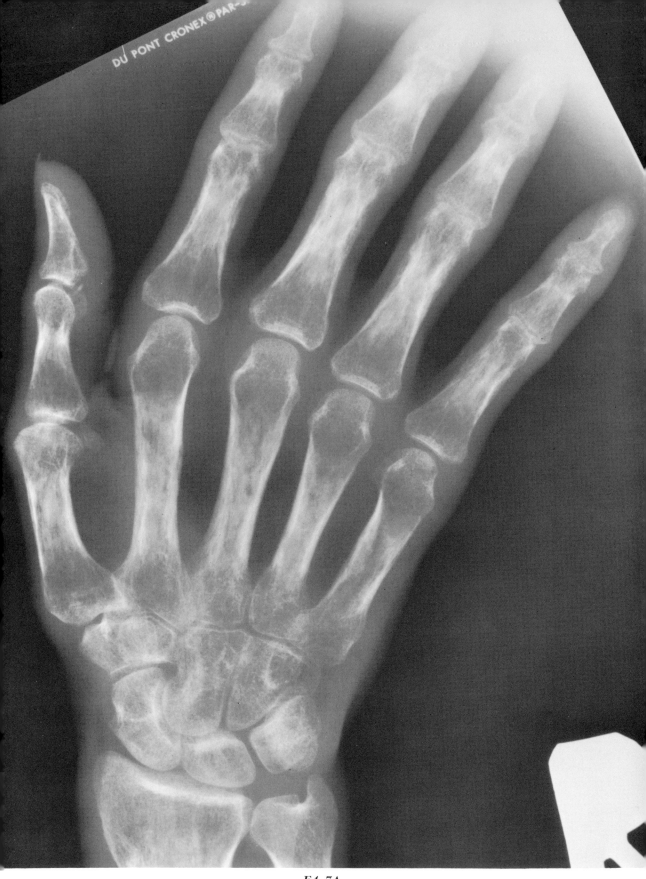

E4–7A.

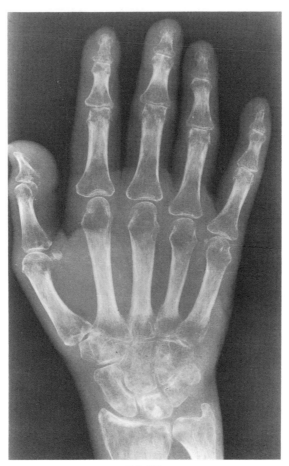

E4-7B.

E4-7. The diagnosis of this condition can be established only by a radiograph. No laboratory test will enlighten the physician in his search for the etiology of his patient's incapacitating pain and soft tissue changes. Although such a precise diagnosis cannot be made from this hand film without corroborative history, *Sudeck's atrophy* should be suggested where severe demineralization and soft tissue wasting are seen together. The concave soft tissue shadows adjacent to the fifth metacarpal bone and the proximal phalanges indicate the severe loss of subcutaneous tissues. Because of wasting and atrophy of the skin, flexion deformities of the fingers develop, and on physical examination the hand looks similar to that involved by scleroderma. However, involvement of a single hand or foot and dramatic mottled osteoporosis (established by a radiograph) eliminates confusion of the two entities.

Rapid demineralization is associated with immobilization and is most commonly seen in the shoulder-hand syndrome, as in this case, or following casting of a fracture of the extremity. The rapidity of mineral loss may give the bone a moth-eaten appearance differing from the ground glass pattern of chronic osteoporosis. It may also cause the shaft of the bone to show a double contour, as seen in the proximal phalanges of this man, erroneously suggesting periostitis.

Despite a history of pain of only two weeks, a second patient has developed the characteristic osteoporosis of Sudeck's atrophy (E4-7B). Diffuse soft tissue swelling precedes the atrophic changes and is apparent in this example. Both patients had bronchogenic carcinomas extending into the brachial plexus, resulting in the clinical and radiographic picture of classic Sudeck's atrophy.

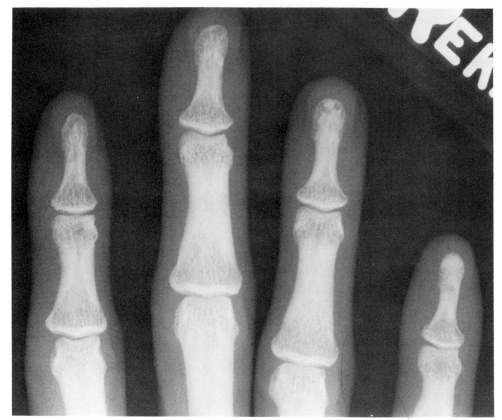

E4–8A.

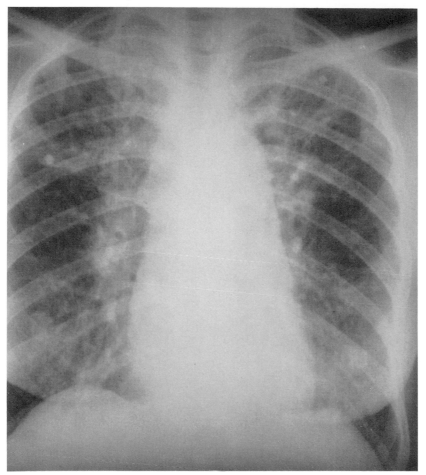

E4–8B.

E4–8. Without the chest film, the discovery of terminal phalangeal sclerosis in a young woman with arthralgias should suggest rheumatoid arthritis. However, mediastinal and hilar adenopathy in conjunction with interstitial lung disease could never be ascribed to a connective tissue disorder and is typical of *sarcoidosis*. Occasionally this disease is associated with a propensity for increased osteoblastic activity and hence producing of thickened cortices or islands of sclerotic new bone. Since a quarter of patients with sarcoidosis will complain of joint pains and yet the vast majority will have perfectly normal radiographs, this hand is a rare find. In its most exaggerated form, endosteal new bone may be combined with a concentric resorption, leading to the changes illustrated in Chapter 3, Figure 3–10.

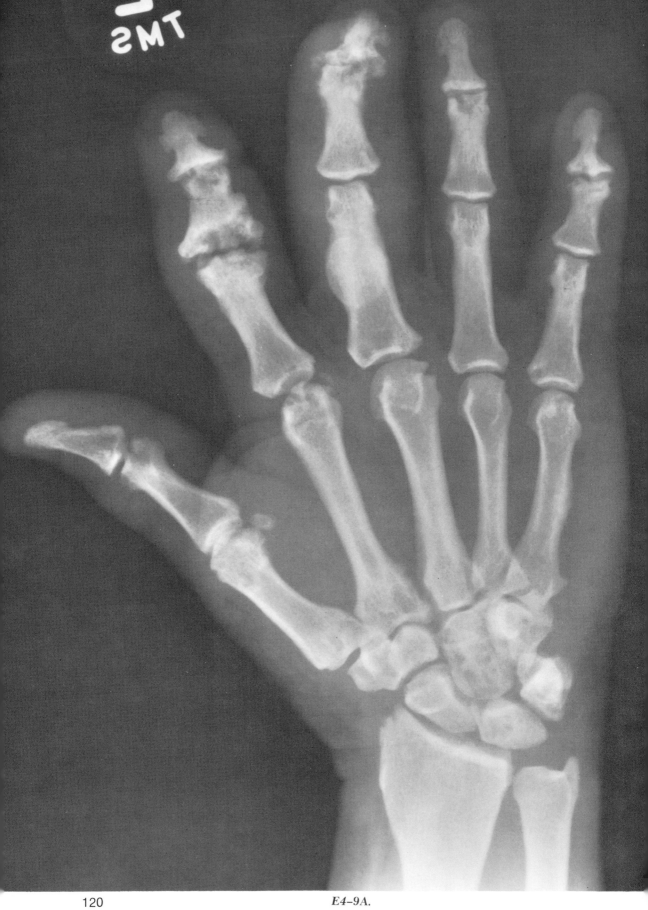

E4-9A.

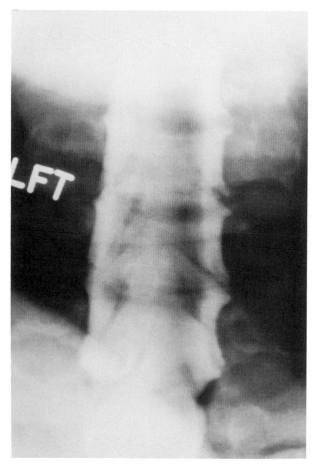

E4–9B.

E4–9. Widened joints are unusual and the diagnostic possibilities are limited. Psoriatic arthritis should always come to mind because of its propensity to deposit excessive amounts of fibrous tissue during the healing phase and its tendency to involve the distal interphalangeal joints. However, the appearance of the wavy, thick periosteal new bone of the third proximal phalanx and fifth metacarpal bone is different from that of the periostitis of psoriatic arthritis. Soft tissue swelling bulges the contours of the palm and third finger of this patient's hand. The combination of soft tissue swelling and periostitis suggests the changes of chronic stasis.

Infection may also destroy a joint in this manner, but multiple sites of involvement are unusual.

This man's occupation gives away the diagnosis of *syringomyelia*. He worked in a "freak show" sticking pins in his hands. Absence of sensation suggested a neuropathic arthropathy as the most likely explanation for the radiographic changes and led to a cervical myelogram (E4–9B).

The spinal cord never takes up more than two thirds of the neural canal, or half the distance between the bony pedicles. A syrinx has expanded the cervical portion of this patient's cord so that it measures two thirds of the interpedicular distance.

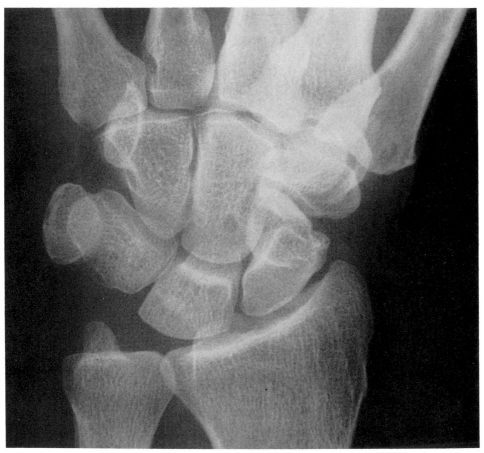

E4–10A. Left wrist.

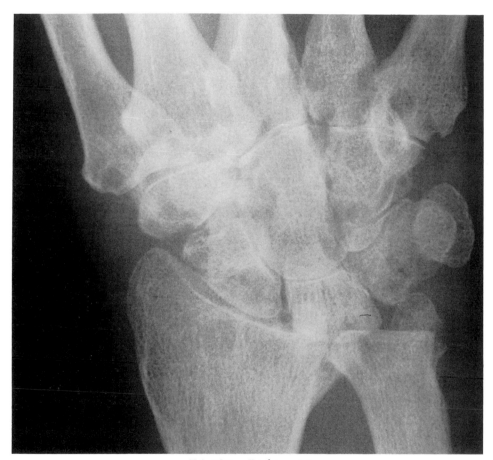

E4–10B. Right wrist.

E4–10. Unilateral wrist involvement should never dissuade one from making a diagnosis of rheumatoid arthritis. It is not unusual for one wrist to be affected, although eventually the contralateral side may reflect inflammatory disease. When cystic changes of the carpal bones are the predominant finding, the question of gout is always raised. Soft tissue swelling and erosion of the ulnar styloid occur in either gout or rheumatoid arthritis and are not distinguishing clues. The most helpful sign is the pattern of change of the joint spaces of the wrist. Uniform narrowing hallmarks the pathologic changes of *rheumatoid arthritis* in any joint, but is a rare occurrence until late in the course of gout. This case offers an excellent opportunity to compare normal and abnormal cartilage width in all three joints of the wrist. Destructive changes of the radioulnar, radiocarpal and intercarpal joints are striking as compared to the normal side. A huge dissecting popliteal cyst brings this same woman back for our attention in Chapter 6 (Fig. 6–7).

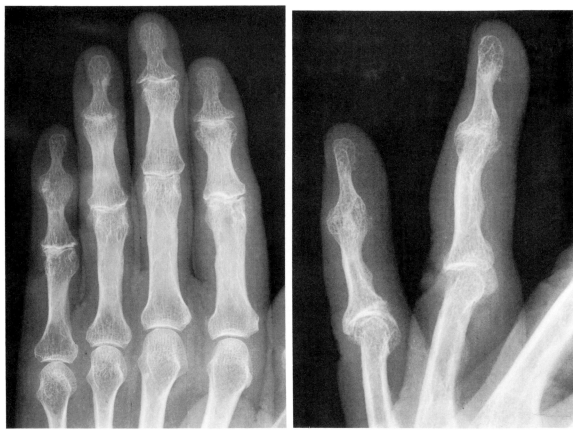

E4–11A.   *E4–11B.*

E4–11. No sooner than one says of a rare condition, "I've never seen it," just such a case will appear, and a second example will follow closely on its heels. Bony ankylosis is very rare in osteoarthritis, and its presence at the distal interphalangeal joint (verified by the oblique view) should first suggest psoriatic arthritis, since this is such a more frequent cause.

Although the distribution of joint involvement seen here is found in psoriatic arthritis, the character of the changes differs in two ways. First, involvement of the distal interphalangeal joints in psoriatic arthritis is always accompanied by changes of the overlying nails; thorough inspection will therefore eliminate this diagnostic possibility. Second, productive rather than destructive bony changes

predominate. Rather than the joint destruction and erosion of the articular margins that would be seen in psoriatic arthritis, eburnation and osteophytes accompany the cartilage loss in this example.

Occasionally metacarpophalangeal joints are narrowed in primary generalized osteoarthritis, and their involvement should never eliminate this as a diagnosis. The narrowing is always inconspicuous as compared to the degenerative changes of the distal and proximal interphalangeal joints, distinguishing the pattern of changes from rheumatoid arthritis.

This woman's age, a postmenopausal 54, her normal sedimentation rate and negative tests for rheumatoid factor complete the classical picture of *Kellgren's arthritis.*

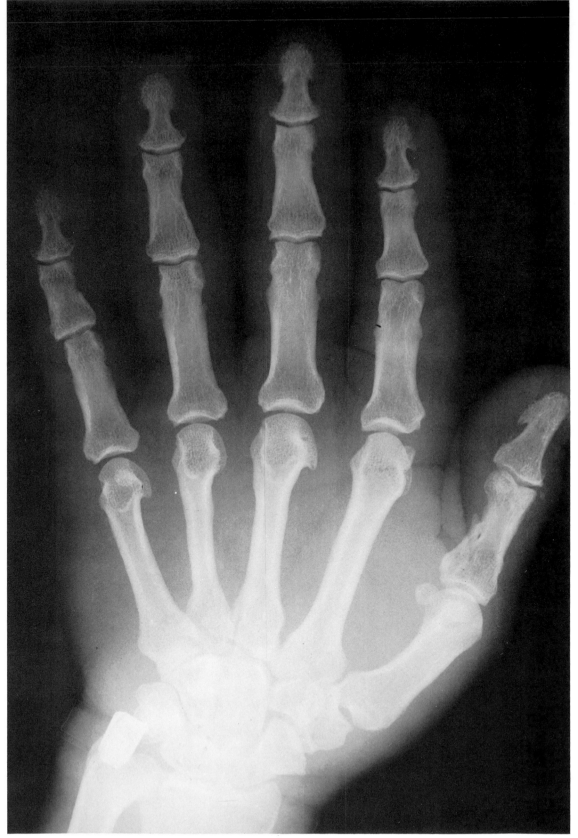

E4–12A.

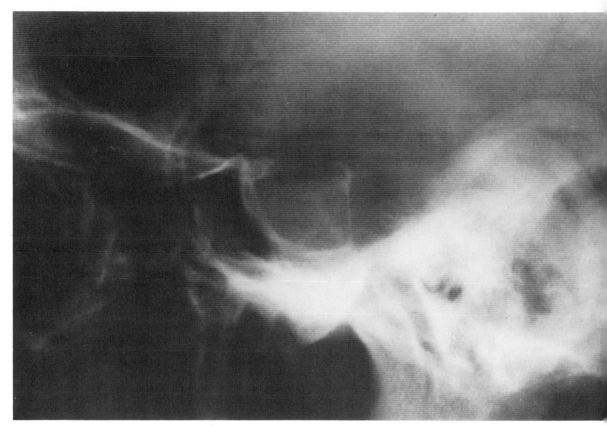

E4–12B.

E4–12. The soft tissues are a little too bulky, the interphalangeal joints a little too widely spaced and the terminal tufts slightly too prominent to be considered normal. Any of these changes by itself could be normal, but taken together they point to *acromegaly*. The most concrete finding is the development of projections of bone along points of tendinous attachment, present on all the proximal phalanges. Although the significance of these minor radiographic findings may be argued, the lateral skull film supports the suspicion of an eosinophilic adenoma. A huge, ballooned sella turcica attests to its presence.

The subtle signs of soft tissue, cartilage and bony overgrowth actually indicate a long-standing adenoma and reflect the generalized changes of acromegaly in all the organ systems.

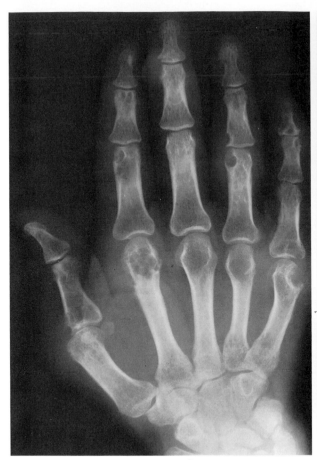

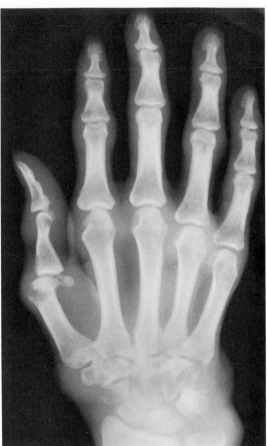

E4–13.   *E4–14.*

E4–13. Whenever cutaneous nodules are seen in association with extensive bony erosions, as in the hand of this 51 year old man, gout is always the prime consideration. However, normal uric acid levels, no history of joint pains and failure to obtain crystals from the "tophus" made it evident that a rare metabolic disorder was the cause of this radiographic picture. Special stains of a biopsy specimen from the wrist revealed foam cells consistent with the diagnosis of *lipoid dermatoarthritis* (reticulohistiocytosis).

This rare disorder may mimic rheumatoid arthritis clinically, but radiographically the pattern of distribution and the type of bone destruction is that of a metabolic disorder. Occasionally the joint destruction may be so severe that a "main-en-lorgnette" hand results, further confusing the picture with that of an inflammatory arthritis.

E4–14. The similarity of radiographic changes from metabolic diseases is apparent when one compares a case of *amyloidosis* with the findings in lipoid dermatoarthritis and gout. The soft tissue masses, bone erosions and periarticular swelling in this illustration are identical. The distribution of the joints affected, the prominence of soft tissue findings and the preservation of cartilage distinguish this pattern from rheumatoid arthritis. The character of the erosions with their overhanging edges and well-defined sclerotic margins indicates a proliferative response of the bone to the presence of this foreign material and offers a critical clue to the correct category of diseases. In amyloidosis, the synovium is infiltrated with amyloid, causing capsular distension which mimics a joint effusion. Pure amyloid deposits may be seen within the bone erosions.

PART II

ARTHRITIS
FROM
HEAD
TO
FOOT

INTRODUCTION

Part I presented a systematic approach to the analysis of joint films and defined the terms that are used in describing radiographic abnormalities. The characteristic appearance of the commonly encountered diseases was illustrated and the radiographic changes that have been found to be most helpful in distinguishing one arthritis from another were underscored. It is apparent that there are specific clues that can be found in the types of soft tissue findings, the manner in which the bones are malaligned, the type and distribution of the demineralization, and the character of periosteal new bone or the type and distribution of erosions that allow one to make a specific diagnosis.

An introduction to any subject, in order to be successful, must be simple and logical and must stress the classical and most distinctive features of diseases. It may be frustrating to a novice to watch an expert in the field immediately zero in on an accurate appraisal of a problem; one should remember that he too has just gone through a logical series of questions and interpretations. His "Aunt Minnie" approach is actually the result of a systematic computer-like analysis with weights on different findings added in light of his experience. For the beginner without the years of experience and in the absence of a methodical approach, it is more painstaking a process. To compound this difficulty, diseases do not always conform to a classical picture. The earlier the patient is seen in the course of his illness, the more nonspecific are his findings, and the more complex the array of possible disease entities becomes.

We hope that any oversimplification in Part I gives you the broad base to a pyramid of experiences that you will add to and modify, learning from your own patients.

Part II is concerned with the same diseases as they occur in different regions of the body and the modifications one sees *because* of the joint affected. The illustrations are grouped according to the joint involved in order to contrast the radiographic findings of the different diseases. By applying the information from Part 1 to the illustrations in each of the subsequent chapters, a sophisticated and logical interpretation can be made.

Chapter 5

THE FOOT AND ANKLE

ANATOMY OF THE FOOT

In the first four chapters of this book we have presented a method of analysis of films of the hand and illustrated the pathologic findings of the commonly encountered arthritides. Because of the basic similarity of the anatomy of the foot, the characteristic features of each disease offer the same clues for diagnosis. There are several important anatomic differences in the foot, however, which alter the manifestations of these same diseases. It is important to be aware of them to avoid the pitfalls of suggesting a serious disease in a patient with a normal foot.

For instance, the anatomic configuration of the proximal phalanges of the foot differs from that of the comparable bones in the hand. The flangelike contour of their shafts is normal and should not be mistaken for periosteal new bone (Fig. 5-1, arrow).

In addition, there are five *important* bursae which respond to pressure. Chronic trauma may cause soft tissue swelling of bursae and, secondarily, degenerative changes of the bony structures beneath them. Two of these frequently involved bursae are located on the outer surfaces of the forefoot, adjacent to the first and fifth metatarsophalangeal joints. Two are associated with the Achilles tendon at the point of attachment to the calcaneus, one lying posterior and one anterior to its insertion. The fifth bursa that plays a prominent role in radiographic abnormalities of the foot is situated along the inferior surface of the calcaneus at the point where the plantar aponeurosis attaches.

Localized swelling in the area of any of these bursae indicates inflammation and excess synovial fluid. Although this may represent the first evidence of rheumatoid arthritis or gout, it may just as easily signify nothing more than man's losing battle with his unyielding environment and be secondary to the repeated trauma of weight bearing.

When the toes are examined carefully on films of normal feet, the soft tissues frequently demonstrate a bulbous appearance to their tips and an absence of the distal tuft, giving the bone a tapered configuration.

The base of the proximal phalanges normally articulates more dorsally on the head of the metatarsal bones than occurs at the metacarpophalangeal joints of the hand. In a similar manner, flexion of the interphalangeal joints is commonly seen on routine dorsoplantar films of the foot, preventing evaluation of the joint spaces.

Fusion of the middle and distal phalanges may occur in any of the toes and is most frequently seen in the fifth toe.

All of these findings are normal variants which, *if present in the hand*, would suggest such important diagnoses as clubbing associated with osteoarthropathy, a resorptive arthritis such as that seen in scleroderma, the malalignment as seen in systemic lupus erythematosus and rheumatoid arthritis (both of which cause laxity of the capsules and ligaments), or the bony ankylosis of psoriatic arthritis. It is evident that correlation with clinical and laboratory findings is

132

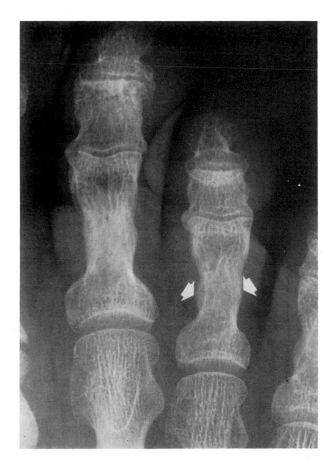

Figure 5–1. Normal toes.
The normal flange of bone that projects from the shafts of the proximal phalanges (arrows) should not be mistaken for the periosteal reaction that accompanies acute inflammatory arthritides.

essential to distinguish the effects of a true arthritis from the hallmarks of a shoeshorne civilized man.

SOFT TISSUE

Generalized Increase in Soft Tissue

The same difficulties in assessing a generalized increase in soft tissues that were encountered in studying the films of the hand are present in the foot. There are two findings that are helpful: (1) If the film is of good quality, there is frequently an appearance of increased overall density of the soft tissue, as in any mass. This is a very subjective evaluation, however, and is fraught with error. (2) A more objective finding is an increase in the soft tissue adjacent to the first and fifth metatarsal bones. Although there is a great deal

of variation from patient to patient, an increase in this dimension and an obvious convex bulge to the contours of the foot is suggestive of an increase in soft tissue.

Acromegaly. The generalized overgrowth of soft tissues in a patient with acromegaly occurs before the characteristic bone changes have developed. This increased soft tissue is extremely difficult to assess on a film of the foot and is more easily *quantitated* on a *lateral view* of the ankle by measuring the thickness of the heel pad.

Figure 5–2 shows a 50 year old woman with acromegaly. The overgrowth of soft tissues is so far advanced that the bulging contours of the foot signal the underlying endocrine disease in this patient and provide the clue to her gradual change of appearance (Fig. 5–2). The changes in the soft tissues differ from the distention of edema. Rather than effacement of the soft

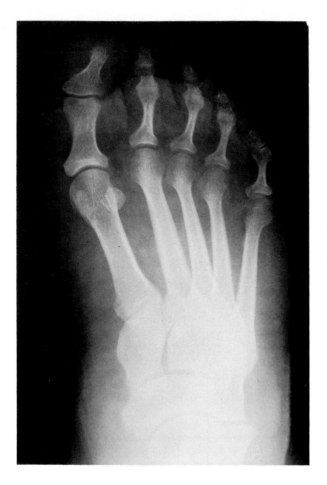

Figure 5–2. Acromegaly.
Before cartilage and bone overgrowth is apparent, diffuse increase in the soft tissues alters the patient's shoe size. The appearance of the redundant skin folds along the medial aspect of the foot distinguishes this from the smooth, effaced configuration of pedal edema.

tissues there is redundancy due to their overgrowth.

Overgrowth of any component of the body, whether soft tissue, cartilage or bone, does *not* occur early in the course of acromegaly. All develop *gradually*, over many years. Diagnosis of this disease is rarely made early. Both the subtle changes in the patient's features and the unreliability of the assay methods for growth hormone at an early stage result in an often undiagnosed condition. Thus, recognition of soft tissue abnormalities on a film often initiates an appropriate diagnostic evaluation.

EDEMA

Chronic edema is frequently seen in patients with neuropathic joints from a variety of causes and is illustrated here in a patient with diabetic neuropathy (Fig. 5–3). There is generalized swelling of the foot with a convex bulging of its borders.

The soft tissues are distended and are *effaced*, in contrast to the thickened, corrugated appearance of the soft tissues in the patient with acromegaly.

Degenerative joint changes are so frequently seen in the first metatarsophalangeal joint that their presence in this patient is unlikely to be related to the neurologic abnormality.

Localized Increase in Soft Tissue

Localized soft tissue masses or effusions are more difficult to detect in the foot than in the hand. When they are a manifestation of inflammation of the bursae associated with the first and fifth metatarsophalangeal joints, they are obvious because they distort the contour of the foot. By contrast, *joint* effusions are much more occult, for two reasons: Because of

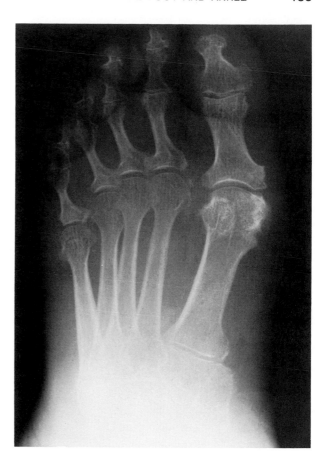

Figure 5-3. Diabetic neuropathy. Chronic effusions often accompany neuropathic conditions and, in the foot, diffusely increase the soft tissues. Secondary degenerative changes of the first metatarsophalangeal joint have resulted in erosions, marginal joint narrowing and hypertrophic bony proliferation.

the thickness of the foot at the level of the metatarsophalangeal joint, the slight increase in mass does not cast a detectable shadow; and, similarly, the flexed position of the toes prevents a precise evaluation of the profile of the interphalangeal joints.

JOINT EFFUSION

Reiter's Syndrome. Occasionally an effusion is so massive that separation of the bones results from the distention of the capsule. This was the earliest radiographic evidence of an inflammatory arthritis in a patient diagnosed as having Reiter's syndrome (Fig. 5–4B). The great toe is an area frequently affected in patients with Reiter's syndrome. In addition, the unilateral distribution in this disease helps to distinguish it from rheumatoid arthritis, which classically affects multiple joints of both hands or both feet simultaneously. The asymmetrical involvement and the grossness of the radio-

logic findings are even more evident when one compares the painful toe with that of the normal foot (Fig. 5–4A). Even without the helpful evidence of the separation of the metatarsal heads, the increased soft tissue along the margin of the foot should be recognized as abnormal.

INFECTION

Gas Gangrene. Localized swelling of the soft tissues is obvious around the first and second toes of a diabetic patient (Fig. 5–5). Its appearance is markedly different from that in the previous examples, however. There is a nonhomogeneity of the soft tissue shadow in this patient. The radiolucent areas indicate the presence of gas. When this is seen, two possible causes must be considered: (1) gas-forming organisms such as clostridia, and (2) the presence of a laceration of the skin and introduction of air into the soft tissues. The latter not uncommonly occurs

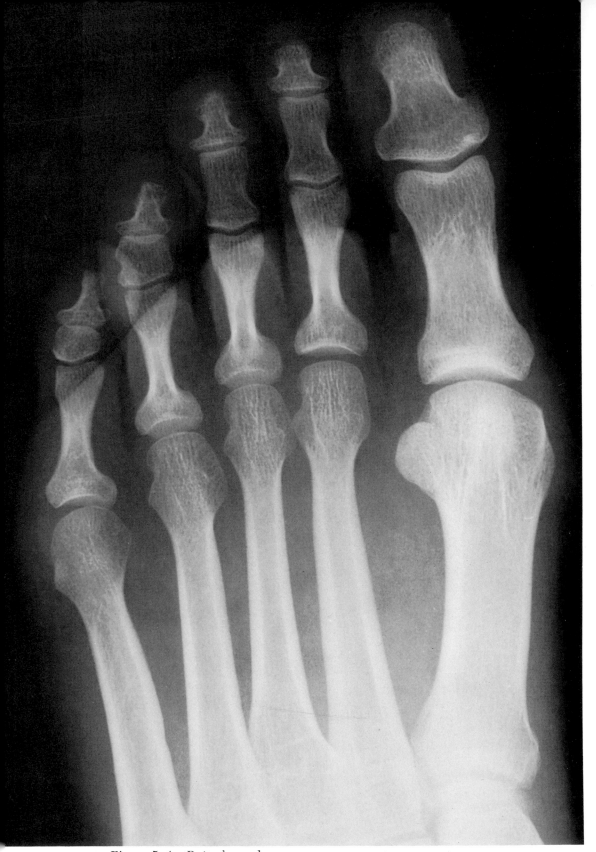

A

Figure 5–4. Reiter's syndrome.
   Massive soft tissue swelling in a patient with acute onset of joint pain has separated the first and second metatarsal heads of the right foot (*B*). This is easily detected when it is compared to the normal left foot (*A*).

Illustration continued on opposite page.

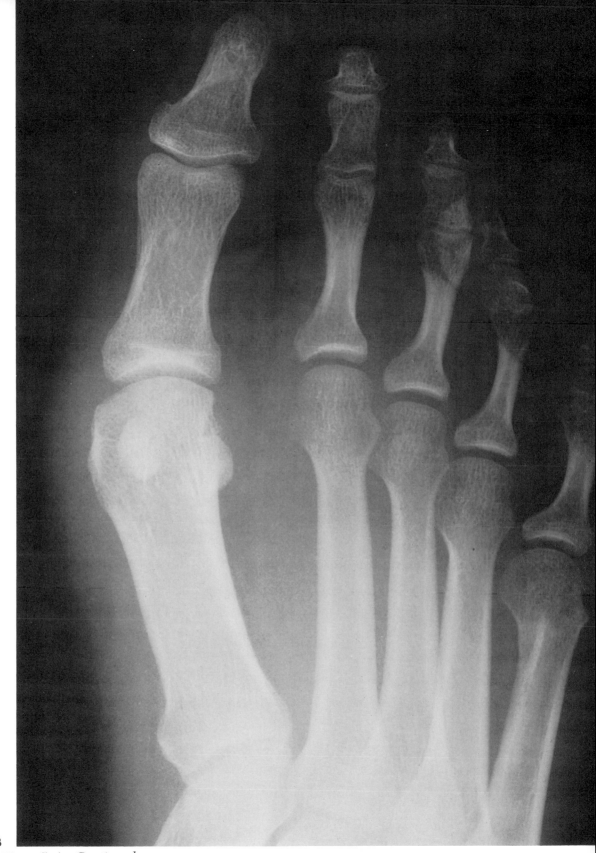

B

Figure 5–4.   Continued.
Capsular involvement of the right second metatarsophalangeal joint is evidenced by demineralization and loss of the sharp cortical margin of the metatarsal head.

137

in the foot if the patient continues to walk with a laceration or plantar ulcer. The bubbly appearance of the gas in this example (Fig. 5–5) is typical of gas gangrene which spreads between the muscle bundles and is not confined to the large tissue planes.

Cellulitis. Infection frequently causes massive distention of the soft tissues adjacent to the fifth metatarsophalangeal joint (Fig. 5–6A). In the example shown, the indistinct appearance of the medial aspect of the metatarsal head indicates demineralization of the bone accompanying the inflammatory process. Five months later (Fig. 5–6B) destruction of the metatarsal head and subluxation of the proximal phalanx substantiates the bony involvement. Persistence of the massive soft tissue swelling indicates continued activity of the infectious process and the presence of a cellulitis. The solid layer of periosteal new bone along the metatarsal bone is commonly seen in osteomyelitis. The progression of

changes indicates a primary infectious arthritis and secondary infection of the bone.

BURSITIS

Hallux Valgus. By definition, hallux valgus is a deviation of the proximal phalanx of the great toe toward the fibular side of the foot. Because of this malalignment, the bursa adjacent to the metatarsophalangeal joint is vulnerable to constant trauma from shoes. The result is a localized soft tissue swelling. Eventually, degenerative changes of the underlying joint may occur as erosions and proliferations of new bone. There are many causes of hallux valgus deformity. It may be primary, or it may be secondary to an inflammatory disease such as gout or rheumatoid arthritis. It may also occur secondary to a primary *varus* deviation of the first metatarsal with the cuneiform. When the first cuneiform has a rounded articular surface the axis of the metatarsal is parallel to that of the midfoot. Not infrequently, the articular surface of the

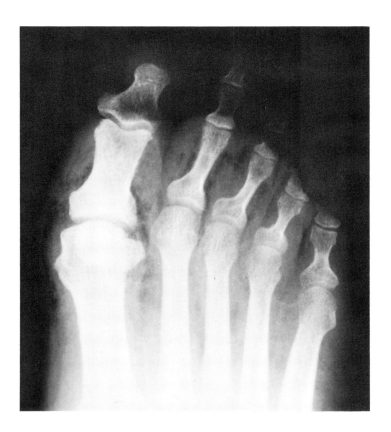

Figure 5–5. Gas gangrene.

The mottled radiolucent shadows surrounding the first three toes represent gas dissecting around the muscles. The appearance of such gas must be distinguished from that of air entering the soft tissue planes through an open wound.

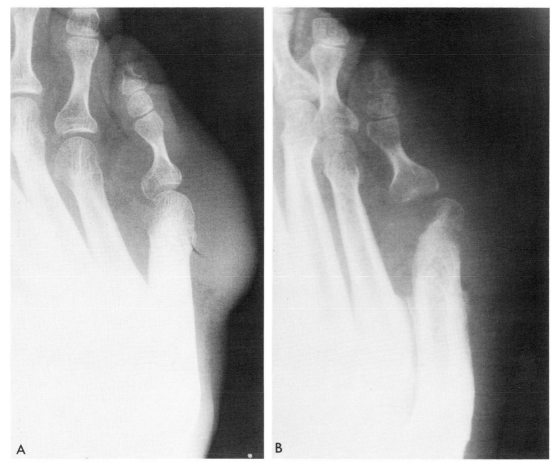

Figure 5–6. Infection.

A. Massive distention of the soft tissues and demineralization of the fifth metatarsal head indicate the presence of inflammation.

B. Five months later, the soft tissue swelling has persisted; in addition, however, destruction of the distal metatarsal, periosteal reaction and disruption of the joint with subluxation of the articulating bone indicate osteomyelitis. Diffuse osteoporosis of the phalanges of the fifth toe accompanies the inflammatory process and may result from hyperemia or disuse.

cuneiform is formed as in the days of the prehensile toe, sloping steeply as in Figure 5–7 (arrow). Because its origin from the protohominids' thumblike great toe, this is termed an atavistic toe. The steep slope results in a varus (medial) angulation of the metatarsal bone. The valgus deformity of the proximal phalanx only adds to the deformity and occurs because the malaligned great toe is chronically wedged into a shoe.

Rheumatoid Arthritis. The bursa adjacent to the fifth metatarsophalangeal joint is frequently involved *early* in the course of rheumatoid arthritis (Fig. 5–8). There is no way to distinguish this in-

volvement from a bunionette (tailor's bunion) unless additional evidence of a more generalized inflammatory disease is present. Fortunately for the clinician, fibular deviation of the proximal phalanges (similar to the ulnar deviation seen in the hand) is also an early manifestation of rheumatoid arthritis in the foot. When it is present, as in the illustration, it substantiates a more generalized inflammatory process with subsequent laxity of the ligaments at the metatarsophalangeal joints. The fifth metatarsal head is often the earliest site of erosion in rheumatoid arthritis, as is seen in Figure 5–8. The combination of soft tissue swelling in the

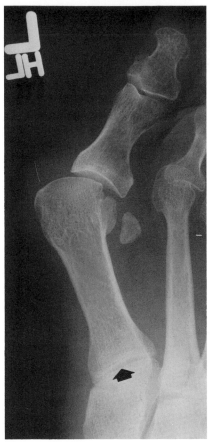

Figure 5-7. Hallux valgus.

A steep slope of the cuneiform (arrow) results in medial deviation of the metatarsal bone. The valgus deviation of the proximal phalanx adds to the deformity, and bursitis accompanies the alignment abnormality, as seen by the soft tissue swelling adjacent to the metatarsophalangeal joint.

area of the bursa and adjacent destructive changes of the bone may be caused by any of a variety of conditions, and although an early manifestation of rheumatoid arthritis in the foot, it is not specific.

Soft Tissue Calcification

The type of calcification that occurs in the soft tissues of the foot is identical to that in the hand; information in Part I concerning this abnormality can be directly applied to similar conditions in the foot.

Calcific Periarthritis. Two types of abnormal calcification are seen in Figure 5-9, which shows the foot of a young man undergoing renal dialysis, and their occurrence together allows the diagnosis of calcific periarthritis to be suggested from the film alone. Tubular calcifications paralleling the metatarsal and proximal phalangeal bones indicate the extent of involvement of the small arteries by arteriosclerosis. An amorphous calcium deposit in the periarticular area of the fifth toe represents calcium apatite. Only by introducing a needle into the bursa and examining the material microscopically could one distinguish between this and a gouty tophus. Since both gout and hyperparathyroidism are complications of intermittent renal failure, it is important to make the correct diagnosis and institute appropriate therapy.

Gout. To emphasize the similarity of the location and radiographic appearance of the calcium deposits in gout with calcific periarthritis, a patient with a tophaceous deposit in the bursa is included for comparison (Fig. 5-10). Prominent erosions deform the head of the fifth metatarsal in a similar fashion to the changes in rheumatoid arthritis. These erosions characteristically are associated with adjacent gouty tophi and, by contrast, have not been seen in calcific periarthritis. The absence of erosions in the latter condition is undoubtedly attributable to the difference in chronicity of the two entities.

Gouty tophi may distend joint capsules as well as soft tissue spaces. They may occur anywhere in the foot but, statistically, are most frequently seen in the forefoot. A lateral view of the first metatarsophalangeal joint shows the typical changes in a patient with chronic tophaceous gout (Fig. 5-11). The cloudlike increased density is from the calcium deposited in the soft tissues. Early erosion of the base of the proximal phalanx and secondary proliferative changes of the metatarsal head are apparent. Preservation of a normal space in the presence of severe destructive changes and *paraarticular* erosions are characteristic of gout and highly unlikely in rheumatoid

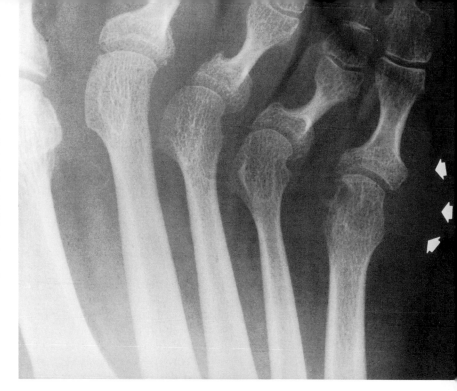

Figure 5–8. Rheumatoid arthritis.

Swelling is confined to the bursa adjacent to the fifth metatarsal joint (arrows). Fibular deviation of the proximal phalanges and erosion of the head of the fifth metatarsal are typical early changes of rheumatoid arthritis and indicate inflammatory involvement of these joints. The dot-dash changes of the subchondral line are evident along the medial side of the third and fourth metatarsal heads, signaling synovitis.

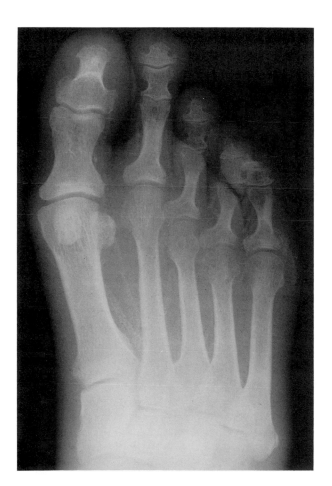

Figure 5–9. Calcific periarthritis.

A 30 year old man on long-term renal dialysis illustrates two abnormal types of calcification in the soft tissues: extensive vascular calcification, and distention of the bursa adjacent to the fifth metatarsophalangeal joint by a large amorphous collection of calcium apatite.

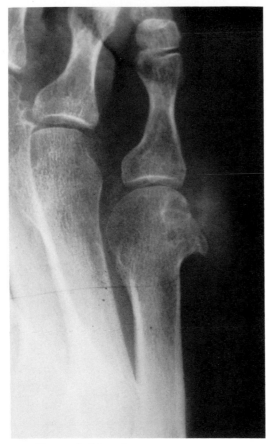

Figure 5–10. Gout.

The radiographic appearance of calcium urate deposits is indistinguishable from calcific periarthritis; the contiguous bony erosion, however, is only seen in chronic tophaceous gout. Often, as in this example, an oblique view is necessary to make the erosion apparent and thereby distinguish the two conditions.

arthritis. Thus, when the helpful sign of calcium urate deposits is absent, it is essential to evaluate the changes in the cartilage space in order to distinguish the two conditions.

ALIGNMENT ABNORMALITIES OF THE FOOT

Malalignment of the bones of the foot is not limited to the forefoot. Mid- and hindfoot anomalies are common and may cause pain and secondary degenerative changes because of the abnormal forces of weight bearing. It is beyond the scope of this monograph to outline the congenital defects of the foot. Rather, *acquired* alignment abnormalities will be reviewed. Long after an acute inflammatory process in the foot has subsided, a patient may be permanently disabled from residual joint deformities. Thus, the aftermath of the disease process in many instances is more disabling than the disease itself.

The characteristic appearances of alignment abnormalities in the foot have led to unique descriptive terms. Deviation or subluxation that results in a hallux valgus deformity of the first toe is popularly called a bunion. The terms hallux flexus and "trigger toe" refer to an abnormality of the interphalangeal joint of the great toe. When flexion contractures deform the proximal interphalangeal joints they cause "hammer toes," and similar flexion at the distal interphalangeal joints results in "mallet toes." Finally, dorsal contraction of the proximal phalanges on the metatarsal heads, combined with flexion of the proximal interphalangeal joints, results in "claw toes."

Rheumatoid Arthritis. The inflammatory involvement of the bursae and capsules in rheumatoid arthritis frequently results in abnormalities of alignment. Clinically, one commonly sees the development of hallux valgus deformity, dorsally contracted toes and hammer toes as manifestations of this systemic disease. The major disabling factor is generally the plantar prominence of the metatarsal heads, which must absorb the force of walking.

An oblique view of the foot of a patient with rheumatoid arthritis demonstrates this alignment abnormality (Fig. 5–12). Progressively more severe dorsal subluxation of the phalanges has led to dislocation. A typical hallux valgus deformity has resulted in overlap of the first and second toes. Erosions are seen only in the heads of the first and the fifth metatarsals, a typical distribution in rheumatoid arthritis. Although eventually erosions may be seen in all of the metatarsal bones, they often begin at the fourth and fifth toes and occur adjacent to an inflamed bursa of the great toe.

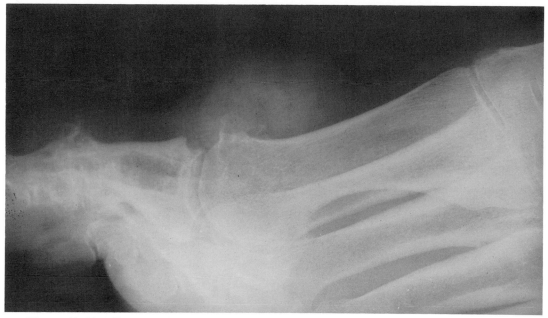

Figure 5–11. Gout.

The para-articular soft tissue mass adjacent to the first metatarsophalangeal joint and its cloudlike increase in density from calcium urate crystals are typical of chronic tophaceous gout. The marginal bony erosions, preservation of the articular cartilage and lack of bony demineralization are also characteristic of this arthritis.

Figure 5–12. Rheumatoid arthritis.

Dorsal dislocations are best appreciated on lateral or oblique views, because the superimposed bony shadows are separated. Diffuse osteoporosis and erosions of the first and fifth metatarsal heads are two additional common findings in rheumatoid arthritis; these are classically demonstrated in this example. Sparing of the tarsal joints of the foot is not uncommon, although the hand frequently exhibits signs of inflammatory destruction of the carpus when its more peripheral joints are affected.

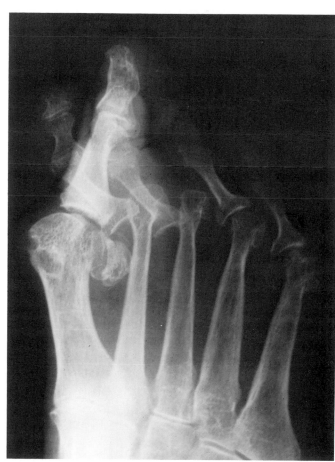

143

Reiter's Syndrome. The bizarre appearance of the toes in Figure 5–13A is due to the severe dorsal contraction of the proximal phalangeal bones. This results in a dramatic visual foreshortening of their image. The "shining white diamond" superimposed on the metatarsal head is the foreshortened projection of the cortical bone of the proximal phalanx.

Although there appears to be complete lack of metatarsophalangeal joint spaces, the oblique view (Fig. 5–13B) demonstrates this to be nothing more than the overlap of the ends of the articulating bones. It is important to know that the cartilage is preserved and that there are no articular erosions. The alignment abnormalities are limited to the metatar-sophalangeal joints. Sparing of the distal interphalangeal joints and absence of erosions and destructive changes distinguish the pathologic findings from both rheumatoid and psoriatic arthritis. Although Reiter's syndrome may cause a mutilating arthritis in the foot, it is extremely rare.

Juvenile Rheumatoid Arthritis. The polyarticular form of juvenile rheumatoid arthritis frequently affects the hands and feet of children. Although it tends to be symmetrical, one foot or one hand may be involved out of proportion to the other. Because of the thick protective cushion of articular cartilage in children and its ability to regenerate, erosions are rarely a primary component of the radiologic pic-

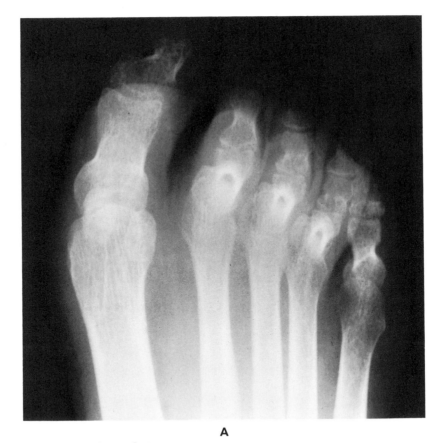

A

Figure 5–13. Reiter's syndrome.

A. Inflammation of the metatarsophalangeal joints causes capsular laxity and subluxations which have this characteristic configuration on the dorsoplantar view. The "shining diamond" that is seen superimposed on the metatarsal heads is the shadow cast by the dorsally angled proximal phalanges.

Illustration continued on opposite page.

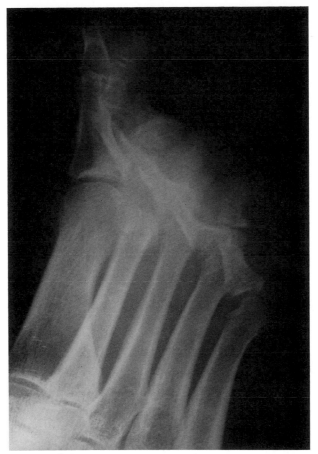

Figure 5–13. *Continued*   **B**

B. Unlike rheumatoid arthritis, Reiter's syndrome has less of a tendency to cause erosions. The smooth round contour of the metatarsal heads is verified by the oblique projection.

ture. Early fusion of epiphyses is frequent and results in cessation of growth as well as distortion of the joint. Occasionally bony ankylosis is seen in a chronic active form of polyarthritis in patients with juvenile rheumatoid arthritis.

A combination of dorsal and fibular dislocation of the proximal phalanges has resulted in the complex overlapping shapes in a patient who had a juvenile onset of rheumatoid arthritis (Fig. 5–14A). As in the film of the patient with Reiter's syndrome (Fig. 5–13), the tubular white shadows are the two-dimensional evidence of the dorsally contracted toes. The severe generalized osteoporosis has reduced the cortex to a pencil-thin white line. Bony ankylosis is seen only in juvenile rheumatoid arthritis after many years of progressive active polyarthritis. In the foot, fusion may occur throughout the tarsal bones, but it

rarely affects the interphalangeal joints and just such a pattern is seen in this example. The findings of severe alignment deformities, extensive osteoporosis and obliteration of the tarsal joint spaces in the absence of severe erosions are characteristic of unremitting juvenile rheumatoid arthritis.

A lateral view of the same foot (Fig. 5–14B) demonstrates to better advantage the flexion deformities of the proximal interphalangeal joints which have resulted in claw toes. An interesting soft tissue finding, frequently apparent clinically but rarely so well demonstrated on a film, is the presence of a plantar keratoma (arrow) beneath the first metatarsal head. Because of the subluxation and abnormal stress to the weight-bearing soft tissue, this is a common complication and often can only be cured by resection of the metatarsal head.

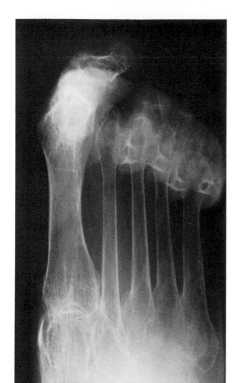

A

Figure 5–14. Juvenile rheumatoid arthritis.

A. Generalized osteoporosis, bony ankylosis of the tarsal bones and severe alignment abnormalities are the residua of juvenile onset rheumatoid arthritis.

B. The dislocated toes have caused a shift in the weight-bearing forces to the metatarsal heads, and a prominent soft tissue plantar keratoma can be seen beneath the head of the first metatarsal (arrow). Flexion at the proximal interphalangeal joints adds to the deformity that results in the clinical picture of claw toes.

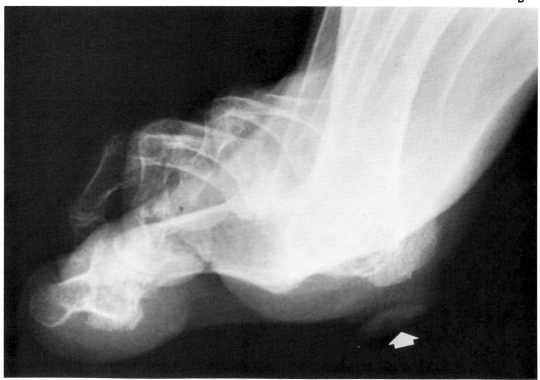

B

ABNORMALITIES OF BONY MINERALIZATION IN THE FOOT

As in the hand, an overview of the condition of mineralization is necessary to provide additional evidence of an underlying arthritis. Therefore, one looks for generalized osteoporosis, juxta-articular demineralization, indicating inflammation within the joint, or subchondral demineralization, suggesting a rapid and acute clinical course.

In addition to signs of loss of bone, evidence of periosteal or endosteal new bone is significant and highly diagnostic.

Periosteal New Bone

Reiter's Syndrome. Two types of mineralization abnormalities are commonly associated with Reiter's syndrome: juxtaarticular demineralization and periosteal new bone. The soft tissue changes have been discussed earlier in this chapter. Swelling is often not limited to the periarticular areas, but diffusely affects the entire toes, causing the "cocktail sausage" configuration so well recognized clinically; this is present in Figure 5–15B.

The prominent frame of periosteal new bone that surrounds the diaphyses of the proximal phalanges and the metatarsal bone (Fig. 5–15B, arrow) is more pronounced than the type seen in the usual case of rheumatoid arthritis. It is easily distinguished from the normal flange of bone if one compares the same toes on a film taken one year earlier (Fig. 5–15A). There is extensive demineralization of the metatarsophalangeal joints, indicating the degree of inflammation within the capsule. Although periostitis and demineralization accompany osteomyelitis as well as the rheumatic dis-

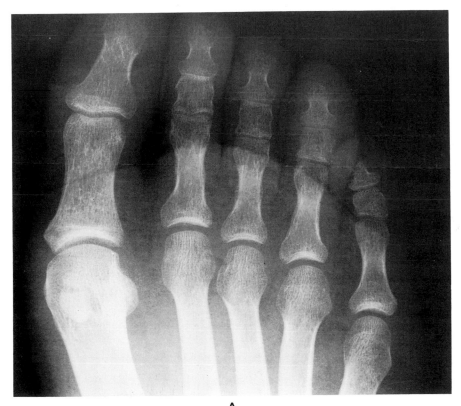

A

Figure 5–15. Reiter's syndrome.
A. At the onset of his symptoms, a film of the foot was normal except for minimal soft tissue swelling of the bursae adjacent to the first and fifth metatarsophalangeal joints.

Illustration continued on following page.

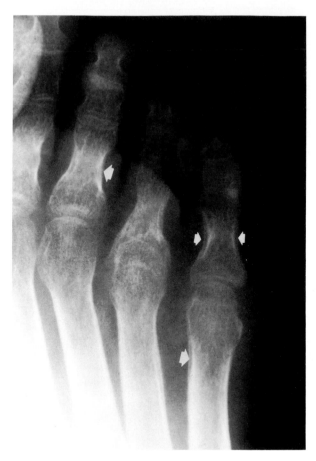

B

Figure 5-15. Continued.
B. A year later, periostitis has altered the contour of the proximal phalanges and the distal fifth metatarsal bone (arrows). The difference between periosteal new bone and the normal flange of the proximal phalanx is evident when comparison is made between the two films. Soft tissue swelling of the toes has given them the "cocktail sausage" configuration.

eases, the great number of bones involved in this patient excludes that diagnosis.

Hypertrophic Osteoarthropathy. Generalized periostitis, synovitis and soft tissue swelling of the distal phalanges are the hallmarks of hypertrophic osteoarthropathy. The soft tissue changes are more localized than in other arthritides, however, and appear as clubbing (Fig. 5-16). Frequently there is an associated loss of the ungual tufts in hypertrophic osteoarthropathy. This may relate to the pressure of the hypertrophied soft tissue. Without the accompanying periosteal new bone to signify an active arthritis, the bulbous toes and absent tufts are indistinguishable from the toes so frequently seen in a normal foot. The juxta-articular demineralization involving all of the joints attests to the generalized state of capsular involvement in this patient. The dramatic periostitis is far more severe than that seen in rheumatoid arthritis or Reiter's syndrome and, together with the clubbing of the soft tissues, is characteristic of hypertrophic osteoarthropathy. In this patient, joint pains

Figure 5-16. Hypertrophic osteoarthropathy.
Thick periosteal new bone frames each metatarsal and phalanx. Although often overlooked because of its subtle radiographic signs relative to periostitis, synovitis is a prominent component of the clinical syndrome and is seen as juxta-articular demineralization and loss of the continuous subchondral line defining the metatarsal heads. Joint pains and the film of the foot led to the discovery of this patient's primary bronchogenic carcinoma.

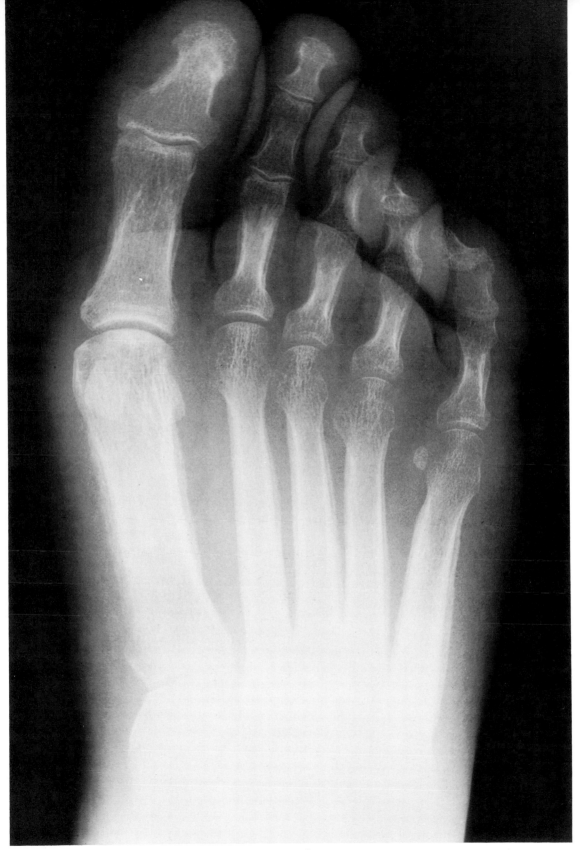

Figure 5–16. See legend on opposite page.

and the film of the foot led to a chest film and the discovery of a primary bronchogenic carcinoma.

ABNORMALITIES OF THE CARTILAGE SPACE

Generalized Widening of the Cartilage Space

An increase in the width of a joint space is unusual and, when the finding is generalized, acromegaly is the only possible cause. Although this makes the diagnosis of this ubiquitous disease sound

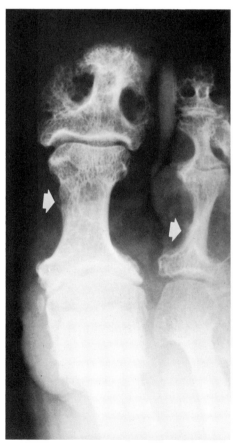

Figure 5–17. Acromegaly.
Proliferation of bone at the base of the phalanges, along the lines of tendinous attachments (arrows) and at the terminal tufts gives a bizarre appearance to the bones in acromegaly.

simple, the difficulty is in assessing whether the joint spaces are actually abnormal. When there is substantiating evidence of acromegaly characterized by bone proliferation, the diagnosis is evident; by this time a film of the foot is usually superfluous.

Acromegaly. The widened cartilage space of both the interphalangeal joint of the great toe and the metatarsophalangeal joint of the second toe is typical of the changes in acromegaly (Fig. 5–17). The soft tissues are massively increased and mimic the clubbing of both hypertrophic and idiopathic osteoarthropathy. Because of the physical similarity, the diseases are frequently confused clinically, and the film may provide a simple means of separating them. The tuft responds in an opposite manner in acromegaly by participating in the general process of tissue overgrowth. Hence, its exaggerated projections are easily distinguished from the resorbed tufts of hypertrophic and idiopathic osteoarthropathy. In this patient, the pronounced overgrowth of the base of the distal phalanx, together with the spur along the diaphysis of the first and second toes (arrows) and the degenerative changes of the first metatarsophalangeal joint, are all signs of the systemic manifestations of this endocrine disorder.

Localized Widening of the Cartilage Space

A single widened joint space, in contrast to the universal change seen in acromegaly, is the result of a localized disease process. Although theoretically it may be due to an acute effusion, practically this is extremely rare in the foot.

Deposition of large amounts of fibrous material within the joint space will appear radiographically as a widened joint. Resorption of both articulating ends of the bones will destroy the joint and result in widening and abnormal alignment.

Collapse of the metatarsal head following avascular necrosis will also result in widening of the joint space and an associated deformity of the metatarsal bone.

Avascular Necrosis. Avascular necrosis or Freiberg's disease is not an infrequent occurrence and is most commonly seen in adolescents. Despite a complaint of foot pain, initial films of the foot are usually normal. Only repeated examination after a suitable period of time will demonstrate the characteristic flattened contour of the metatarsal head, the sclerotic new bone formed as a part of the reparative mechanism and the widened joint space, as seen in the third metatarsophalangeal joint (Fig. 5–18). Periosteal new bone often accompanies the changes and alters the shaft by converting it to a more rectangular shape in a fashion similar to that in idiopathic osteoarthropathy. The most frequent bone involved is the second metatarsal. Less commonly, it occurs in the third and fourth metatarsals, and very rarely is the fifth metatarsal head affected.

Psoriatic Arthritis. Rarely does one see separation of a joint space in the foot due to an acute effusion. This may be due to the more limiting overlying soft tissues. Occasionally a joint space is widened late in the course of an inflammatory arthritis by virtue of extensive deposition of fibrous tissue. When this occurs, it is said to be characteristic of psoriatic arthritis; its appearance is illustrated in Figure 5–19. Because this is a late change, it is accompanied by erosions and therefore is easily distinguished from an acute effusion.

Narrowed Cartilage Space

Narrowing of the joint space is a much more common manifestation of arthritis than widening. The pathophysiologic mechanisms are identical to those seen in the hand.

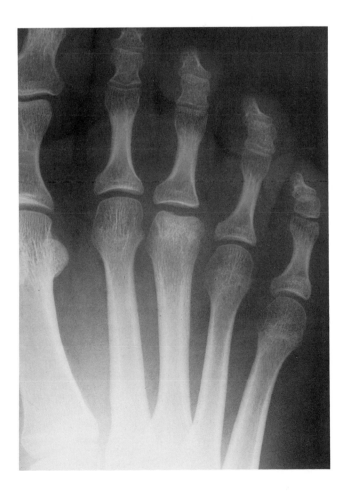

Figure 5–18. Freiberg's disease.

Widening of a joint space is rare. When it occurs in a single metatarsophalangeal joint it is most likely caused by flattening of the metatarsal head from avascular necrosis. Signs of healing are the presence of sclerotic new bone in the metatarsal head and periosteal new bone along the shaft of the third metatarsal, which has a squared appearance.

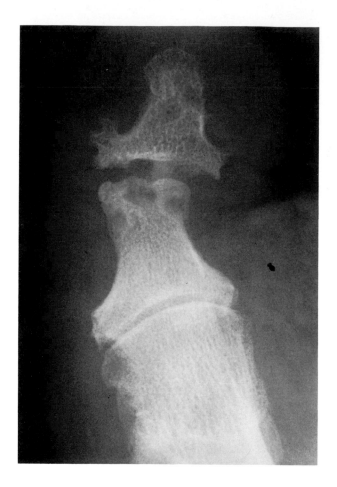

Figure 5-19. Psoriatic arthritis. Widening of the interphalangeal joint from deposition of fibrous tissue, erosions of the articular surfaces of bone and proliferation of the base of the distal phalanx are characteristic of psoriasis but may also be seen in patients with Reiter's syndrome. The picture differs from acromegaly in two ways: the terminal tufts are not prominent and the widening of the joint space is not universal throughout the joints of the foot.

THE EROSIONS OF RHEUMATOID ARTHRITIS

Although the fourth and fifth metatarsophalangeal joints are often involved first in rheumatoid arthritis, symmetrical loss of cartilage throughout the metatarsophalangeal joints of the foot, when present (as in Fig. 5-20A), is characteristic of this connective tissue disorder. The flexion deformities of the third and fourth toes are the typical hammer toes that so often follow the inflammatory changes of rheumatoid arthritis. A later film of the same patient demonstrates progressive destruction and erosions of the metatarsal heads and further joint space narrowing (Fig. 5-20B). A severe hallux valgus deformity has developed, and surgical resection of the base of the proximal phalanx and the hypertrophied medial side of the metatarsal head (Keller procedure) has been performed to alleviate the symptoms. Fibular deviation of the second, third, and fourth toes is

Figure 5-20. Rheumatoid arthritis.

A. Uniform narrowing of the metatarsophalangeal joints and small erosions on the fibular sides of the third and fifth metatarsal heads are typical of the changes of rheumatoid arthritis. The thin layer of periosteal new bone along the proximal phalanx of the third toe is more extensive than the normal anatomic flange of bone (note the appearance of the fourth toe) and reflects the periostitis present in many bones of this patient.

B. Progressive deformities from the inflammatory arthritis are seen. The thick periosteal new bone along the shaft of the second metatarsal bone indicates healing of a stress fracture, a frequent accompaniment of hallux valgus deformity. The irregular contour of the articulating bones of the first metatarsophalangeal joint indicates a previous Keller procedure performed to correct the severe hallux valgus deformity that had developed.

C. An oblique view prior to surgery documents the presence of three stress fractures and delineates the two at the base of the third and fourth metatarsal bones to better advantage (arrows).

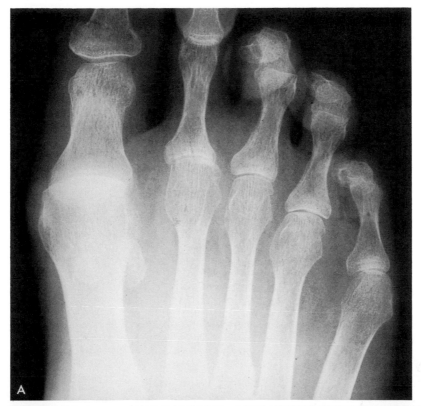

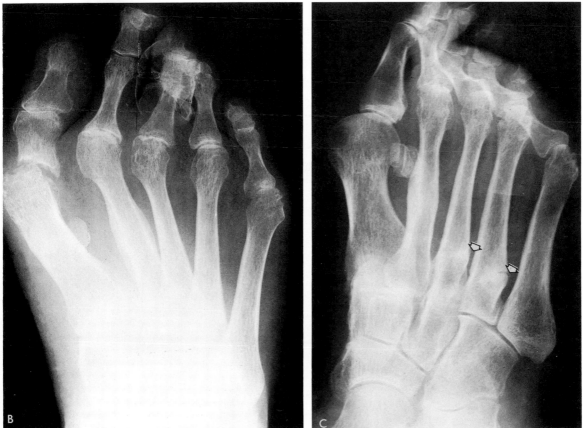

Figure 5-20. *See legend on opposite page.* 153

frequently seen in rheumatoid arthritis and is equivalent to ulnar deviation in the hand. The fifth toe rarely deviates laterally despite extensive capsular involvement from inflammation, as is illustrated by this example.

Narrowing and erosions of the metatarsophalangeal joints tend to appear simultaneously, whereas narrowing precedes visible erosions in the proximal interphalangeal joints in just the same manner as occurs in the hand. In addition, inflammatory arthritis leads to capsular laxity and imbalance of musculature and will therefore cause deviation and subluxation of the articulating bones.

A frequent and often overlooked complication of rheumatoid arthritis is also observed in this patient. The development of the severe hallux valgus deformity in this 22 year old woman has caused a shift in the weight-bearing forces, and the typical thick periosteal new bone that is seen along the shaft of the second metatarsal bone attests to the healing process in an underlying stress fracture (Fig. 5–20B).

An earlier film documented that this complication *preceded* her surgery (Fig. 5–20C). Stress fractures are often missed unless serial films are taken. Sometimes only slight irregularity of the cortex indicates their presence. Later, the signs of healing become apparent and make the diagnosis obvious. When the fracture is through the diaphysis, thick periosteal new bone develops. If the fracture is at the base of the metatarsals, only a sclerotic horizontal line indicates the healing fracture. The oblique view demonstrates two additional stress fractures at the base of the third and fourth metatarsals, hidden on the dorsoplantar view (arrows). Their presence is much more subtle than the healed stress fracture through the midshaft of the second metatarsal bone.

Stress fractures are a common occurrence in army recruits, where the abnormal stress is the number of miles marched rather than a shift of the weight-bearing forces to a different metatarsal. They may accompany hallux valgus deformities from any cause as changes in alignment shift the weight-bearing forces. Podiatric surgeons acknowledge the occurrence of stress fractures following corrective procedures for hallux valgus deformities. Resection of the base of the proximal phalanx reduces the propulsive force of the great toe by detachment of the intrinsic muscles; secondarily, alteration of the biomechanical forces result in a stress fracture. Acute onset of pain following corrective surgery is disheartening to the patient and should suggest the possibility of a secondary stress fracture.

THE EROSIONS OF GOUT

When erosions accompany gouty tophi there is often evidence of new bone formation, in either an overhanging edge or a sclerotic base to the erosion. This evidence distinguishes the condition from rheumatoid arthritis, which characteristically provides no stimulus to the production of new bone.

Because 85 per cent of the patients with gout have arthritis in the foot, it is important to know the spectrum of changes that may occur. Pain and swelling localized to the first metatarsophalangeal joints occur in hallux valgus deformity due to pressure, in rheumatoid arthritis due to bursitis and in gout when irritating monosodium urate crystals are present; therefore, all three conditions may show inflamed bursae clinically and soft tissue swelling radiographically. Erosion of the adjacent bone, unfortunately, may also be present in all three of these entities. Thus, other criteria must be used in making the diagnosis of gout.

Early nonspecific changes of soft tissue swelling and contiguous erosions are both seen in a patient with gout and, on the dorsoplantar view, are indistinguishable from the findings in rheumatoid arthritis (Fig. 5–21A). An oblique view (Fig. 5–21B) projects the erosions tangentially, revealing their punched-out configuration.

The pathologic appearance of early gouty erosions is evident in Figure 5–22. Two well-defined punched-out lesions are present in the head of a resected metatarsal, demonstrating destruction of the articular cartilage and the underlying subchondral bone. At this stage there is no evidence of new bone, and the sclerotic margin and overhanging edge that

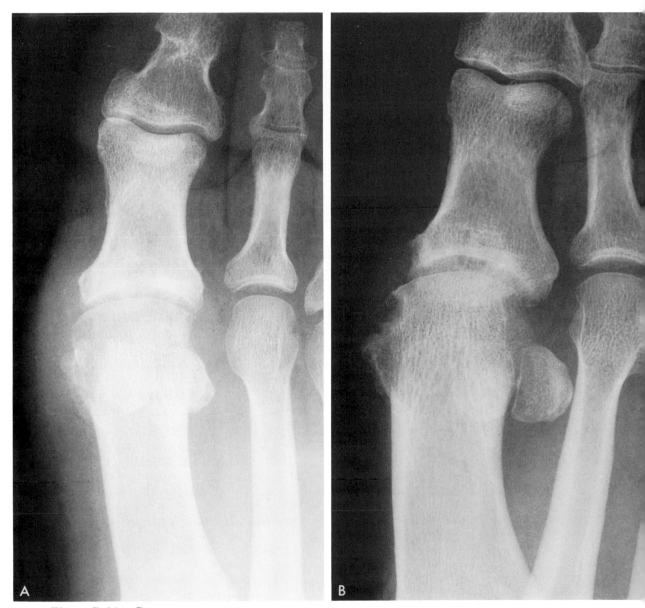

Figure 5–21. Gout.

A. Minimal soft tissue swelling adjacent to the first metatarsophalangeal joint and faint radiolucencies of the medial margins of the articulating bones are evident in this relatively nonspecific and unremarkable film.

B. The usefulness of the oblique view becomes apparent as the radiolucencies are revealed to be sharply defined cortical erosions. Although the soft tissue swelling is transient, the bone destruction is a permanent record of the previous attacks of podagra.

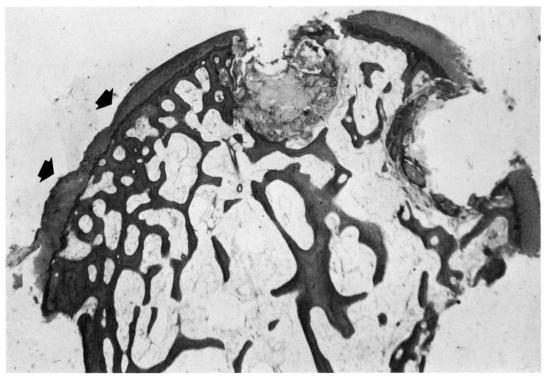

Figure 5–22. Gout.
Two cysts have destroyed articular cartilage and subchondral bone and are sharply circumscribed, as in the preceding radiograph. Irregular loss of cartilage is also present at the periphery (arrows), suggesting a diffuse inflammation within the joint. (Courtesy of The Arthritis Foundation.)

typify the erosions of gout have not developed. Irregular destruction of the articular cartilage along the lateral aspect of the joint is also present (arrows).

Sometimes a film is so typical of gout that other erosive arthritides are excluded by the radiographic picture alone. The localized soft tissue swelling of the tophus, in association with erosion and an overhanging edge, allows the diagnosis of gout to be made with confidence in a second patient with this disease (Fig. 5–23).

Involvement of the third metatarsophalangeal joint in a third patient with gout is suggested by capsular distention, which is seen as a slight increase in the periarticular density (Fig. 5–24). The erosion has a suggestion of an overhanging edge to distinguish it from rheumatoid arthritis, but these two findings alone are far from diagnostic of gout. The strongest clue against the diagnosis of rheumatoid

arthritis, however, is the preservation of the articular cartilage in the face of extensive inflammatory changes, similar to the preceding example. Joint *narrowing* and *erosions* coexist at the metatarsophalangeal joints in patients with rheumatoid arthritis. The erosions of gout, on the other hand, tend to be marginal or periarticular, and the uninvolved cartilage maintains its width.

A severe deforming or mutilating arthritis can occur with extensive soft tissue involvement and bone destruction in patients with gout (Fig. 5–25). Massive deposits of tophaceous material surround the great toe. Erosions of both articulating bones and destruction of the joint have resulted in a mutilating arthritis.

The severe destruction that is seen in the previous pathologic specimen is illustrated radiographically in Figure 5–26. There is much more proliferation of bone than was present in the specimen,

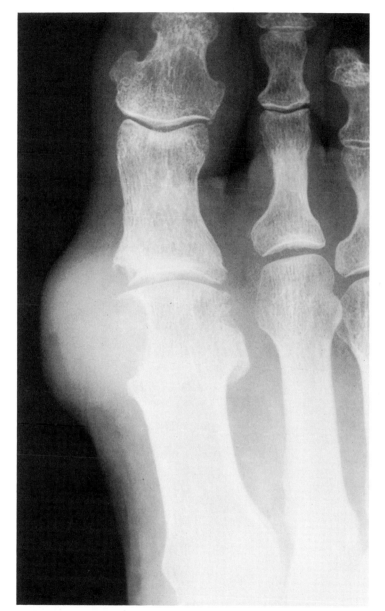

Figure 5–23. Gout.
Massive soft tissue swelling and well-circumscribed marginal erosions associated with a relatively normal joint are characteristic of the periarticular changes of gout.

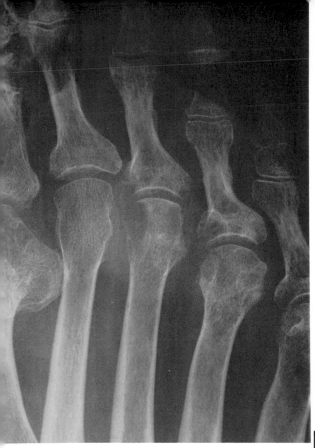

Figure 5–24. Gout.
The well-circumscribed erosion of the third metatarsal head, the adjacent soft tissue mass and the normal bony mineralization and joint space typify the destructive changes in gout.

Figure 5–25. Chronic tophaceous gout.
Huge tophi surround the great toe, causing well-circumscribed erosions of the bones and complete destruction of the joint. The "overhanging edge" characteristic of the proliferative bony changes of gout encompasses the proximal margins of the large plantar tophus (arrow). (Courtesy of The Arthritis Foundation.)

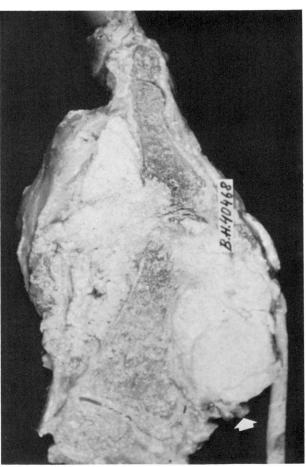

158

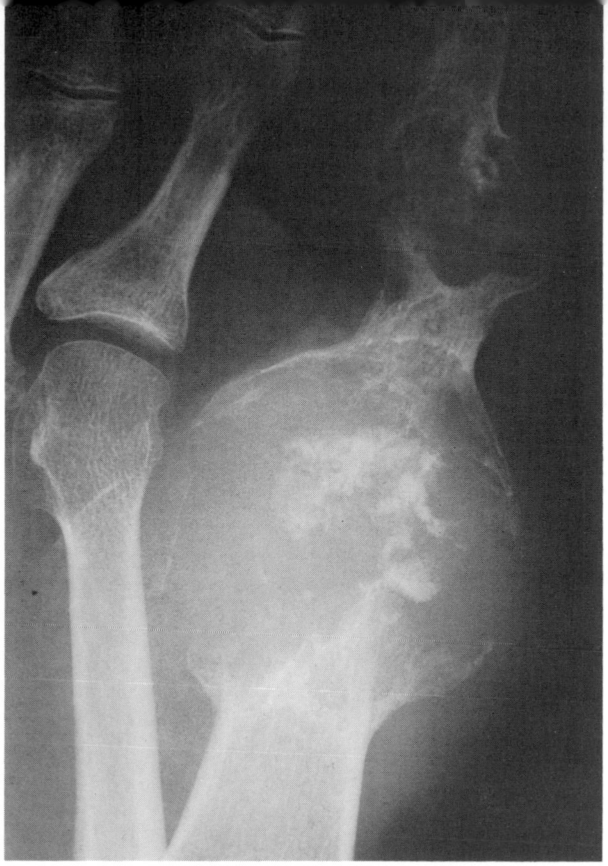

Figure 5–26. Gout.
Huge tophaceous masses have destroyed both joints of the great toe and have splayed the articular ends of the bones, forming the typical "over hanging edge" of gout. The bony mineralization is normal.

however. Both joints of the great toe have been completely destroyed, and the wide shell-like expanse of new bone surrounding the intracapsular tophus is a graphic demonstration of the proliferative response of bone to the deposition of tophaceous material.

Large erosions may rarely occur in the tarsal bones from contiguous tophi, and these may be difficult to distinguish from the erosions of rheumatoid arthritis (Fig. 5–27). It is helpful in making a diagnosis of gout to find preservation of the cartilage between the tarsal bones, as in this example. In rheumatoid arthritis, uniform loss of cartilage in the joint space usually accompanies such extensive erosions of the bones.

THE EROSIONS OF DEGENERATIVE JOINT DISEASE

Hallux Valgus. Although pain in the great toe is a hallmark of gout, the more mundane condition of hallux valgus or bunion is far more commonly a cause of discomfort. Surprisingly, it is often difficult to distinguish this local phenomenon from systemic diseases, because it too may cause erosions and degenerative changes with proliferation of new bone,

as in Figure 5–28. The presence of an atavistic cuneiform with its consequent malalignment of the first metatarsal bone does not exclude gout, since this is such a common congenital deformity that it is frequently seen in patients with this metabolic disease. The multiple areas of rarefaction in the metatarsal head, similarly, do not help to distinguish one inflammatory arthritis from another. The overgrowth of bone, both adjacent to the bursa and involving the sesamoid bone of the flexor tendon, is typical of the degenerative change superimposed on a malaligned toe in primary hallux valgus but may also occur as an end stage of long-standing gouty arthritis.

A section through the first metatarsal joint demonstrates similar changes (Fig. 5–29), characterized by non-uniform loss of cartilage and bony overgrowth of both the metatarsal head and the sesamoid bone. The thickened subchondral line in the area of cartilage loss (arrows) is the microscopic change that results in the radiographic appearance of eburnation.

RESORPTIVE ARTHROPATHY

Resorptive arthropathies occur in the foot in the same manner as in the hand.

159

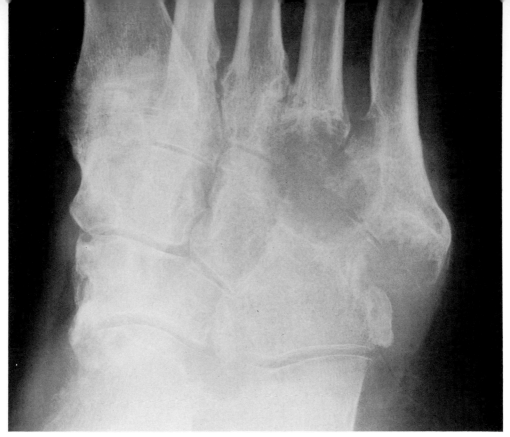

Figure 5-27. Gout.

Occasionally the tarsal bones may be destroyed by adjacent tophi which cause large areas of erosion. The destruction is localized, and normal articulation of many of the tarsal bones can be seen; this contrasts with the symmetrical narrowing of the cartilage spaces seen in rheumatoid arthritis.

The whittled end of a bone on the proximal side of a joint may invaginate into the base of the articulating bone, resulting in a "pencil-in-cup" configuration. Resorptive changes may also affect both articulating ends of bones, and rather than a pencil-in-cup appearance, a pencilling of both bones will result. The condition causing these extensive destructive changes has been termed "arthritis mutilans" but more properly should be called "resorptive arthropathy" to distinguish it from arthritides which cause severe mutilation by other mechanisms (i.e., gout and lipoid dermatoarthritis with pressure erosions from adjacent masses).

In the foot, the *radiographic* picture of resorptive arthropathies is seen most frequently in rheumatic diseases (rheumatoid arthritis, psoriatic arthritis and occasionally Reiter's syndrome), neuropathies and infection.

It seems apparent that some common pathophysiologic mechanism may be brought into play to cause similar radiographic changes in such widely diversified pathologic conditions. Such a mechanism might involve the rich glomus network of vessels that surrounds the joint. Vascular instability from loss of neurogenic control or excessive stimulation directly from a localized inflammatory process might result in an uncontrolled resorption of bone.

Rheumatoid Arthritis. Figure 5–30 demonstrates the typical pencil-in-cup deformity of the fourth and fifth metatarsophalangeal joints and illustrates the early changes that may eventually result in a mutilating arthritis in a patient with rheumatoid arthritis.

Psoriatic Arthritis. Two pathologic findings characterize resorptive arthropathy: concentric *resorption of bone* and *primary joint destruction.* Figure 5–31 illustrates these findings in a finger. All three phalanges have been whittled down from loss of bone along the perios-

160

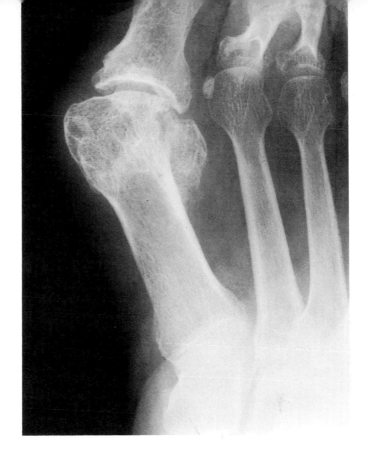

Figure 5–28. Hallux valgus. The atavistic cuneiform, a metatarsus varus deformity and hallux valgus preceded the degenerative changes of the metatarsophalangeal joint. Irregular narrowing of the joint and proliferative changes of the metatarsal head and sesamoid bone, as well as deviation of the second phalanx, are complications of the primary alignment abnormalities.

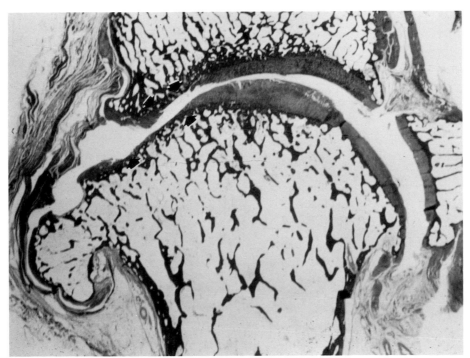

Figure 5–29. Degenerative joint disease.
Degenerative changes are frequently seen at the first metatarsophalangeal joint. A sagittal section shows non-uniform loss of cartilage and osteophytes of both the metatarsal head and the sesamoid bone. The thickened subchondral line in the area of cartilage loss (arrows) would appear as eburnation on a radiograph. (Courtesy of The Arthritis Foundation.)

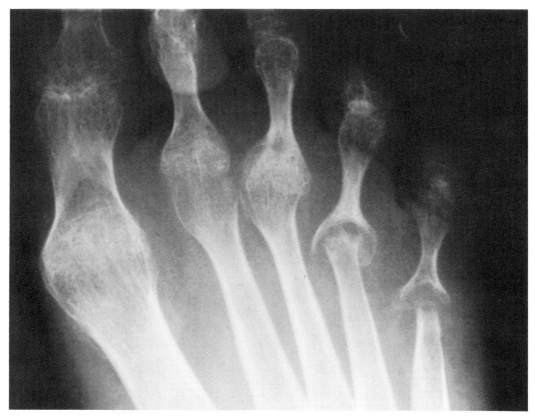

Figure 5–30. Rheumatoid arthritis.
Progressive degrees of involvement illustrate the development of the pencil-in-cup deformity. Narrowing and erosions of the first, second and third metatarsophalangeal joints mimic bony ankylosis on this view. Concentric resorption of the distal fourth and fifth metatarsal bones and invagination into the base of the proximal phalanges have resulted in cuplike deformities. Diffuse osteoporosis is typical of rheumatoid arthritis.

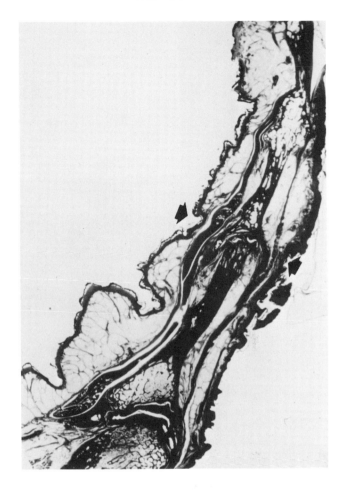

Figure 5–31. Pencil-in-cup deformity.

Concentric resorption of bone from the periosteal surface and endosteal new bone formation have converted the phalanges of a finger to thin, solid "toothpicks" of bone. Invagination of the base of the middle phalanx where it meets the proximal phalanx has caused a cuplike configuration (arrows). Bony ankylosis has fused the distal interphalangeal joint. Minimal volar subluxation of the metacarpophalangeal joint adds to the deformity. (Courtesy of The Arthritis Foundation.)

teal surface. New bone produced on the endosteal surface has resulted in a solid shaft of cortical bone of both the proximal and distal phalanges and is beginning to transform the middle phalanx in a similar fashion. Telescoping of the pointed end of the proximal phalanx into the base of the middle phalanx (arrow) produces a pencil-in-cup deformity similar to that seen in the previous radiograph. Bony ankylosis has fused the distal interphalangeal joint. Minimal subluxation of the metacarpophalangeal joint adds to the severe deformity.

Because of the uneven involvement of the four toes, a single film demonstrates the step-by-step changes that result in the mutilating deformity of psoriatic arthritis (Fig. 5–32). The fifth metatarsophalangeal joint demonstrates a pencil-in-cup deformity. The fourth, third and

second metatarsophalangeal joints manifest progressively more severe alteration of the articulating bones. Resorption is so severe at the second metatarsophalangeal joint that a major portion of the proximal phalanx has disappeared.

Although rheumatoid arthritis and psoriatic arthritis may be identical in appearance, in this patient there are four characteristic features of psoriatic arthritis that distinguish it from rheumatoid arthritis.

1. The *preservation* of relatively *normal mineralization* is more commonly seen in psoriatic arthritis and contrasts with the severe generalized osteoporosis that usually accompanies rheumatoid arthritis.

2. The *pattern of distribution* of the joint involvement with severe destructive changes primarily of the distal in-

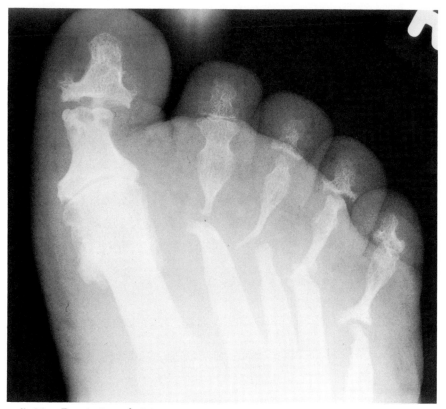

Figure 5–32. Psoriatic arthritis.

Concentric resorption of bone and formation of endosteal new bone have whittled the ends of the metatarsal bones and proximal phalanges in a similar fashion as the previous microscopic specimen. Bony ankylosis of the proximal interphalangeal joints and widening and destruction of the distal interphalangeal joints and the interphalangeal joint of the great toe are characteristic findings in psoriatic arthritis.

terphalangeal joints is rarely seen in rheumatoid arthritis.

3. The excessive fibrous tissue that has been deposited in the interphalangeal joint of the great toe and the distal interphalangeal joint of the fourth toe has resulted in *widening* of the joint spaces. Where this widening is seen in the chronic stage of rheumatoid arthritis it is associated with severe resorptive changes of the articular bones.

4. Although *bony ankylosis* occurs in rheumatoid arthritis, it is usually limited to the tarsal bones and rarely occurs in the phalanges. Psoriatic arthritis, on the other hand, frequently causes obliteration of the *interphalangeal* joint spaces and bony fusion, as is seen in the second through the fifth proximal interphalangeal joints.

Although irregularly eroded articulating surfaces of the interphalangeal joint of the great toe, proliferative new bone at the base of the distal phalanx and an associated widened interphalangeal joint space are sometimes said to be pathognomonic of psoriatic arthritis, an identical picture may occur with Reiter's syndrome.

Leprosy. The destructive changes of leprosy are most commonly due to the neuropathic condition rather than to direct invasion of the bone by the lepromatous bacilli; hence, these changes are indistinguishable from those produced by such neuropathic diseases as lues and diabetes. It is unusual to find severe destruction of the bones of the feet without coexistent plantar ulcers and infection, and the contribution from each

condition to the final mutilating picture is academic. The brunt of the trauma in the feet is at the metatarsophalangeal joints, since the major weight-bearing forces during walking are at this point. For this reason destructive changes in the foot differ in location from those in the hand, where the tips of the fingers absorb the majority of trauma.

The resorptive changes at the metatarsophalangeal joints in a patient with leprosy (Fig. 5–33) are similar to those in the patient with psoriatic arthritis (Fig. 5–32). However, lack of proliferative changes at the base of the distal phalanges helps to distinguish the two diseases. Resorption of the distal phalanges is also evident. Generally, bone mineralization is maintained in neuropathic conditions as in psoriatic arthritis. The generalized osteoporosis in this foot, however, is con-

sistent with that of a 60 year old female.

A second patient with leprosy demonstrates less advanced changes (Fig. 5–34). As in the previous example, the tufts of the distal phalanges are destroyed. In addition, resorption of the proximal phalanges of the fourth and fifth toes has whittled them and caused destruction of the proximal interphalangeal joints. Plantar ulcers were present beneath the involved bone and appear to have accelerated the resorptive changes that occur in a primary neuropathic disease.

INFECTION

Fungal infections or low-grade bacterial infections may occasionally mimic the mutilating arthritis of a connective tissue disease or a neuropathic disorder.

The appearance of a film of a patient with diffuse fungal involvement of his

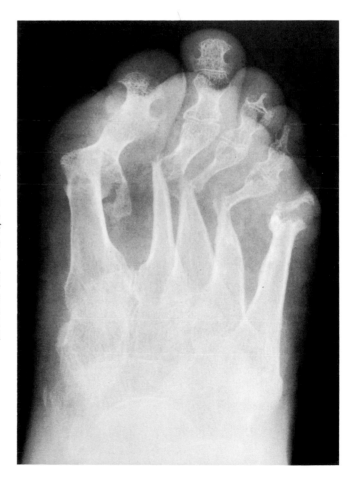

Figure 5–33. Leprosy.

When the foot is involved, resorptive changes in neuropathic arthropathies most frequently destroy the metatarsophalangeal joints and the distal phalanges. The "licked candy stick" appearance of the bones is contributed to by the combination of cortical resorption and endosteal new bone formation, making them solid white and spindle-shaped. This is seen in the third, fourth and fifth distal phalanges and, in a transitional stage, at the distal end of the second metatarsal bone.

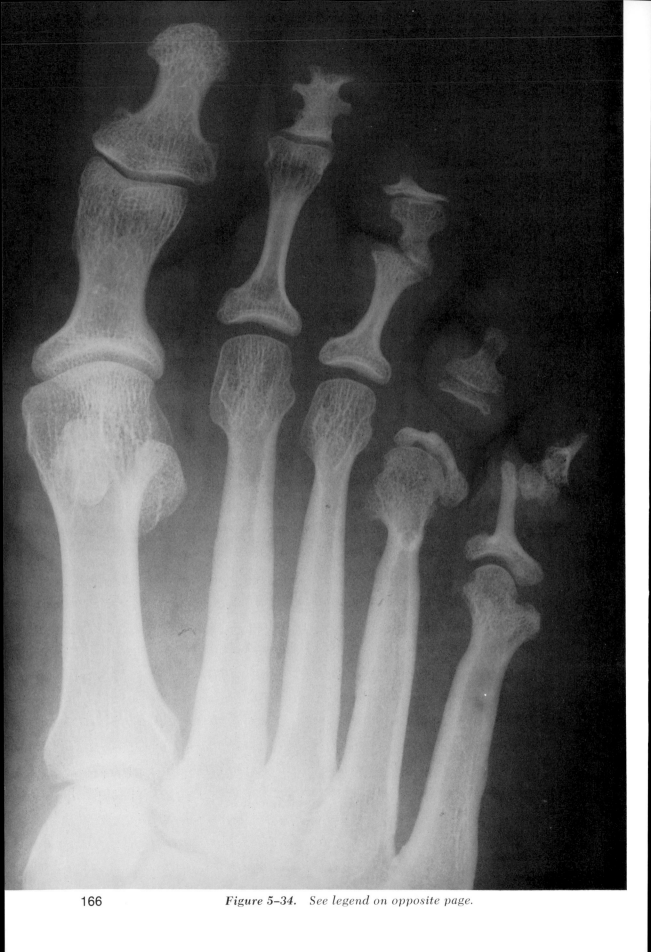

Figure 5–34. *See legend on opposite page.*

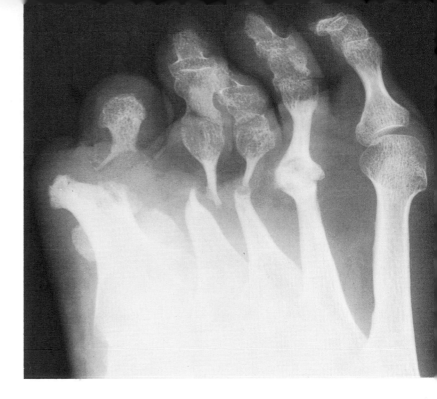

Figure 5–35. Infection.
Chronic soft tissue infection of the foot and draining sinuses have led to secondary changes in the bones and a typical resorptive arthropathy. The mutilating changes are at the metatarsophalangeal joints and are identical to the changes in neuropathic conditions.

foot and *no* neuropathy (Fig. 5–35) differs from the preceding example only by virtue of the distortion of the soft tissues of the great toe from draining sinuses. The pencilling at the metatarsophalangeal joints and filling in of the spongiosa by endosteal new bone have converted the phalanges to thin white "toothpicks." The appearance here differs little from that in previous examples and necessitates clinical correlation before a specific diagnosis can be suggested.

Bony Ankylosis

Bony ankylosis, in which there is union of the bones of a joint, is the opposite phenomenon from resorption. When it is seen in the tarsal bones it most commonly is associated with rheumatoid arthritis. If it occurs in the interphalangeal joints, it is usually associated with psoriatic arthritis. It may be seen as an isolated phenomenon in any joint as the end stage of an infectious process.

Infection. The hallmarks of a pyogenic arthritis are all present in Figure 5–36. There are soft tissue swelling, bony demineralization, periosteal new bone and rapid destruction of the cartilage with narrowing of the joint space (Fig. 5–36A). Over a three month interval, complete destruction of the joint cartilage occurred (Fig. 5–36B). Bony ankylosis not infrequently is the end result of the healing phase of an infectious arthritis and is seen in this patient one year later (Fig. 5–36C). The rapidity of the process and its localization to one joint makes this cause of bony ankylosis easily distinguishable from psoriatic arthritis.

Suppurative infections rapidly destroy the articular cartilage by means of pro-

Figure 5–34. Leprosy.
Resorption of the second, third and fifth distal phalanges and the fourth and fifth proximal plalanges illustrates the pathologic changes in a neuropathic disorder leading to a resorptive arthropathy. The destruction differs from that in the connective tissue disorders. It does not necessarily begin at the joint but, as in this example, may be related to adjacent plantar ulcers and may begin in the middle of the phalanges.

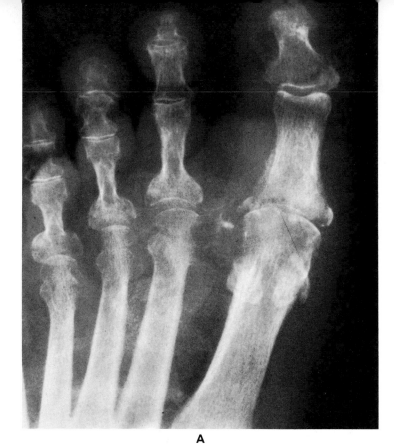

A

Figure 5–36. Pyogenic arthritis.

A. Diffuse soft tissue swelling, rapid destruction of the joint space and periosteal new bone along the proximal phalanx are characteristic of suppurative infections.

B. Three months later, a contiguous osteomyelitis has contributed to the joint destruction.

C. A year after the onset of the infection there has been healing with complete bony ankylosis of the two bones.

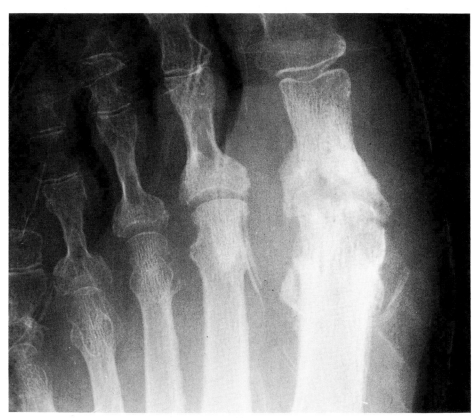

B

Illustration continued on opposite page.

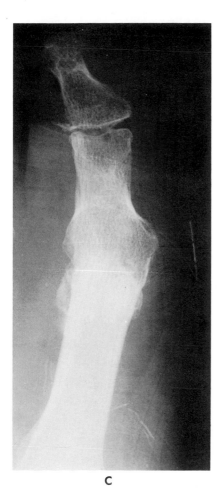

C

Figure 5-36. Continued.

teolytic enzymes produced by the bacteria. Rapid and complete loss of a joint is characteristic of a pyogenic infection, and contiguous osteomyelitis of the articular bones contributes to the destruction. Figure 5–37 illustrates the microscopic counterpart of the findings seen on the previous film. Total destruction of the proximal interphalangeal joint (arrows) and the articular bones is seen.

ANATOMY OF THE LATERAL ANKLE

The lateral view of the ankle demonstrates soft tissue changes of the heel and alignment abnormalities and the cartilage space between the tarsal bones. In addition, specific alterations associated with the calcaneus are useful in suggesting a

systemic disease and can be seen only on this view.

An arthrogram of the normal ankle joint delineates the extent of the capsule and its anterior and posterior dimensions (Fig. 5–38).

SOFT TISSUE ABNORMALITIES OF THE ANKLE

Generalized Increase in Soft Tissue

Acromegaly. As an example of the usefulness of the lateral view of the ankle, the thickened heel pad of acromegaly reflects the generalized increase in soft tissues in this endocrine disorder. It is far more easy to quantitate these changes from this view than from the AP (anteroposterior) views of the hands and feet. It has been found that the normal heel pad is no larger than 23 mm in men and 21.5 in women when measured perpendicularly from the lowest point of the calcaneus. Since the heel is placed directly on the film, there is no magnification to complicate this measurement. The measurement must be made in the non-weight-bearing foot in order not to flatten the soft tissue. Because of the increase in soft tissue in obesity, an additional 1 mm is allowed for every 25 pounds of weight over 150 pounds.

Any increase in soft tissue is a reliable indicator of acromegaly, although the rare condition of pachydermoperiostosis (idiopathic osteoarthropathy) may also cause infiltration of the subcutaneous tissues of the heel. Edema, myxedema and infection will also increase the heel pad measurement, but these entities may be easily excluded clinically.

The overgrowth of soft tissue is apparent in a lateral view of the heel in a patient with well-documented acromegaly (Fig. 5–39); it measures 30 mm. Degenerative changes of the calcaneus which commonly accompany the natural progression of acromegaly are present at the attachment of the Achilles tendon and the plantar aponeurosis along the inferior calcaneal margin (arrows).

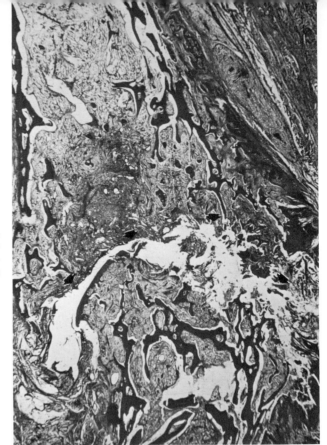

Figure 5–37. Pyogenic arthritis.
A photomicrograph illustrates total destruction of a proximal interphalangeal joint (arrows) as well as the adjacent bone. (Courtesy of The Arthritis Foundation.)

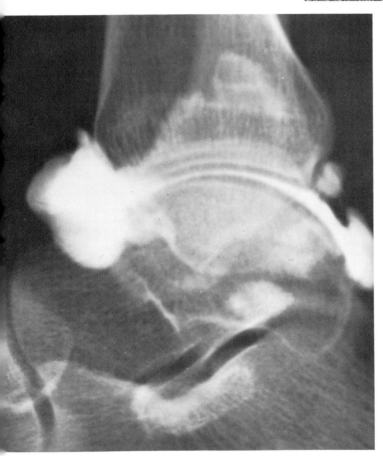

Figure 5–38. Arthrogram of normal ankle.
The anterior and posterior extent of the joint is delineated by contrast material.

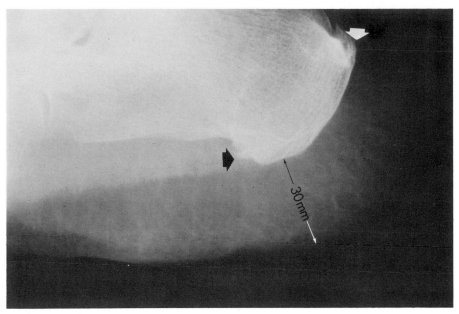

Figure 5–39. Acromegaly.
Overgrowth of soft tissues is easily quantitated on a lateral view of the heel. The overgrowth measures 30 mm on the original film. Bony spurs project into the Achilles tendon and the attachment of the plantar aponeurosis (arrows).

Localized Increase in Soft Tissue

SOFT TISSUE NODULES

Localized soft tissue changes are occasionally seen in the ankle as rheumatoid nodules, tophaceous deposits, abscesses associated with inflammatory disease and xanthomatous deposits in patients with Type II hypercholesterolemia.

Rheumatoid Arthritis. The nodule seen adjacent to the Achilles tendon in Figure 5–40 reflects one of many subcutaneous nodules in a patient with rheumatoid arthritis. It is indistinguishable from a "pump bump" secondary to chronic pressure from high heels and by no means is pathognomonic of rheumatoid arthritis. The inflammatory arthritis is extensive and has involved the area of the Achilles tendon so that the normal triangular fat lucency between the posterior tibia and the tendon has become edematous and blends imperceptibly with the surrounding water density structures.

Generally, rheumatoid arthritis is not accompanied by proliferative new bone in areas of inflammatory involvement. However, in the heel, bony spurs charac-

teristically develop adjacent to inflamed bursae. In this patient new bone is forming within the Achilles tendon at its point of attachment to the calcaneus.

Gout. The huge soft tissue mass posterior to the tibia and displacing the Achilles tendon is a massive tophaceous deposit in a patient with long-standing disease involving all the joints of his body (Fig. 5–41). Although this film shows only a small part of the midfoot, the bones that are included are deformed by erosions from deposits within the joint capsule.

Tuberculosis. Not infrequently, tuberculous osteomyelitis is accompanied by a cold abscess. The soft tissue mass characteristically is well defined and overlies the involved bone, in contrast to the diffuse soft tissue swelling of cellulitis that accompanies a suppurative bacterial osteomyelitis. The abscess of tuberculosis does not destroy the surrounding soft tissue planes, and the skin and subcutaneous fat are preserved as distinct radiographic entities. These findings are illustrated in Figure 5–42.

This example of tuberculous os-

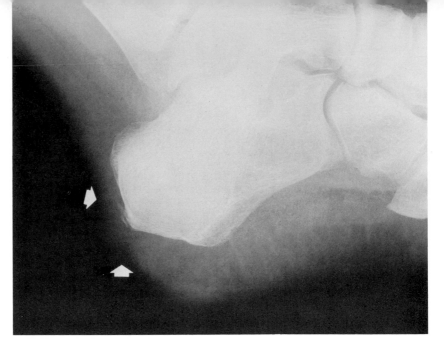

Figure 5–40. Rheumatoid arthritis.

The soft tissue mass posterior to the calcaneus is one of many rheumatoid nodules present in this patient (arrows). Edema has obliterated the triangle of fat anterior to the Achilles tendon (posterior to the tibia). A calcific spur is forming at the attachment of the tendon to the calcaneus.

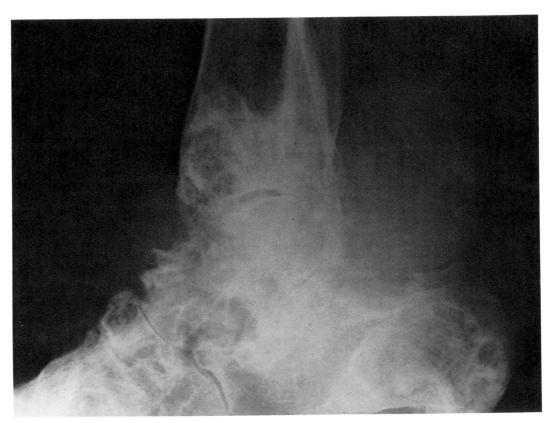

Figure 5–41. Gout.

A huge tophus distorts the soft tissue posterior to the ankle, and distention of the joint capsule is evident anteriorly, indicating an active arthritis.

Multiple subchondral cysts are present in all the tarsal bones.

172

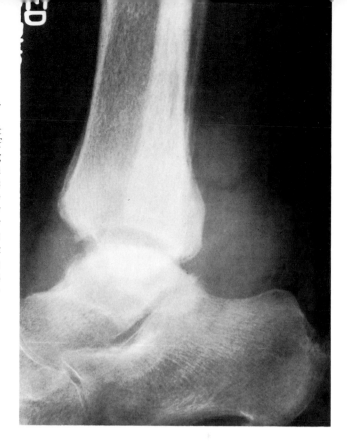

Figure 5–42. Tuberculous arthritis.

Massive distortion of the soft tissue is evident, and a slight bulge of the anterior joint space, indicating capsular effusion, can be seen. An erosion of the posterior calcaneus reflects inflammation of the pre-Achilles bursa. Thick periosteal new bone along the shaft of the tibia may occur from a primary infectious arthritis but must always suggest intraosseous infection. Permeative changes throughout the distal fibula and tibia indicate extensive osteomyelitis.

teomyelitis demonstrates permeative changes throughout the distal tibia as well as periosteal new bone. It must be remembered that tuberculosis and other granulomas often are well-circumscribed within the bone, but occasionally, as in this patient, they show the changes of a more virulent infection spreading throughout a large area of bone.

CHARCOT JOINT

Whenever there are severe destruction and disorganization of a joint, as seen in Figure 5–43, an underlying neuropathy must be suspected. The vascular instability that accompanies a neuropathic condition results in intermittent massive effusions. The complete disorganization of the joint and destruction of the articulating ends of the bones are seen in this lateral view. Both resorption of bone and simultaneous new bone formation within the soft tissue compartment of the joint capsule mark the pathologic changes of a Charcot joint. The presence of periosteal new bone along the anterior tibial shaft suggests the possibility of a superimposed infection. However, subperiosteal bleeding may occur from trauma. In addi-

tion, thick periosteal bone may be produced wherever there is vascular stasis. Although the diagnostic possibility of infection must be considered when periosteal new bone is seen, it is not pathognomonic of this complication.

Figure 5–44 illustrates the microscopic changes at the periphery of a Charcot joint. Complete destruction of the articular cartilage and deposition of fibrous material have widened the distance between the bones. A prominent projection of new bone extends into the para-articular soft tissues (arrow).

BONY OVERGROWTH (SPURS)

New bone is commonly deposited as spurs adjacent to the three bursae in the heel. They frequently accompany rheumatoid arthritis, Reiter's syndrome and ankylosing spondylitis; thus, when spurs are seen these disease entities must be considered. Most *commonly*, however, a spur represents nothing more than a proliferative change due to stress from the tendon or attachment of the aponeurosis;

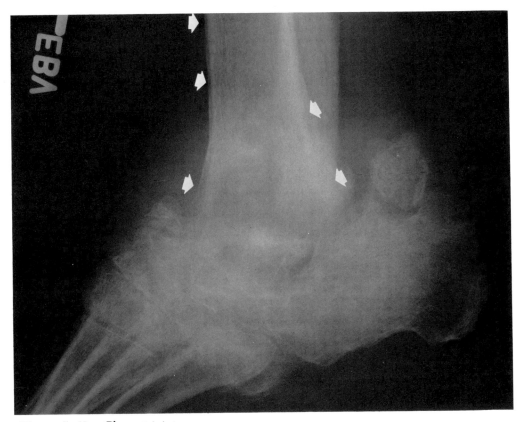

Figure 5–43. Charcot joint.
Massive distention of the joint capsule, total destruction of the joint and ectopic new bone within the capsule are characteristic of a neuropathic joint. The thick periosteal bone along the anterior and posterior tibia (arrows) may be seen as a component of a Charcot joint and, as in this example, may not reflect a superimposed infection.

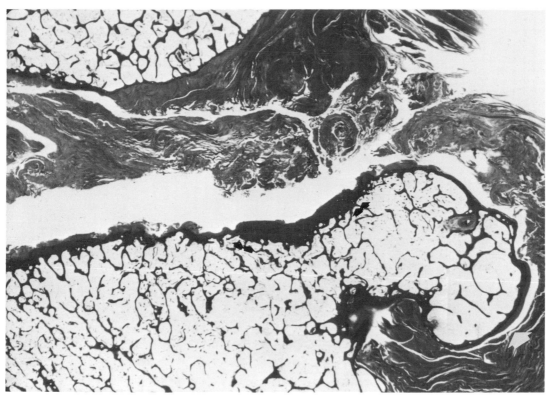

Figure 5–44. Charcot joint.

A close-up of the margin of a Charcot joint reveals total destruction of the articular cartilage, deposition of fibrous tissue between the bones and proliferative new bone distorting the articular bone (arrow). Marked thickening of the subchondral line is evident (double arrows). (Courtesy of The Arthritis Foundation.)

it need not be a harbinger of a connective tissue disorder.

Proliferative Spur. An example of the solid, well-defined shelf of bone that develops along the attachment of the plantar aponeurosis is seen in Figure 5–45A. Because it is viewed in profile on a lateral projection, its shadow appears as a triangular spur. Bony projections occur in response to stress and are frequently seen in hypermobile feet such as pes cavum, or associated with flat feet (Fig. 5–45B).

Reiter's Syndrome. It has been stated in the literature that the periostitis that accompanies Reiter's syndrome is distinctive, appearing fluffy and less sharply defined than that of rheumatoid arthritis. In practice, this distinction is not valid enough to merit a specific diagnosis from a film finding. When it is accompanied by extensive reactive sclerosis of the entire

calcaneus, however, Reiter's syndrome is the most likely cause.

A patient with Reiter's syndrome (Fig. 5–46) has radiographic changes in the calcaneus that are sharp and well-defined, at the attachment of both the plantar aponeurosis and the Achilles tendon. Inflammatory erosions not infrequently affect the spur itself and appear as radiolucent defects altering the sharp contour as in this example. The orientation of the spur toward the base of the calcaneus rather than along the axis of the plantar aponeurosis is helpful in distinguishing it from the proliferative spur that develops in response to stress.

Rheumatoid Arthritis. A patient with rheumatoid arthritis (Fig. 5–47) has developed periosteal new bone at the attachment of the plantar aponeurosis and the Achilles tendon. The configuration of the spur is solid and sharply defined as in

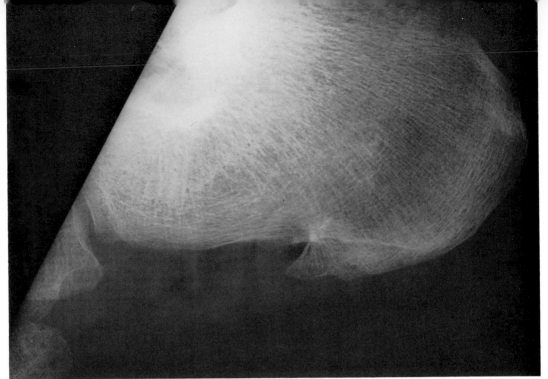

A

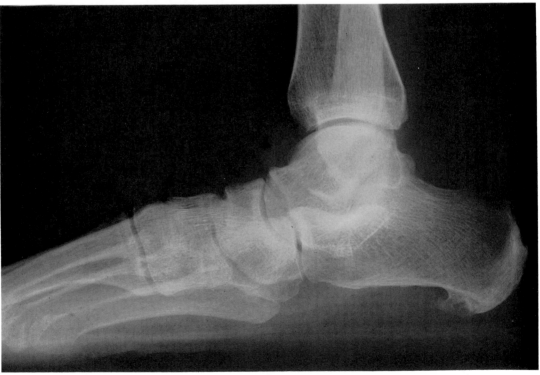

B

Figure 5–45. Plantar spur.

    A. The thick, solid wedge of new bone at the attachment of the plantar aponeurosis reflects localized periostitis along the inferior calcaneus.

    B. Whenever the foot is hypermobile and the plantar aponeurosis is excessively stretched, spurs tend to develop. They are commonly associated with pes planum, as in this example.

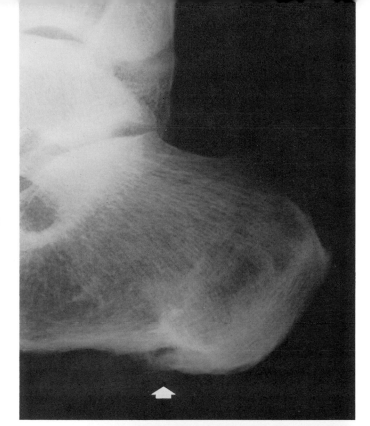

Figure 5–46. Reiter's syndrome.

Frequently, inflammatory involvement of the bursa in Reiter's syndrome results in the development of a spur (arrow). Unlike degenerative spurs, they are less sharply defined and often project upward toward the base of the calcaneus, as in this example.

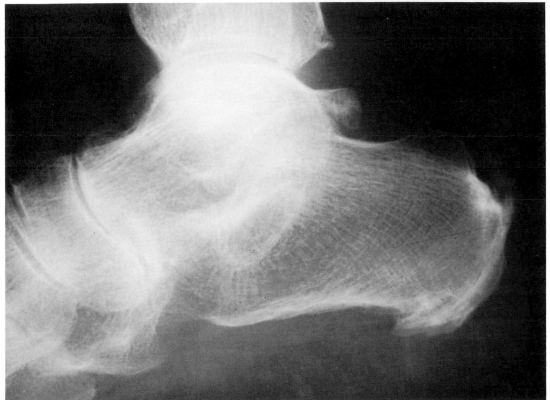

Figure 5–47. Rheumatoid arthritis.

Bony proliferation at the attachment of the Achilles tendon and the plantar aponeurosis occur in rheumatoid arthritis, reflecting adjacent bursitis. The character of the spurs is frequently indistinguishable from Reiter's syndrome.

177

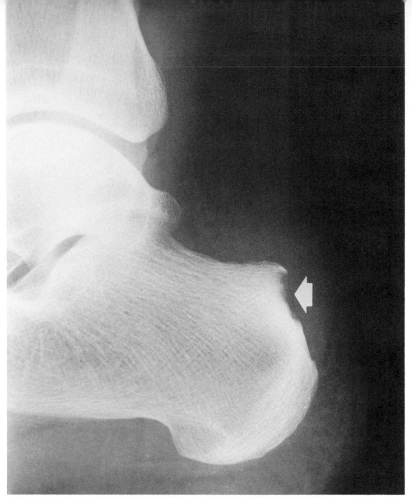

Figure 5–48. Rheumatoid arthritis.

Bursitis may be reflected by an erosion as well as by new bone formation. The typical "rat-bite" erosion of rheumatoid arthritis anterior to the Achilles tendon indicates localized inflammation (arrow). Edema of the adjacent fat pad can be seen just above the calcaneus.

the film of the patient with Reiter's syndrome (Fig. 5–46). The difficulty in distinguishing these two conditions by radiographic criteria alone is evident.

Bone erosion adjacent to an inflamed bursa is not as common an occurrence in the heel as new bone proliferation in patients with rheumatoid arthritis. Figure 5–48 illustrates the typical rat bite erosion with ill-defined margins adjacent to the pre-Achilles bursa that may occasionally be seen.

THE ANKLE EN FACE

Since the articulation of the tibia and fibula with the tarsal bones cannot be evaluated on the projection that is taken for the foot, additional views must be ob-

tained in order to project the ankle joint tangentially. Involvement of the ankle by inflammatory disease causes soft tissue swelling and destruction of the cartilage and articulating bones in a fashion similar to that in the previously described joints.

The extent of the joint capsule that encloses the distal tibia and talus is defined by an arthrogram (Fig. 5–49). Immediately above the attachment of the capsule, the periosteum of the tibia begins.

Rheumatoid Arthritis. In about five per cent of patients with rheumatoid arthritis, periostitis will be a prominent component of the disease. Most frequently it is seen along the distal tibia and femur and in the small bones of the hands and feet. It appears in Figure 5–50 as a thin line of periosteal new bone

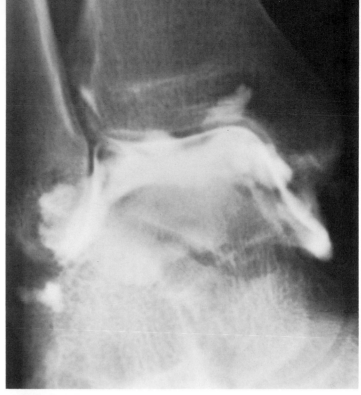

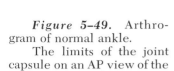
Figure 5–49. Arthrogram of normal ankle.

The limits of the joint capsule on an AP view of the ankle are defined by contrast material.

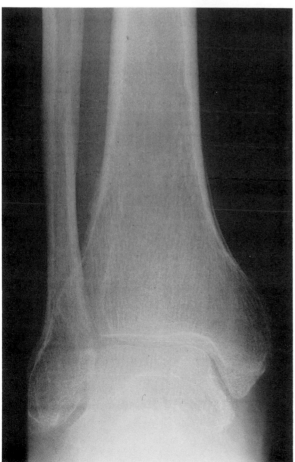

Figure 5–50. Rheumatoid arthritis.

The thin line of periosteal new bone along the outer surfaces of the tibia and fibula signal the presence of an inflammatory arthritis before joint destruction is evident.

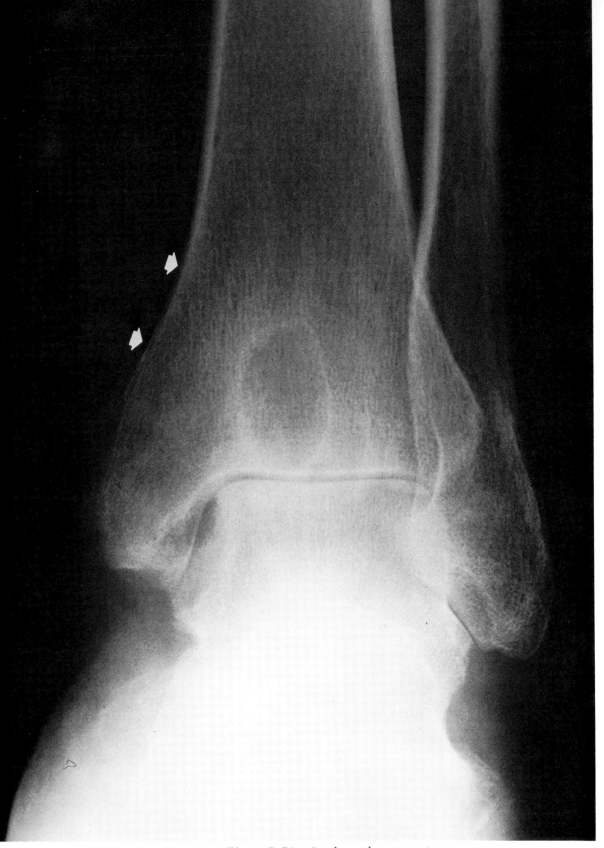

Figure 5–51. See legend on opposite page.

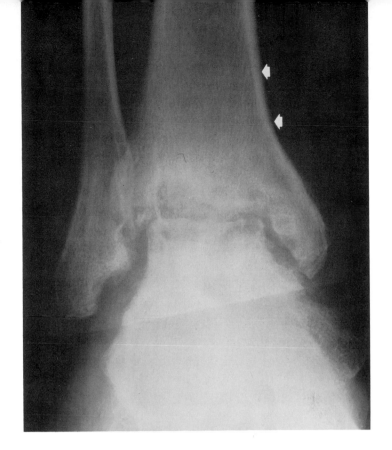

Figure 5–52. Rheumatoid arthritis.

In addition to joint narrowing, large erosions are seen in the articulating bones. Separation of the fibula from the talus indicates either synovial proliferation or a joint effusion. A wispy layer of periosteal new bone is evident along the outer margin of the tibia (arrows).

along the outer surface of the distal tibia and fibula. There is, in addition, a thicker layer of periosteal new bone along the fibular side of the tibia. This should not be confused with the periostitis that accompanies an inflammatory arthritis. Such a layer is normally seen along the attachment of the interosseous membrane and is a response of the underlying bone to the attachment of the membrane itself. At this early stage in the patient's disease process, the periostitis is the only clue that the ankle is involved with rheumatoid arthritis. The cartilage space is normal.

Uniform narrowing of the joint is as characteristic of rheumatoid arthritis in the ankle as it is in the joints of the foot and hand. Figure 5–51 emphasizes the symmetry of cartilage destruction as well as the frequency of periosteal new bone accompanying an inflamed joint in this condition. The well circumscribed radiolucent shadow in the tibial epiphysis is typical of the subchondral cysts that occur in rheumatoid arthritis. It must be distinguished from benign bone cysts, which do not occur in epiphyses, and low grade infection, which rarely affects the ends of the bones and more commonly occurs in the metaphyses. An identical picture may be seen in hemophiliacs who have had multiple episodes of intra-articular bleeding.

The final stage in the destructive process of rheumatoid arthritis is seen in Figure 5–52. There are soft tissue swelling adjacent to the medial and lateral malleoli and actual separation of the distal fibula from the talus. The separation may be due to an acute effusion; however, loss of cartilage and extensive erosions of all the bones suggest that the separation may be due to synovial proliferation in a chronic arthritis. A wispy layer of periosteal new bone is present along the outer

Figure 5–51. Rheumatoid arthritis.

Uniform joint narrowing and periosteal new bone (arrows) are typical of the inflammatory changes of rheumatoid arthritis. A well-defined subchondral cyst is present in the tibial epiphysis.

margin of the tibia, again emphasizing how frequently periostitis occurs in rheumatoid arthritis.

Hemophilia. The radiographic changes of hemophilia are similar to those of juvenile rheumatoid arthritis. Both diseases produce a synovial hypertrophy, and it is not surprising that their radiographic pictures may be identical. In hemophilia, the process is initiated by bleeding into the joint. Massive swelling of the joint capsule results and is much more excessive than in other arthropathies. Repeated episodes of hemorrhage cause synovial hypertrophy with subsequent destruction of the cartilage and pressure erosion of the articular cortices. The presence of blood in the capsule results in hemosiderin deposits, and with excellent film techniques the slight increase in density from the iron may be visible.

Villous hypertrophy can be seen in a microscopic section of synovium from a patient with hemophilia (Fig. 5–53). In addition, the dark stained superficial synovial cells indicate the presence of hemosiderin.

The joint space in a patient with hemophilia (Fig. 5–54) is asymmetrically destroyed. The subchondral cysts in the articular surfaces of the bone may be due to either invagination of synovium or hemorrhage in the bone itself. Because of the hyperemic state that accompanies the capsular irritation, irregular overgrowth and early fusion of the tibial epiphysis result. There is subsequent distortion of the ends of the growing bone. Juvenile rheumatoid arthritis, because of its time of onset, results in the same deformities for the same reasons. In the ankle, the distortion often causes a slanted tibiotalar joint. In this example, the medial aspect

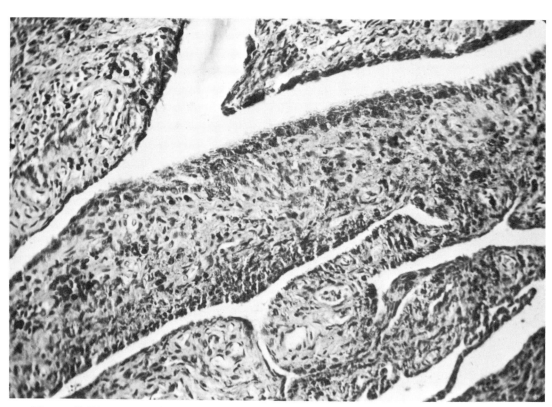

Figure 5–53. Hemophilia.
A microscopic examination of a synovial biopsy specimen reveals villous hypertrophy. The dark-staining cells indicate the presence of hemosiderin. (Courtesy of The Arthritis Foundation.)

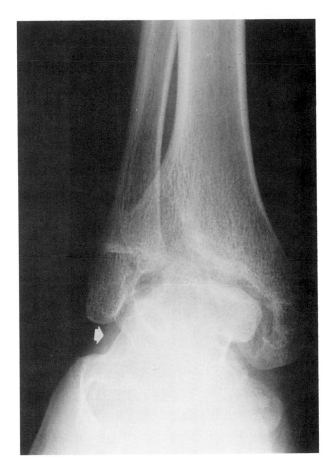

Figure 5-54. Hemophilia. Destruction of the joint and erosions of the articular bones are similar to the changes seen in rheumatoid arthritis. Overgrowth of the medial malleolus has caused a tibiotalar slant, a common occurrence when an inflammatory arthritis begins in childhood. The slight increase in density of the joint capsule (arrow) may be from hemosiderin deposits.

of the tibia is greater than 0.5 cm lower than the lateral aspect. Hyperemia and disuse contribute to the osteoporosis of the bone. Continued weight bearing may result in degenerative changes superimposed on the basic destructive process, but these are not apparent as yet in this patient.

SUGGESTED READINGS

Blankenhorn, D. H., and H. I. Meyers. Radiographic determination of Achilles tendon xanthoma size. Metabolism *18*:882 (1969).

Bywaters, E. G. L. Heel lesions of rheumatoid arthritis. Ann. Rheum. Dis. *13*:42 (1954).

Calabro, J. J. A critical evaluation of the diagnostic features of the feet in rheumatoid arthritis. Arthritis Rheum. 5:19 (1962).

Callaghan, J. E., E. C. Percy, and R. O. Hill. The ankle arthrogram. J. Canad. Ass. Radiol. *21*:74 (1970).

Cochrane, R. G., and T. Davey. *Leprosy in Theory and Practice.* Baltimore, Williams and Wilkins Co., 1964, pp. 425–461.

Coste, F., S. Braun, J. Moutounet, and F. Panahi. Rheumatoid forefoot. Ann. Radiol. (Paris) *11*:1 (1968).

Gamble, F. O., and I. Yale. *Clinical Foot Roentgenology.* Baltimore, Williams and Wilkins Co., 1966.

Kho, K. M., A. D. Wright, and F. H. Doyle. Heel pad thickness in acromegaly. Brit. J. Radiol. *43*:119 (1970).

Marmor, L. The rheumatoid foot. Geriatrics *21*:132 (1966).

Mehrez, M., and S. E. Ganeidy. Arthrography of the ankle. J. Bone Joint Surg. (Brit.) *52*:308 (1970).

Paterson, D. E. Radiologic bone changes and angiographic findings in leprosy with special reference to the pathogenesis of "atrophic" conditions of the digits. Clin. Radiol. 7:35 (1955).

Peterson, C. C., and M. L. Silbiger. Reiter's syndrome and psoriatic arthritis. Their roentgen spectra and some interesting similarities. Amer. J. Roentgen. *101*:860 (1967).

Seminars in Roentgenology. The Foot. Vol. 4, No. 4, Oct. 1970, Henry M. Stratton, Inc.

Sturgill, B. C., and J. H. Allan. Rheumatoid-like nodules presenting as "pump bumps" in a patient without rheumatoid arthritis. Arthritis Rheum. *13*:175 (1970).

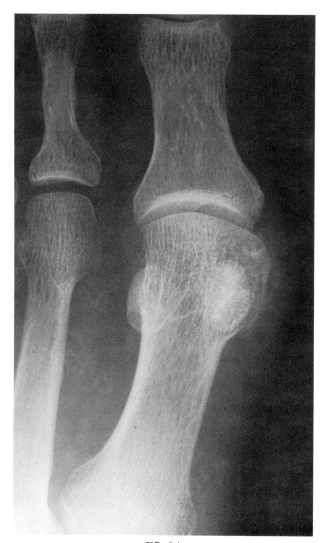

E5–1A.

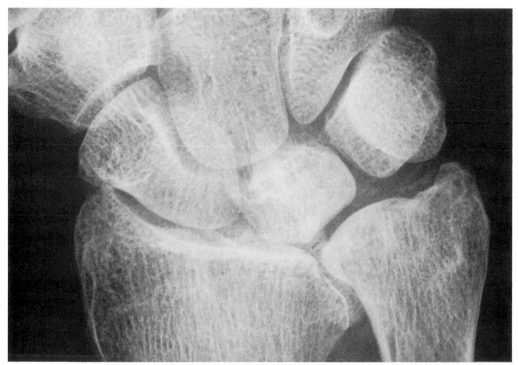

E5–1B.

E5–1. "Of the affections of the joints, the most dangerous are those seated in the hand and great toe."*

Bulging of the soft tissue shadow adjacent to the first metatarsophalangeal joint indicates bursitis. In the absence of a hallux valgus deformity a more far-reaching cause of the swelling must be suspected.

———————————
*Hippocrates

The film of the wrist alone is of no help. The list of causes of chondrocalcinosis is extensive—but in combination with faint calcification within the distended bursa of the great toe, a diagnosis of gout or pseudogout can be made with confidence. In this case, the serum uric acid was normal, and calcium pyrophosphate crystals were aspirated from the joint, establishing the diagnosis of *pseudogout.*

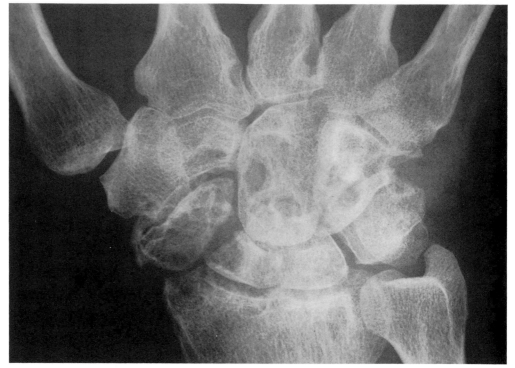

E5–2A.

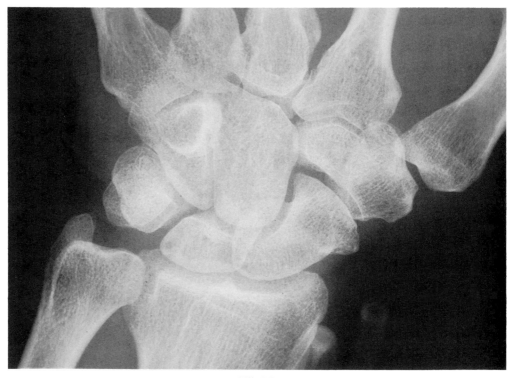

E5–2B.

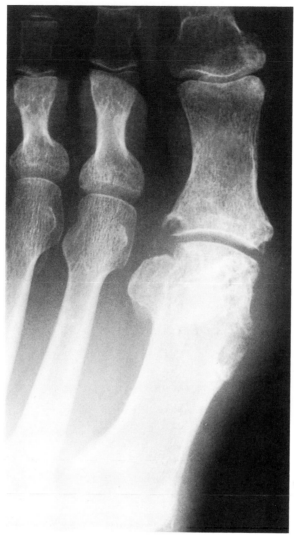

E5–2C.

E5–2. "Oh, the leers and sly winks implying I am a glutton and drunkard! Abject ignoramuses, of course."*

— It has long been a basic tenet among medical men and the lay public alike that lechery is the bridesmaid of gout, and gluttony its wet nurse.

This man's renal disease was severe enough to require dialysis; his Scribner shunt can be seen adjacent to the radial styloid process of the left wrist (E5–2B).

The diagnosis of *podagra* is aided by the evidence of overhanging edges of the erosions and preservation of the cartilage space of the first metatarsophalangeal joint. Whenever *gout* affects the carpal bones, the question of rheumatoid arthritis versus gout arises. Subchondral cysts and soft tissue masses characterize both conditions, and the only helpful radiographic finding is the preservation of the cartilage space between the carpal bones and in the radiocarpal joint. Such extensive erosions in rheumatoid arthritis are always accompanied by cartilage loss and uniform joint space narrowing. (See also E4–10).

---

*John Kobler

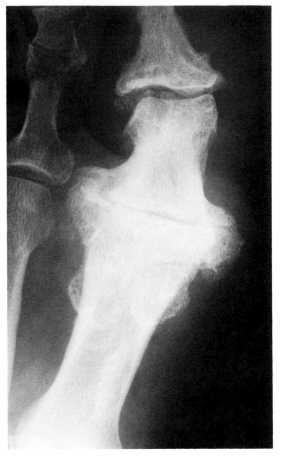

E5–3A.

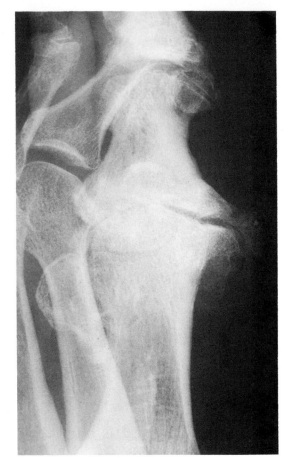

E5–3B.

E5–3. By any other name, this is degenerative arthritis and it fulfills all the criteria: a narrowed joint, associated with eburnation and osteophytes, and absence of erosions. As is traditional in the foot, special conditions have earned descriptive eponyms, and this is no exception. The name *hallux rigidus,* or hallux limitus, is applied to severe osteoarthritis of the first metatarsophalangeal joint. Depending on the degree of limitation of motion, one or the other term is given to the condition afflicting the great toe. The condition is usually associated with prominent dorsal bunions, as can be seen in this example on the oblique view (E5–3B). The rigidity is a mechanical phenomenon, as osteophyte wedges against apposing osteophyte, and neither fibrous nor bony ankylosis contributes to the limitation of motion.

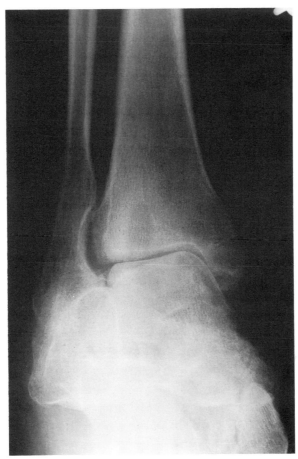

E5–4.

E5–4. Uniform narrowing of the tibiotalar joint, a prominent subchondral cyst in the tibial epiphysis and a scooped-out erosion of the fibula could as easily be hemophilia as *rheumatoid arthritis,* and only a history or laboratory evidence will distinguish the two.

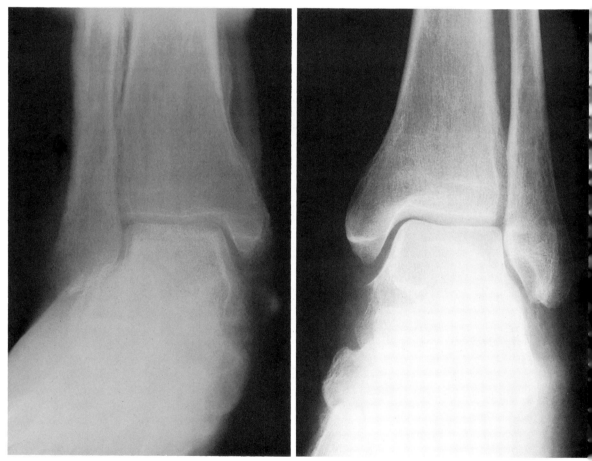

E5–5A.   *E5–5B.*

E5–5. The sign of prominent periosteal reaction at the ends of long bones in the absence of joint destruction should almost always wave a red flag toward an underlying bronchogenic carcinoma, but not when it is limited to one extremity, as in this case. Thick periosteal new bone is produced when there is stasis; for this reason it is seen in Charcot joints as well as where there is venous insufficiency. As is so frequently the case, appreciation of the soft tissue abnormalities provides the concrete clue toward a specific diagnosis—here, a large soft tissue defect abruptly narrows the shadows of the skin and subcutaneous tissues over a distance of several centimeters, giving evidence of the chronic stasis ulceration so frequently associated with *venous insufficiency.*

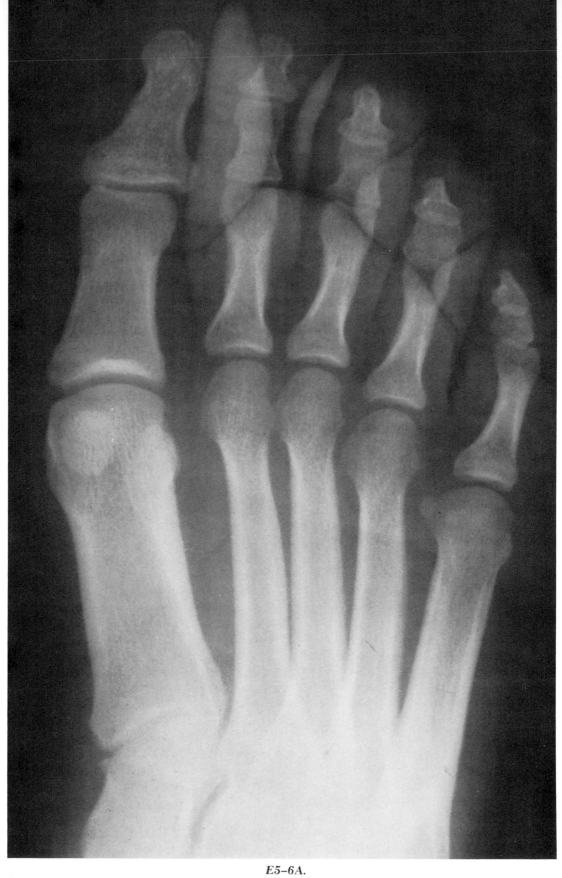

E5–6A.

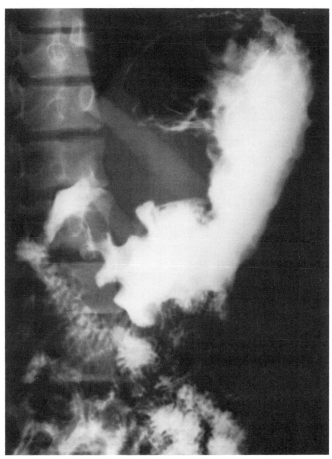

E5–6B.

E5–6. Normal? This adolescent boy complained of discomfort in his hands and feet that was sufficient to stop him from playing basketball. The seriousness of his symptoms warranted a second look at his films. The toes are bulbous and the first and fifth metatarsal bones very rectangular in appearance, suggesting the apposition of periosteal new bone. Even the fibular sides of the third and fourth metatarsal bones show thickening of the diaphysial cortex. *Idiopathic osteoarthropathy* is a difficult diagnosis to prove, however, when it hangs on such flimsy radiographic criteria.

The stomach is infiltrated in a similar manner to the skin in this disease: A barium study of this boy's stomach shows the exaggerated rugal pattern so frequently seen in idiopathic osteoarthropathy (E5–6*B*).

It is important to note that a similar combination of findings can occur in hypertrophic osteoarthropathy as well, although the periostitis is generally more distinctly separate from the underlying bony cortex. An underlying malignancy in this teenage boy, however, would be a highly unlikely find.

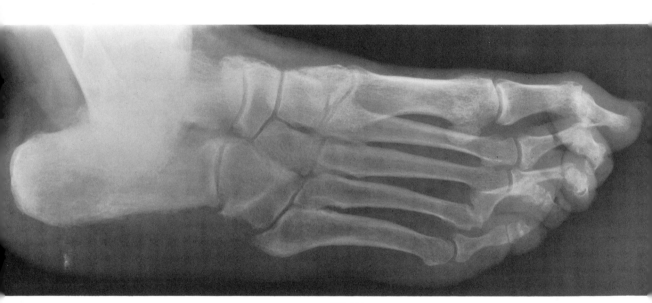

E5–7A.

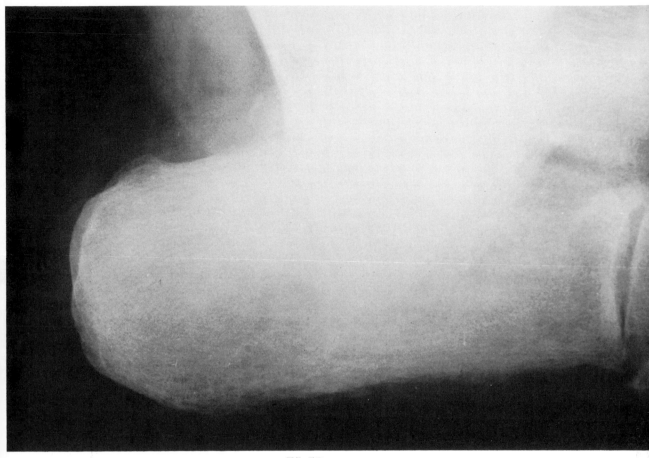

E5–7B.

E5–7. The price of promiscuity is implied by the expression "lover's heels." There are many causes of heel pain, however, with such diverse etiologies as stress fractures (commonly seen in soldiers), and plantar fasciitis associated with a hypermobile foot. Both Reiter's syndrome and rheumatoid arthritis may cause inflammation at the attachment of the plantar aponeurosis; this is also an occasional finding in ankylosing spondylitis. The radiographic changes seen in these three diseases are frequently indistinguishable. Rarely, as in this heel, the entire calcaneus may reveal a reactive sclerosis; when this occurs it is diagnostic of *Reiter's syndrome* or the frequently indistinguishable case of *psoriatic arthritis*. A generalized inflammatory process is revealed by the erosive changes of the fourth metatarsophalangeal joint. The calcaneal changes alone, without this additional finding of inflammatory arthritis, might otherwise suggest Paget's disease or even an osteosarcoma.

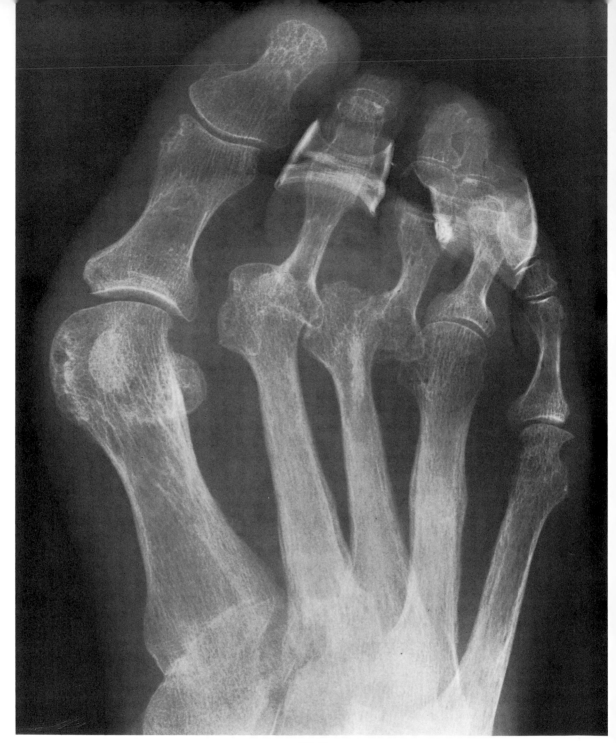

E5–8.

E5–8. There are many reasons for pain in this foot: the subluxed second and third metatarsal heads, the hammer toes of the second and fourth digits (protected by surrounding bandages), and the inflammatory synovitis of the metatarsophalangeal joints. How frustrating for the physician and patient when a new site of discomfort suddenly appears! With this complex of alignment abnormalities a new pain should suggest the possibility of a *stress fracture* secondary to a shift in the weight-bearing forces. The thick periosteal bone paralleling the shafts of the second, third and fourth metatarsal bones reveals this new source of pain.

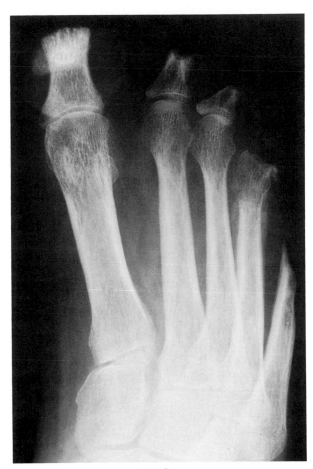

E5–9.

E5–9. It is rare to see *Raynaud's phenomenon* involving the feet, and it is even more unusual to see a case so severe as to cause autoamputation of an entire digit. This unfortunate girl with systemic lupus erythematosus developed gangrene and suffered consequent amputation of her digits on all four extremities.

The periosteal bone surrounding the distal fourth metatarsal bone may reflect an osteomyelitis or a stress fracture, but there is no clue from radiographic appearance of the adjacent bone to indicate either a fracture or pus.

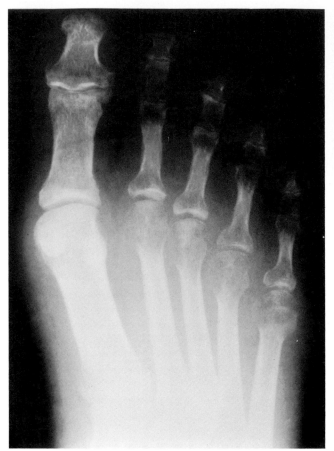

E5–10A.

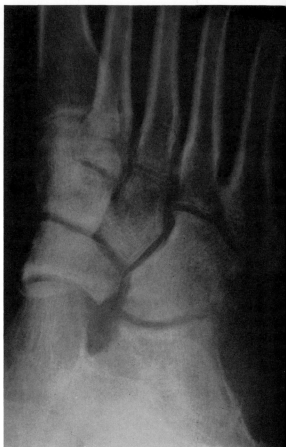

E5–10B.

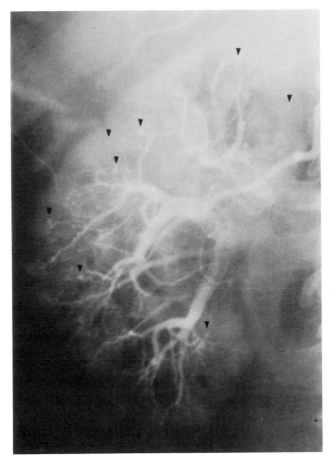

E5–10C.

E5–10. Juxta-articular demineralization of the toes and subchondral demineralization of the tarsal bones indicate rapid loss of calcium. Such generalized involvement of the foot is seen in three conditions: immobilization, Sudeck's atrophy and an acute inflammatory arthritis.

This 23 year old man was first seen because of an acute onset of arthritis of multiple joints, including his hands, feet and knees. His latex fixation was the highest ever recorded by the laboratory, which leaned toward a diagnosis of rheumatoid arthritis. Vasculitis and skin ulcerations complicated the course, and the patient died within a month. Occasionally periarteritis nodosa may com-plicate this malignant form of rheumatoid arthritis.

An arteriogram (E5–10C) demonstrated multiple microaneurysms in the kidneys (the beadlike collections of contrast). This finding was once thought to be pathognomonic of periarteritis nodosa but in fact represents any severe vasculitis. It is now seen most commonly in the large group of patients with a history of intravenous drug abuse, particularly the injection of "speed." Since this patient had no such background, a connective tissue disease culminating in a severe *malignant vasculitis* and death gave a mixed picture of rheumatoid arthritis and periarteritis nodosa.

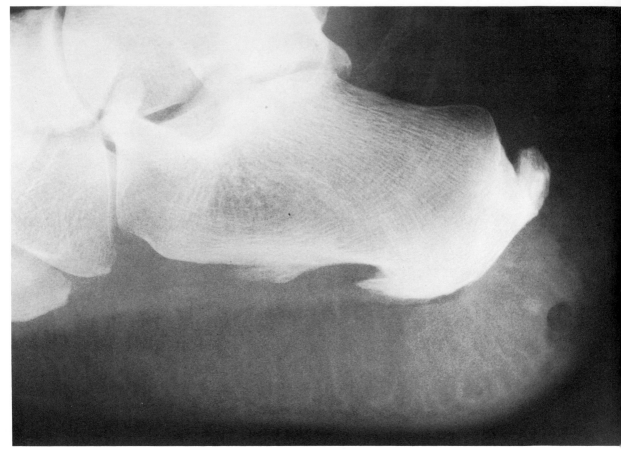

E5–11.

E5–11. A thick heel pad and exaggerated degenerative changes of the calcaneus suggest acromegaly. Without a history the correct diagnosis could not be made. Two suspicious findings are present, however, that should prompt the consideration of infection: a "hole" in the soft tissues of the heel, and severe vascular calcification reflecting a possible compromised blood supply.

Edema from any etiology may increase the heel pad dimension, and an expensive endocrine workup should never be undertaken on the basis of this measurement alone. The patient had *diabetes and an infection* of his heel that resulted in diffuse inflammation and localized ulceration.

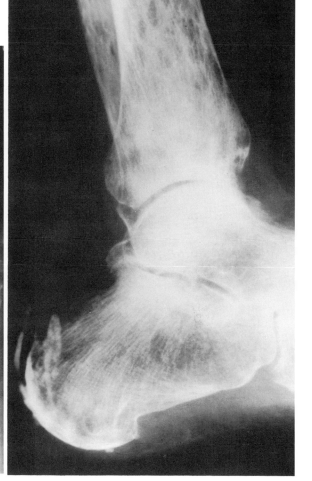

E5–12A.

E5–12B.

E5–12. The complex of subcutaneous calcification, resorption of the distal phalanges, and atrophy of the skin resembles progressive systemic sclerosis, but a glance at the patient's short stature and wizened features should suggest the rare condition of *progeria*. Profound osteoporosis may be a component of this generalized tendency toward early aging, and therefore the films are helpful in establishing the diagnosis. In this example, the moth-eaten appearance of the bones is so severe as to mimic multiple myeloma. Because of an increased incidence of osteosarcoma in patients with progeria, recognition of the condition is important if confusion with a rheumatic disease is to be avoided.

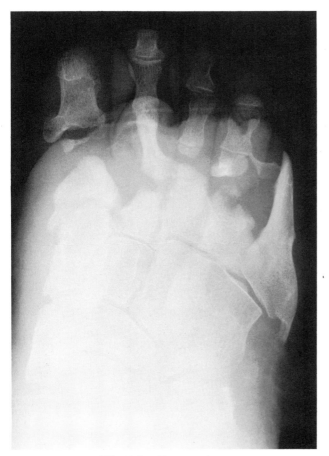

E5-13A. Patient A.

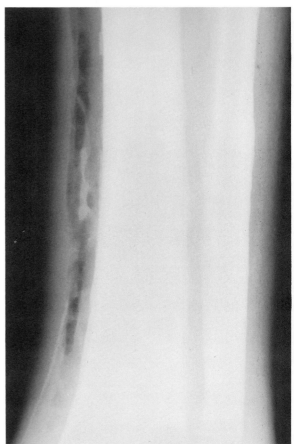

E5-13B. Patient A.

Exercise continued on opposite page.

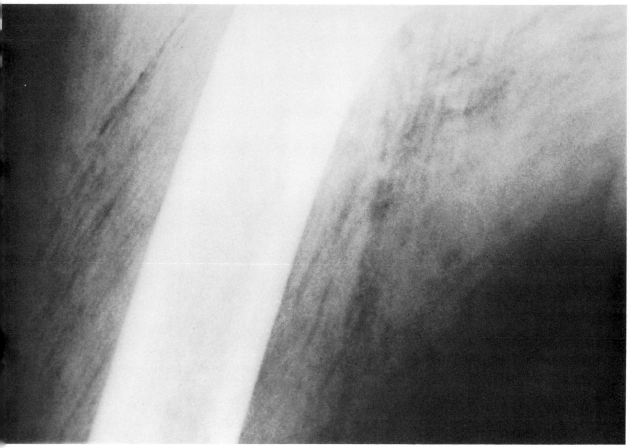

E5–13C. Patient B.

E5–13. Both a peripheral neuropathy and a chronic infection contributed to this resorptive arthropathy. Destruction of all the metatarsophalangeal joints and resorption of the metatarsal heads in conjunction with normal bony mineralization typify the *Charcot foot*. A patch of gas adjacent to the talus and creeping up the leg had the surgeons sharpening their saws.* But the diagnosis of gas gangrene

*"Unreasonable haste is the direct road to error"—Moliere.

was erroneous. Dissection of gas up the *major* tissue planes should never be mistaken for gas gangrene. It usually represents ambient air tracking in from an open wound. This is especially true in the foot, as continued walking on a laceration (or as in this case, a *chronic ulcer*) sucks the air in. The changes from such gas-producing organisms as Clostridium are very distinctive. The gas dissects around the muscle fibers, as in E5–13C.

While the patient lay in bed gathering his courage to face an amputation, the gas resolved spontaneously.

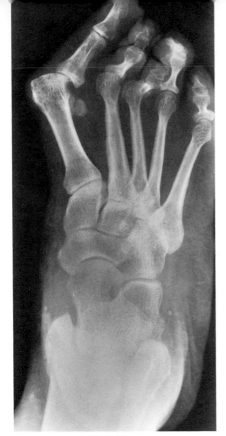

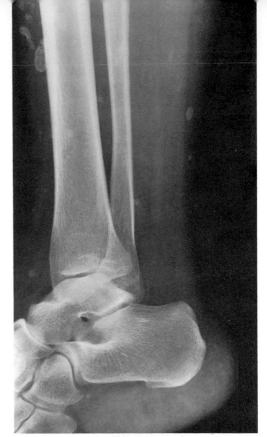

E5-14A.

E5-14B.

E5-14. At first glance this looks like a run-of-the-mill hallux valgus, severe enough to deviate the second and third toes but not exciting enough to warrant inclusion as an Exercise. The presence of extensive subcutaneous calcification, very different in appearance from parasites and phleboliths, should suggest that this might not be an ordinary problem. This type of soft tissue finding is thought to represent fat necrosis and is a prominent component of *Ehlers-Danlos syndrome*. Joint laxity not uncommonly leads to subluxations and secondary degenerative joint disease—one of the rarest causes of hallux valgus.

E5-15. "Hell hath no fury like a woman's corns."*

Plebian, unembroidered by fancy systemic disease, the lowly *bunion* can be of prime import to the patient who is afflicted therewith, deforming her mood as well as her foot.

The radiographic triad of findings is illustrated by this film: an atavistic cuneiform, metatarsus primus varus and a hallux valgus deformity.

*Sunday *Times*, London.

204

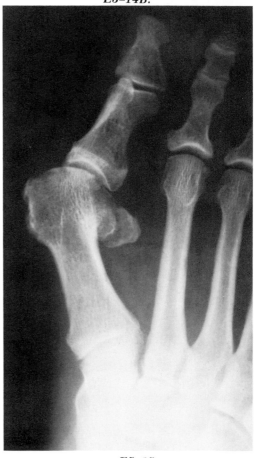

E5-15.

Chapter 6

THE KNEE

The shadows that one sees on a film of the knee consist of the articulating ends of the femur and tibia, the proximal end of the fibula, and the patella, a sesamoid bone within the quadriceps tendon. Adjacent to the bones, the numerous muscles of the thigh and leg are delineated by sharp black lines of fat (Fig. 6–1).

The joint space in a normal knee appears as a homogeneous water density shadow between the femur and tibia. Anatomically it contains the articulating hyaline cartilages which cover the femoral and tibial condyles, the wedge-shaped fibrocartilaginous menisci that act as cushions or shock absorbers during walking, the thin layer of synovium that lines the capsule and the joint capsule it-

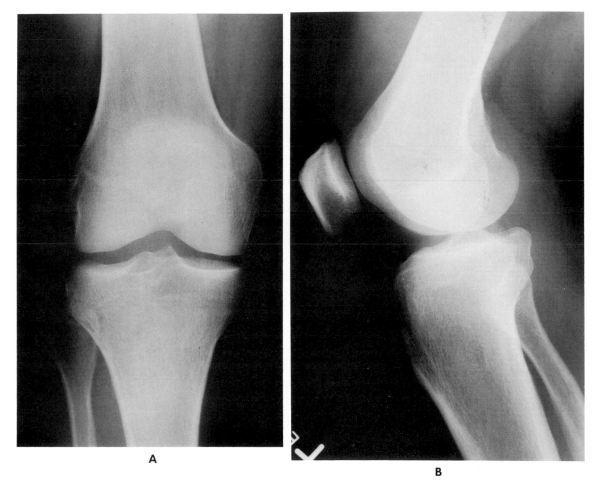

A

B

Figure 6–1. Normal knee.

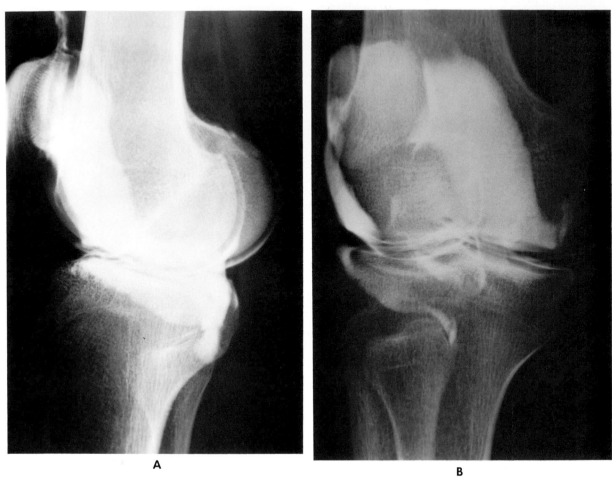

A   B

Figure 6–2. Arthrogram of normal knee.
 The extent of the joint space, the width of the articular cartilage and the shape of the medial and lateral menisci are delineated by the opaque contrast material on a lateral and an oblique view of the knee.

self. Its limits are best delineated by an arthrogram (Fig. 6–2). The capsule attaches to the epiphyses of the femur and tibia and has a capacity to distend in response to massive increases in its contents. The large suprapatellar pouch tends to accumulate excess fluid, and joint effusions are best detected in this region, both clinically and radiographically.

 There are numerous bursae in the knee. The largest is the semimembranosus bursa, located in the medial popliteal space. It is superficial in position, and deep to it is the medial gastrocnemius bursa. A lateral gastrocnemius bursa communicates with the joint space. A prepatellar bursa separates the patella from the subcutaneous tissues and has no communication with the joint space.

SOFT TISSUE ABNORMALITIES

Capsular Distention

 It is much easier to detect the presence of small effusions clinically than radiographically. Since fluid tends to accumulate in the suprapatellar pouch, the straight fat lines which outline the joint capsule are displaced away from the femur as the ballooning capsule expands. Experimentally, as little as five ml of fluid may be detected in the joint capsule on a frontal projection of the knee, but this small amount of fluid is not evident in the usual clinical situation.

The radiographic detection of small effusions depends on the presence of a well-defined layer of fat outlining the capsule. A small effusion appears as a convex black line crossing the vertical fat lines that separate the muscles; by this sign it may be recognized on a frontal projection. The fullness of the suprapatellar pouch is usually more easily detected on the lateral view.

Hemophilia. *Massive* joint effusions are frequently seen in children with hemophilia. The capsule fills with blood after minor trauma, distending the joint space and often spreading the articulating ends of the bones apart as seen in Figure 6–3C. The opposite knee is included to compare the normal soft tissue shadows and width of the joint (Fig. 6–3A). The convex line of fat that outlines the suprapatellar pouch crosses the muscle planes laterally (Fig. 6–3C) indicating the extent of the swelling superiorly. The increase in periarticular soft tissue width and the separation of the articulating bones further demonstrate the large amount of blood lost into this joint.

The lateral view (Fig. 6–3D) illustrates the increased density anteriorly and posteriorly, demarcating the anatomic boundaries of the distended joint capsule. A lateral view of the opposite knee (Fig. 6–3B) illustrates the appearance where there is not excess fluid. The effusion seen in Figure 6–3D has displaced the patella anteriorly along with the quadriceps tendon, which bows convexly around the bulging suprapatellar accumulation of fluid. In a similar fashion, the patellar tendon and infrapatellar fat pad continue the arc of this massively ballooned joint capsule. Fluid has also dissected into the popliteal fossa. When effusions are more subtle, comparison with the contralateral knee is often essential to distinguish minor abnormalities in the popliteal fossa. On the lateral projection there is normally a prominent soft tissue shadow in the posterior compartment due to the overlapping shadows of the bulky gastrocnemius and semimembranosus muscles. To the uninitiated this may suggest a pathologic condition such as a Baker's cyst (fluid in the popliteal bursa) or a soft tissue mass.

In addition to the soft tissue abnormalities in the patient with hemophilia, there are overgrowth and irregularity of the epiphyses. This occurs in diseases that cause an active hyperemia at a stage when the bones are rapidly growing; hence, epiphyseal overgrowth is commonly seen in hemophilia and juvenile rheumatoid arthritis.

Lipohemarthrosis. Massive effusions are easily detected clinically; a radiograph is helpful only to reveal additional important information. In Figure 6–4, a subtle break in the cortex along the posterior lateral femoral condyle indicates the traumatic nature of the effusion (arrow). This radiograph was taken with the X-ray beam perpendicular to the knee and the film placed against the side of the leg (a transtable lateral view). By this method two abnormal densities are separated in the suprapatellar pouch—the soft tissue shadow indicative of the accumulation of blood and, floating on its surface, a black crescent cast by fat. This phenomenon is termed lipohemarthrosis and can only be demonstrated by positioning the knee with the patella uppermost, so that the two types of body tissue will separate according to their specific gravity. The extreme capsular distention is indicated by the forward displacement of the patella away from the femur.

Hypertrophic Osteoarthropathy. Massive distention of the knee joint is occasionally associated with the synovitis of hypertrophic osteoarthropathy (Fig. 6–5). The homogeneous appearance of the tissues adjacent to the distal femur represents the distended suprapatellar pouch. In addition, there is soft tissue swelling anterior to the patella. This space does not communicate with the capsule, and its participation in the soft tissue enlargement indicates inflammation and fluid within the prepatellar bursa and the more inferiorly situated superficial patellar tendon bursa. The additional finding of thick periosteal new bone is more drama-

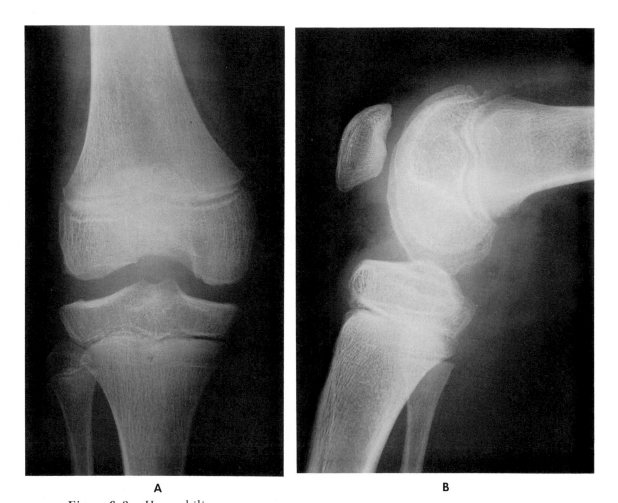

A   B

Figure 6–3. Hemophilia.
A and *B*. The right knee shows bony overgrowth and irregularity of the femoral epiphysis, but the soft tissues and joint space appear normal.

Illustration continued on opposite page.

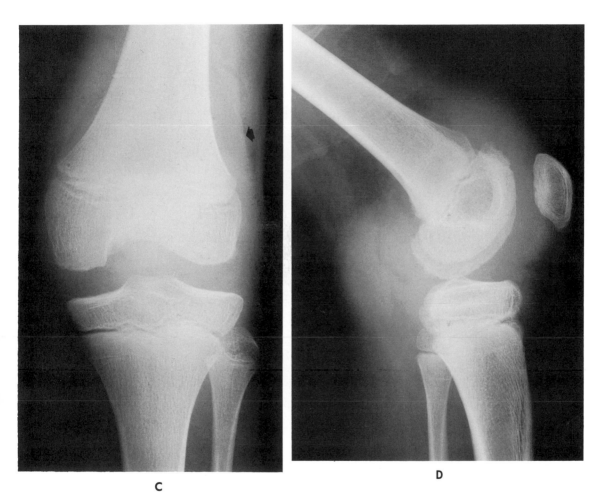

C

D

Figure 6–3. Continued.
C. Massive capsular expansion from acute hemorrhage distends the soft tissues and separates the femur from the tibial plateau.

D. The fluid has dissected posteriorly into the popliteal bursa and has filled the supra-patellar pouch, displacing the patella anteriorly.

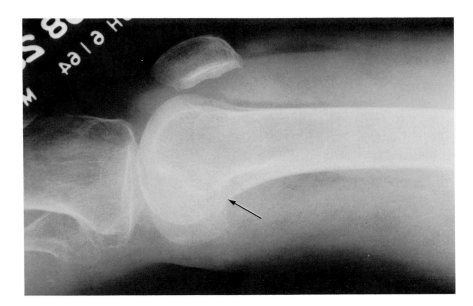

Figure 6–4. Lipohemarthrosis.
A transtable lateral view illustrates the black crescent of fat floating on the intracapsular fluid. A subtle break in the cortex of the femoral condyle (arrow) indicates the source of the fluid: hemorrhage following trauma and a nondisplaced fracture.

tic than the joint effusion. It surrounds the distal femur and extends to the point of capsular attachment. Joint effusions and periosteal new bone are the radiographic manifestations of synovitis and periostitis and are the primary components of hypertrophic osteoarthropathy. Recognition of the significance of this type of periosteal new bone as the harbinger of an underlying lung tumor is essential, as it separates this picture from the remaining causes of capsular distention.

Villonodular Synovitis. Villonodular synovitis is a monarticular disease of young adults that most commonly involves the knee. Although the abnormal synovium may cause pressure erosions of the articulating bones, this is rarely seen in the knee because of the marked distensibility of the joint capsule. Its usual appearance is that of a soft tissue mass, filling the joint capsule and hence mimicking a joint effusion.

The difficulty in estimating the degree of distention of the capsule from a film becomes evident with Figure 6–6A. The frontal view shows a soft tissue fullness lateral to the femur that could as easily represent the musculature of a healthy male as a distended joint capsule. The swelling is more convincing on the lateral view (Fig. 6–6B), since the soft tissue

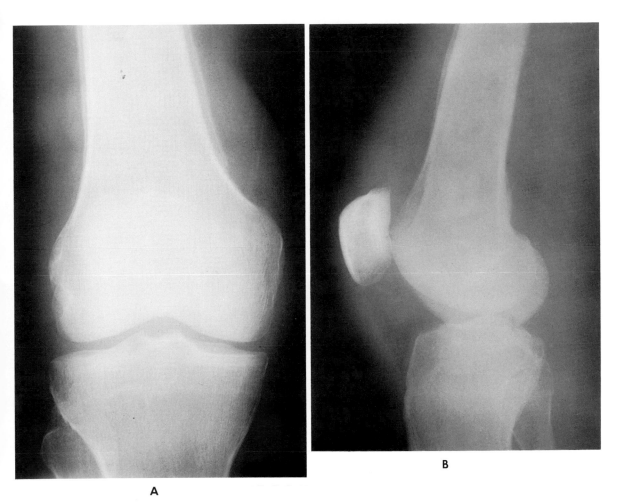

Figure 6-5. Hypertrophic osteoarthropathy.
Massive distention of the knee joint occasionally is as dramatic as the thick periosteal new bone that is so characteristic of this condition.

planes above the patella are obliterated and a homogeneous shadow is present. Contrast material injected directly into the joint capsule defines the limits of the joint space and documents the presence of a prominent soft tissue mass (Fig. 6–6C). The capsular distention in this patient is caused by proliferation of synovium rather than fluid and appears as nodular masses within the suprapatellar pouch surrounded by contrast material (arrow). Synovial hypertrophy with an inflammatory etiology is identical in ap-

pearance, and biopsy is necessary to establish a diagnosis.

Bursal Distention

Communication between the joint capsule and the popliteal bursae occurs most frequently in patients with chronic knee effusions. They are seen particularly in patients with trauma and with rheumatoid arthritis.

Rheumatoid Arthritis. The amazing

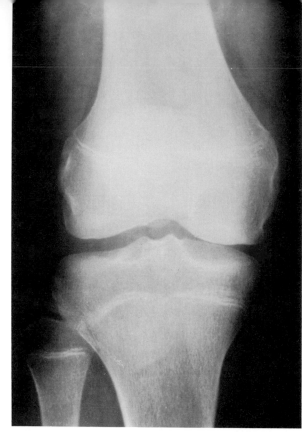

Figure 6–6. Villonodular synovitis.

A. Capsular distention is difficult to detect on the frontal view.

B. Obliteration of the tissue planes superior to the patella suggests an abnormality on the lateral view.

C. The arthrogram demonstrates expansion of the normal suprapatellar pouch and irregular filling defects (arrow). Although it indicates abnormal synovium, a specific diagnosis from the film alone is unwarranted.

A

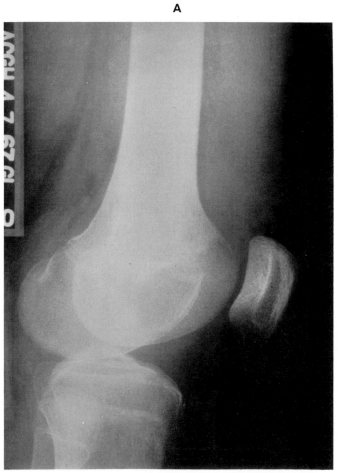

B

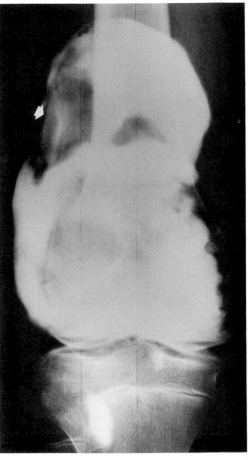

C

capacity of the intercommunicating bursae of the knee to distend with fluid is most dramatically demonstrated in patients with rheumatoid arthritis. Such patients occasionally develop a leg mass which may extend to the calf or even the ankle. When the synovial fluid leaks out of the bursa into the surrounding muscles, severe pain, mimicking thrombophlebitis, occurs.

Figure 6–7 illustrates this clinical problem. Pain and swelling of the calf suggested the presence of thrombophlebitis in a patient with a long history of rheumatoid arthritis. The exact etiology was established by an emergency arthrogram which demonstrated the communication of the leg mass with the joint. The striated appearance of the contrast material documents the extravasation into the muscle.

This arthrogram shows the remarkable distensibility of the joint capsule and intercommunicating bursae of the knee. It is easy to understand why the underlying bones are spared the erosive pressure changes from intracapsular masses until late in the disease.

Prepatellar Bursitis. Figure 6–8 illustrates a localized infection limited to the superficial tissues. It involves the bursae anterior to the patella and the infrapatellar tendon (arrows) and spares the joint capsule. A cellulitis involving the soft tissues would have a similar radiographic appearance on the lateral view, but its

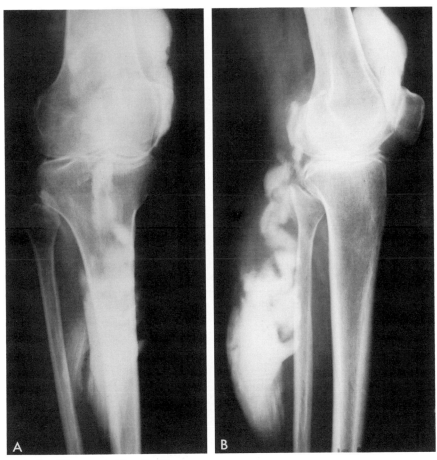

Figure 6–7. Rheumatoid arthritis.
Chronic knee joint effusions may dissect into the popliteal bursae, and the consequent massive calf swelling and pain mimic the findings in thrombophlebitis. The striated configuration of the contrast material indicates extravasation into the muscle.

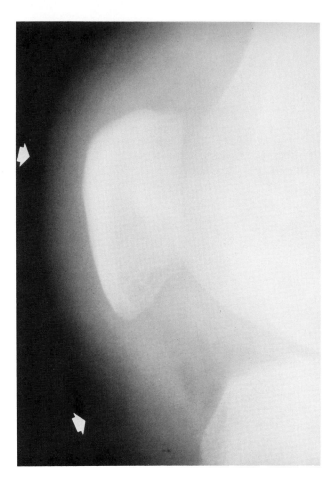

Figure 6–8. Prepatellar bursitis. Infection has caused fluid to distend both the suprapatellar and infrapatellar bursae (arrows).

circumferential involvement would probably distort the soft tissues in all projections. The anterior location of this collection distinguishes it, in addition, from a suprapatellar collection of fluid within the joint space.

Periarticular Soft Tissue Calcification

All of the soft tissue components of the knee may calcify: the subcutaneous tissues, muscles, tendons, cartilage and the synovium. Although on film these structures normally blend imperceptibly into each other, precise localization of the abnormal calcium on a frontal and lateral radiograph identifies the anatomic structure and narrows the list of diagnostic possibilities.

Progressive Systemic Sclerosis. The superficial location of the calcium as seen in Figure 6–9 places it in the subcutaneous tissues. Calcification in this region may result from *localized* disease such as trauma, or it may signal a *systemic disorder* such as hypoparathyroidism, pseudohypoparathyroidism, Ehlers-Danlos syndrome or one of the rheumatic diseases. Although amorphous calcification may be seen in systemic lupus erythematosus, it is much more common in patients with scleroderma, as in this example. Since the amorphous appearance and superficial location of the calcium deposits are so similar radiographically in all these conditions, a precise diagnosis cannot be made from a film alone.

Dermatomyositis. In striking contrast to the previous examples of subcutaneous

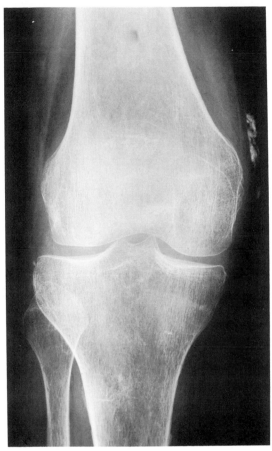

Figure 6–9. Progressive systemic sclerosis.

A prominent subcutaneous collection of amorphous calcium lies medial to the femoral condyle. Diffuse osteoporosis reflects the long-term steroid therapy in this patient. The joint space itself is normal.

calcification is the diffuse scattered calcification in a patient with childhood dermatomyositis (Fig. 6–10): this spares the superficial tissues and is localized to the region of the muscle. In addition to extensive calcium deposits there are osteoporosis, severe atrophy of the soft tissues and flexion deformities, which distort the normal alignment. The abnormal bone texture reflects the high dosage of adrenocorticosteroids given to this young patient as well as the immobilization necessitated by her contractures. The position of the calcium deposits in dermatomyositis usually easily distinguishes it from the subcutaneous involvement in scleroderma.

Pellegrini-Stieda Calcification. The knee is a vulnerable joint and is subjected to constant traumatic insults which may result in permanent damage and arthritic changes. Figure 6–11A demonstrates swelling along the medial side of the joint, well-demarcated by this patient's excessive subcutaneous fat. The calcification adjacent to the medial femoral condyle is in the proximal attachment of the medial collateral ligament. Because of its frequent occurrence, this condition has been given a special designation—the cumbersome name of Pellegrini-Stieda calcification.

Depending upon associated degenerative changes of the menisci, the joint may be widened on the side of the damage (from collateral ligament tears) or narrowed (from degenerative changes of the cartilage). In this example there is narrowing of the medial side of the joint. Since there is a wide variation in normal knee joint width (normally three to five mm in width) asymmetry of the space reflects an abnormality of the knee but does not indicate whether one side is too wide or the other too narrow. Comparison with the contralateral knee is helpful. Weight-bearing views may be confusing, since the patient automatically flexes *or* locks his knee, thus spuriously giving the impression of a narrowed joint.

Verification of medial joint space abnormalities is demonstrated on a film of the same knee eight years later (Fig. 6–11B). In addition to the persistent joint space narrowing, small osteophytes have developed on the articular surfaces of the tibial and femoral condyles, indicating degeneration of cartilage.

Progressive degenerative changes of the tibial eminences have also occurred in the interim. Their normal round contour is lost and they have become sharp and pointed.

Intra-articular Soft Tissue Calcification

When calcification occurs *within* the joint space it may represent any of four entities: calcification of synovium, calcification of cartilage, calcification of cruciate ligaments or the presence of a frag-

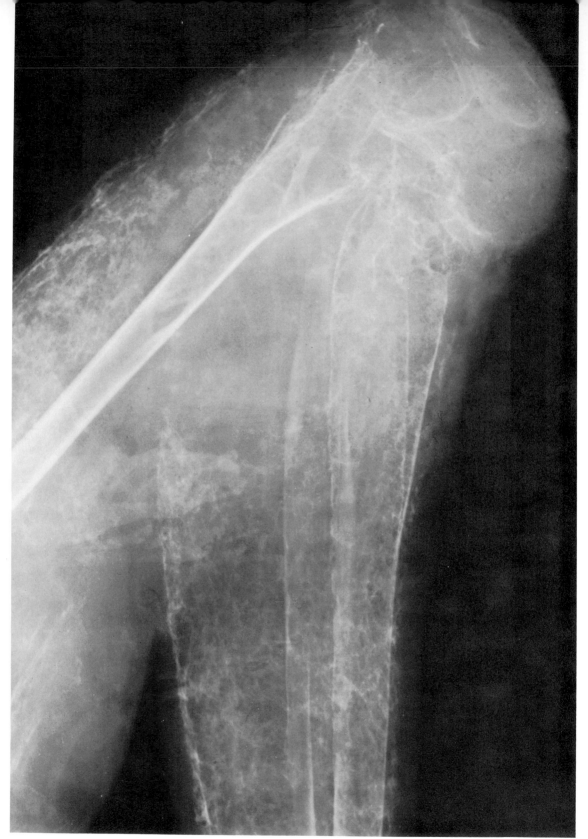

Figure 6–10. Dermatomyositis.

The location of the soft tissue calcification differs from that in progressive systemic sclerosis. It lies within the muscle, rather than in the subcutaneous tissues. The severe soft tissue and bone atrophy, diffuse demineralization and grotesque subluxations reflect both steroid medication and disuse.

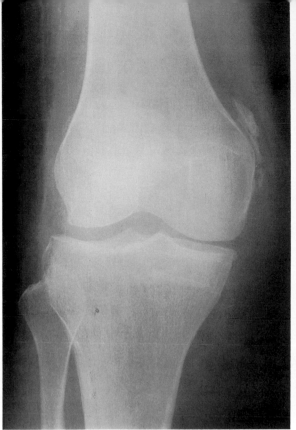 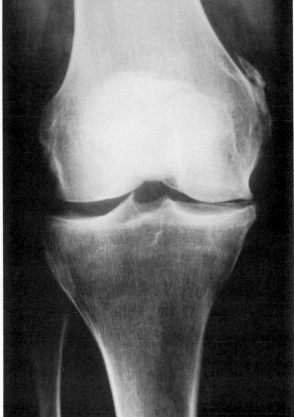

A **B**

Figure 6–11. Pellegrini-Stieda calcification.

A. There are calcification within the proximal portion of the medial collateral ligament and narrowing of the medial joint space.

B. Eight years later, small osteophytes attest to the degenerative changes of the adjacent cartilage in the medial joint space.

ment of bone that has broken off the articulating end of the tibia or femur. The location as well as the pattern of calcification distinguishes these possibilities.

Synovial Osteochondromatosis. The oval densities of synovial osteochondromatosis represent ossification and calcification of synovial fragments, as the name implies. Because they are bone, the appearance of synovial fragments is more structured than that of the amorphous calcium collections seen in the connective tissue disorders. Cortex and trabeculae are easily identified. Examples from two different patients emphasize the similarity of their appearance (Figs. 6–12 and 6–13). Because these calcifications are solid structures within the joint space, they interfere with the normal function of the knee. Patients often complain of locking of the knee or limitation of motion or of a clicking sensation as the articulating surfaces glide over this

bony "joint mouse." The normal sesamoid bone in the lateral head of the gastrocnemius muscle, called the fabella, should not be confused with synovial osteochondromatosis. One is seen in Figure 6–12, partially superimposed on the calcified synovium (arrow).

Synovial Chondromatosis. Hyaline cartilage in the center of a hypertrophied synovial villus is seen in Figure 6–14, which shows a representative piece of tissue from a synovectomy of the knee. Since no elements of bone are present, the cartilaginous loose body would be invisible on a film. Unlike the previous example of synovial *osteochondromatosis*, diagnosis of synovial *chondromatosis* is not made radiographically.

Osteochondrosis Dissecans. The oval ossification in the joint space of an adolescent boy is similar in appearance to synovial osteochondromatosis. The frontal view of the knee (Fig. 6–15*B*) reveals

217

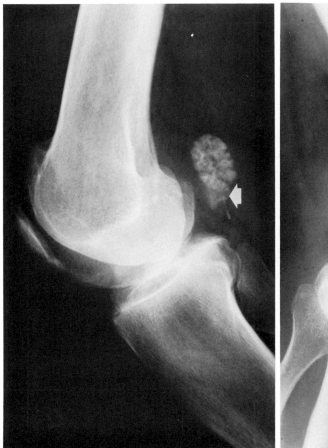

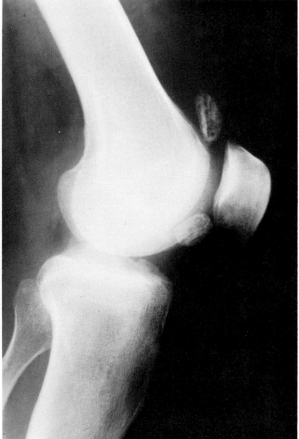

Figure 6–12. Synovial osteochondromatosis.

A large, ossified loose body is partially superimposed on the fabella (arrow) in the popliteal space.

Figure 6–13. Synovial osteochondromatosis.

Two ossified fragments of synovium are evident in the anterior joint space.

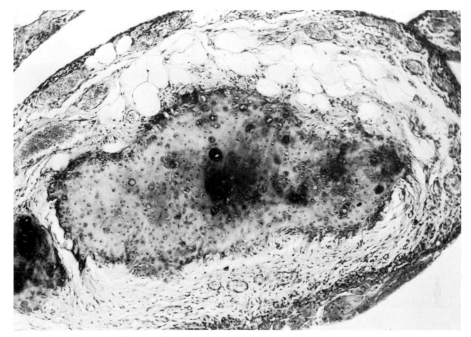

Figure 6-14. Synovial chondromatosis.

The elliptical shape of a hypertrophied synovial villus containing cartilage is similar to the preceding two examples of osteochondromatosis. The absence of bone however, would make this loose body invisible on a radiograph. (Courtesy of The Arthritis Foundation.)

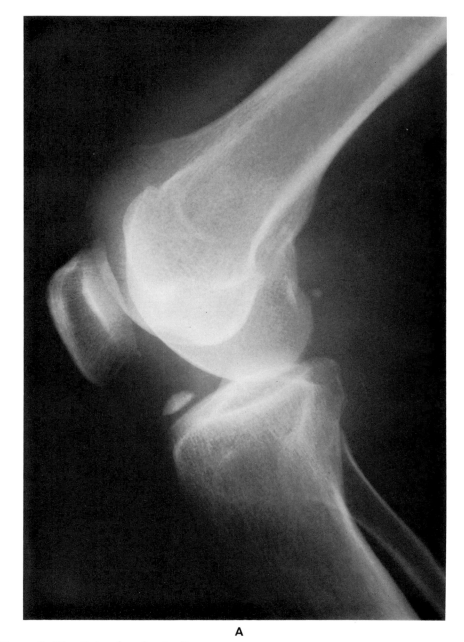

A

Figure 6–15.   Osteochondrosis dissecans.
An ellipse of bone within the joint space (*A*) is exactly the same size and configuration as the radiolucent defect in the lateral femoral condyle (*B*).

Illustration continued on opposite page.

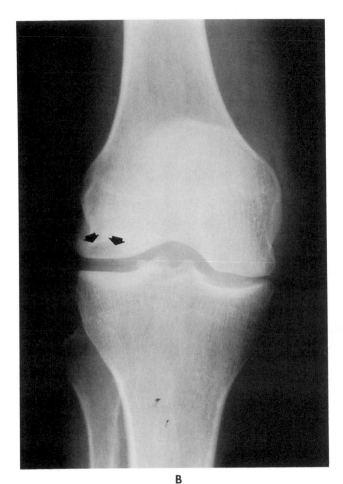

B

Figure 6–15. Continued.

the origin of this joint mouse to be quite different, however. An identically sized *radiolucent* defect (arrows) is present in the medial aspect of the lateral femoral condyle. This is the site of origin of the free-floating bony fragment. Debate as to its pathogenesis has resulted in two different labels for this condition. Those who feel it has an etiology of localized inflammation call the condition osteochondritis dissecans, whereas a second school feels it is a localized area of avascular necrosis resulting from trauma and call the condition osteochondrosis dissecans. The phenomenon is most commonly seen on the medial condyle of the femur. Less often it occurs on the inner surface of the lateral condyle, as in this patient. The button of necrotic bone becomes covered with cartilage before it separates from the femur; therefore, a radiolucent line around it is evident.

A pathologic specimen demonstrates the elliptical fragment of bone covered by a cartilaginous cap (Fig. 6–16).

A film of a second patient with osteochondrosis dissecans demonstrates the fragment of bone and its sharp border of cartilage in place in the femoral condyle (Fig. 6–17). Although the usual

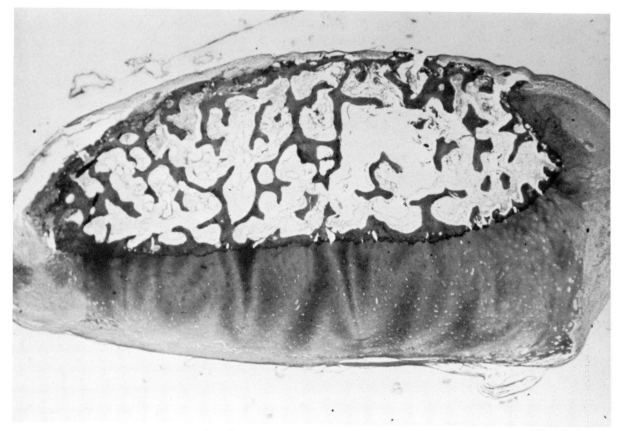

Figure 6–16. Osteochondrosis dissecans.
A pathologic specimen illustrates the bony fragment covered with a thick layer of cartilage. (Courtesy of Roger Terry, M.D.)

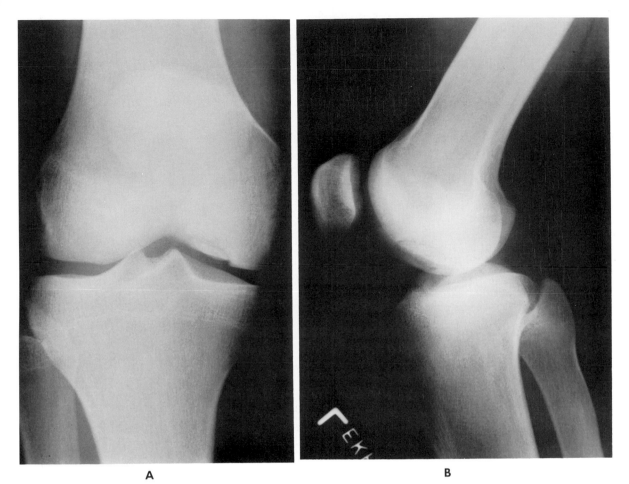

| A | B |

Figure 6–17. Osteochondrosis dissecans.
Cartilage surrounds the bony fragment, forming a radiolucent line prior to its separation from the femur (*A* and *B*).

course of events results in separation of the fragment, it may either remain attached to the femur or be completely resorbed, leaving only a shallow depression in the condyle as evidence of the previous abnormality.

Hyperparathyroidism. After reviewing the anatomy of the joint space as outlined by the arthrogram (see Figure 6–2) it is easy to determine the nature of the abnormal calcification in Figure 6–18. The thin linear calcific line that parallels the femoral and tibial condyles is in the hyaline articular cartilage. The wedge-shaped peripheral collections are in the fibrocartilage of the medial and lateral menisci (arrows). Chondrocal-

cinosis is a common finding in patients with primary hyperparathyroidism and often provides the clue that initiates the search for the parathyroid adenoma.

ABNORMALITIES OF ALIGNMENT

The axes of the femur and the tibia should be on a 180 degree line with each other; any deviation from this is abnormal. When the tibia is angled laterally, too close an approximation of the distal thighs results in knock knees. This valgus deformity is called genu valgum. In the opposite condition, genu varum (bowlegs), there is separation of the distal

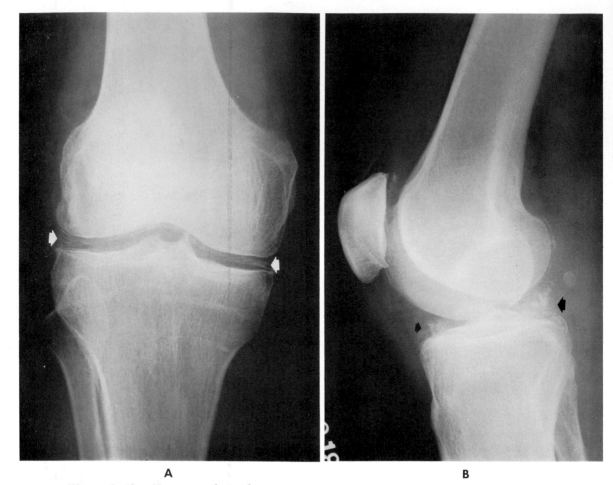

A　　　　　　　　　　　　　　　　　　　　**B**

Figure 6–18. Hyperparathyroidism.
Calcification outlines both the hyaline articular cartilage of the femoral and tibial condyles and the wedge-shaped menisci (*A* and *B*, arrows).

femora. Flexion and hyperextension abnormalities may also occur: abnormal hyperextensibility of the knee is called genu recurvatum.

Although alignment abnormalities may be secondary to destructive processes from a primary arthritis, they will not be dealt with separately.

ABNORMAL BONY MINERALIZATION

Normal mineralization, with thin, sharp, closely packed trabeculae and a well-defined cortex, may be seen in the films of the two young patients of Figures 6–15 and 6–17.

Osteoporosis

The classic appearance of osteoporosis, with its pencil-thin cortex and ground glass matrix is contrasted by the film of the patient with dermatomyositis (Fig. 6–10). Severe osteoporosis may also be seen in patients with juvenile rheumatoid arthritis.

Juvenile Rheumatoid Arthritis. The thin white cortical margin and lack of fine trabeculae within the spongiosa attest to the severity of bone atrophy in a patient with juvenile rheumatoid arthritis (Fig. 6–19). The oversized and irregular epiphyses are similar to the changes that were seen in the patient with hemophilia

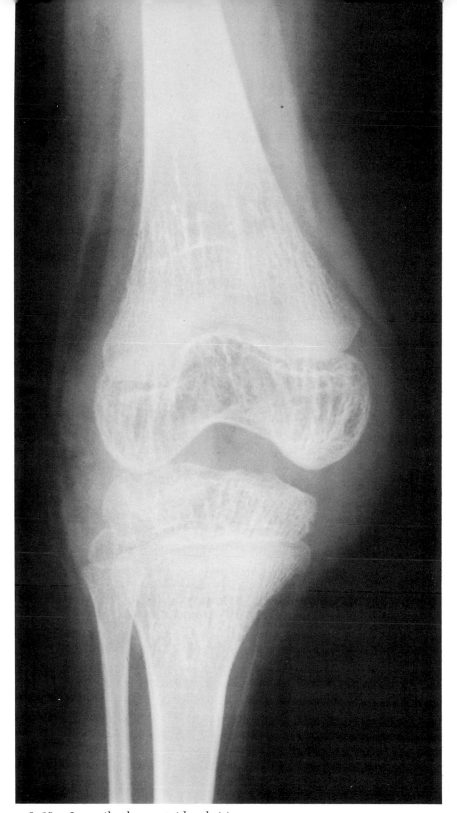

Figure 6-19. Juvenile rheumatoid arthritis.
Severe osteoporosis and overgrowth of the epiphyses are common residual stigmata of the juvenile onset of rheumatoid arthritis. Soft tissue wasting is also evident.

and reflect the onset of his arthritis prior to epiphyseal fusion.

Subchondral Demineralization

Pyogenic Arthritis. Pyogenic arthritis is marked by soft tissue swelling, rapid bone demineralization and destruction of the cartilage by proteolytic enzymes. The acute and rapid loss of calcium in a septic joint results in subchondral demineralization, which appears as a black line paralleling the sharp white cortical margin. This typical radiographic finding is seen in Figure 6–20 (arrows).

Reiter's Syndrome. Identical changes of subchondral demineralization are present in a patient with Reiter's syndrome (Fig. 6–21). The sharp white contour of the bone is exaggerated because

of the presence of the parallel black line beneath it—the radiographic sign of rapid demineralization (arrows).

Periostitis

Radiographic evidence of bone repair is frequently seen in conjunction with the destructive changes from an inflammatory process. Its presence is not pathognomonic, since new bone also accompanies many malignant processes. Reparative new bone may be manifested in three ways: as sclerosis within the medullary cavity, as thickening along the endosteal surface of the cortex or as new bone applied to the surface of the cortex.

Tuberculous Arthritis. Periosteal new bone observed on a radiograph indicates repair from an underlying de-

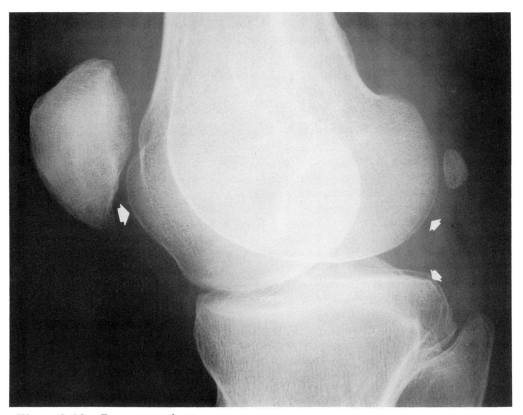

Figure 6–20. Pyogenic arthritis.
Subchondral demineralization signifies an acute and rapid loss of mineral and is easily detected in this example along the femoral condyles and tibial plateau (arrows). A concomitant joint effusion is present but is not seen in this close-up projection.

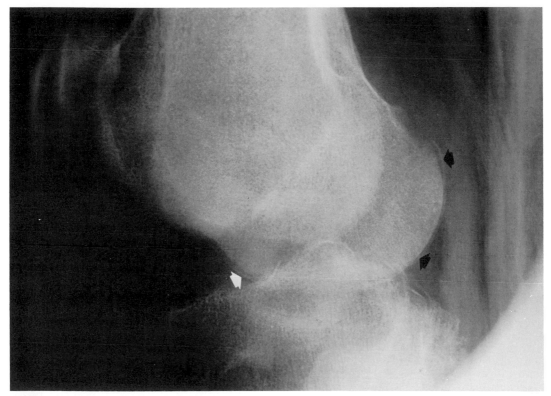

Figure 6–21. Reiter's syndrome.

Joint effusion and subchondral demineralization may occur in any acute inflammatory arthritis. The radiolucent line paralleling the cortex indicates the severity of the joint involvement (arrows). A break in the cortex suggests synovial proliferation and a marginal erosion at the vulnerable point where the protective articular cartilage ends.

structive process. Figure 6–22A demonstrates this finding in the knee of a patient with tuberculous arthritis, the new bone paralleling both sides of the distal femur (arrows).

Additional signs of an active infectious process are best appreciated on the lateral view (Fig. 6–22B). A large joint effusion is present, distending the capsule. The accompanying juxta-articular demineralization reflects the hyperemia. Marginal erosions of the tibial plateau are typical of tuberculosis and are seen on both views (double arrows). These destructive changes reflect the granulomatous involvement of the synovium.

Rheumatoid Arthritis. The presence of periosteal new bone may accompany any acute inflammatory process and is not pathognomonic of infection. Figure 6–23 demonstrates the fine line of new bone

identical in appearance and location to that seen in the previous example of tuberculosis (arrows). Accompanying the changes in the periosteum is a symmetrical narrowing of the joint space. The uniformity in cartilage loss is typical of rheumatoid arthritis and differs from granulomatous diseases.

Although periosteal new bone is present in a small percentage of patients with rheumatoid arthritis, it is always subtle, as in this example, and must be diligently searched for. In our experience it is most frequently seen along the distal tibia and femur and in the small bones of the hands and feet. Solid, thick periosteal new bone should never be erroneously mistaken for that associated with rheumatoid arthritis; when it is seen, other significant diagnostic possibilities must be excluded.

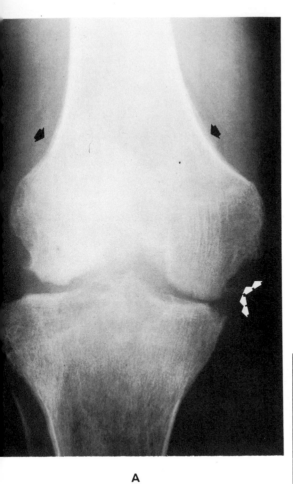

A

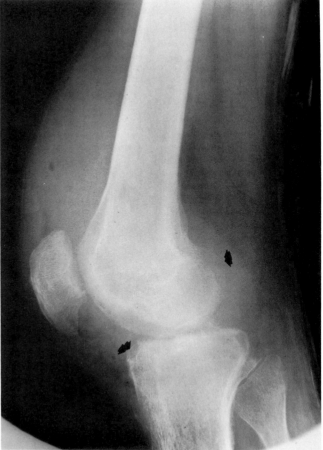

Figure 6–22. Tuberculous arthritis.

A. Periosteal new bone (arrows) and marginal erosions (double arrows) are best seen on the frontal view in this case.

B. The joint effusion is appreciated only on the lateral view. It distends the suprapatellar pouch and widens the soft tissue shadow beneath the femoral condyles.

B

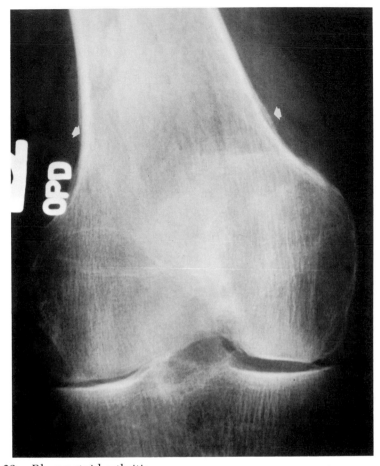

Figure 6–23.   Rheumatoid arthritis.
Symmetrical narrowing of the joint space and periostitis (arrows) attest to the inflammatory involvement of the knee.

ABNORMALITIES OF THE CARTILAGE SPACE

Any process which destroys the articular cartilage or alters the synovium may secondarily cause changes in the vulnerable, denuded bone. Hence erosions and deformities are nonspecific findings. There are patterns of change, however, which characterize the different arthritides and help distinguish confusing clinical entities. Symmetry or asymmetry of cartilage loss, location and configuration of erosions and evidence of rapidity of destruction may aid in differentiation of rheumatoid arthritis from osteoarthritis or of low-grade infections from more virulent ones.

Inflammatory Disease

INFECTIOUS ARTHRITIS
Tuberculous Arthritis. Destruction of bone from an inflammatory process characteristically begins at the margins of the joint where the protective cap of articular cartilage ends. This finding reflects synovial proliferation from any cause and is not a specific sign of tuberculosis. A sharp marginal erosion of the medial tibial condyle is seen in Figure 6–24 (arrow). Its well-defined edge and the absence of a sclerotic margin are similar to the changes that are seen in rheumatoid arthritis. The nonspecificity of the radiographic finding is emphasized by this example.

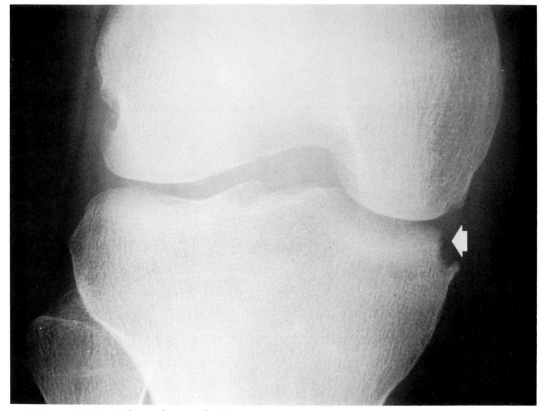

Figure 6–24. Tuberculous arthritis.
   Marginal erosions may be seen in any inflammatory arthritis when synovial proliferation occurs. The small erosion of the medial tibial condyle (arrow) is sharply defined but without a sclerotic margin.

OSTEOMYELITIS

Coccidioidomycosis. The changes in the joint that have just been illustrated are secondary to infectious arthritis. The latter should not be confused with osteomyelitis, where the infection is within the bone rather than the joint. The next case demonstrates the difference between an erosion from a process within the joint and a primary bone infection.

Figure 6–25, a lateral view of the knee in a patient with disseminated coccidioidomycosis shows two areas of involvement—the metaphysis of the femur and the tibia. The sclerotic margins of the radiolucent lesions are typical of the radiographic pattern seen in low-grade infections; they are frequently seen in tuberculosis and fungal osteomyelitis as well as in a "Brodie's abscess." It is obvious, when one compares the findings here with those in preceding examples, that the joint space in this patient is normal and the erosions reflect granulomatous change from a primary process within the bone rather than extension of pathologic changes of the synovium.

CONNECTIVE TISSUE DISEASES

Psoriatic Arthritis. Psoriatic and rheumatoid arthritis are indistinguishable when they affect the knee. The pathophysiologic events may best be understood when serial films are available to show the progression of changes leading to destruction of the joint. Three films which span a six year period demonstrate this progression in a patient with psoriatic arthritis.

A radiograph of the earliest change (Fig. 6–26A) demonstrates a synovial effusion bulging the soft tissue shadows along the medial side of the knee. Uni-

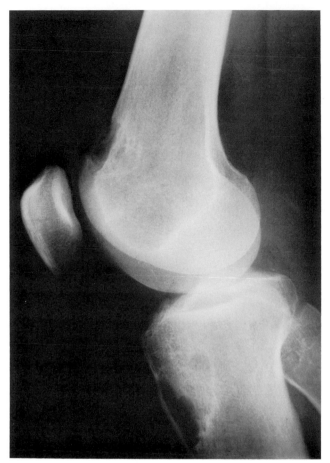

Figure 6–25. Coccidioidomycosis.
Granulomatous involvement of the femur and tibia in a patient with disseminated osseous coccidioidomycosis is sharply defined by a sclerotic margin, mimicking the appearance of cortical defects.

form narrowing of the joint space attests to the cartilage destruction concomitant with the inflammatory synovitis. The irregularity of the bone along the lateral tibial condyle is due to early erosion of the cortex. Four years later (Fig. 6–26B) the joint has narrowed further, and the mechanical stress on the unprotected articular bone has resulted in sclerosis or eburnation—new bone in the weight-bearing area (arrow). Osteoporosis is present, and is even more pronounced two years later (Fig. 6–26C). In addition to the cartilage loss and joint narrowing, there are subchondral cysts, indicating the presence of synovial proliferation through the disrupted cortex into the epiphysis. Widening of the intercondylar notch, another manifestation of synovial proliferation, is not uncommon in psoriatic and rheumatoid arthritis. It is not pathognomonic, however, and is seen

just as frequently with hemophilia, juvenile rheumatoid arthritis and occasionally granulomatous diseases.

Bony Ankylosis

Total destruction of the cartilage and healing by bony ankylosis may occasionally occur as the end stage of an inflammatory arthritis.

Juvenile Rheumatoid Arthritis. Severe soft tissue wasting and osteoporosis attest to the chronicity of the arthritis in a patient with juvenile rheumatoid arthritis (Fig. 6–27A). The joint space between the patella and femur (Fig. 6–27B), as well as the tibia, has been destroyed, and the vulnerable articulating surfaces, denuded of their protective cartilage, are fused into a continuous immobile structure. Because bone is laid down along

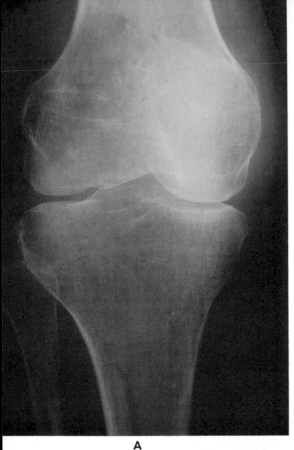

Figure 6–26. Psoriatic arthritis.

A. Increase in the soft tissue adjacent to the medial femoral condyle indicates an acute joint effusion.

B. Four years later, uniform joint narrowing and a subchondral cyst of the tibia reflect extensive cartilage destruction. Eburnation of the adjacent bone is evident (arrow).

C. After two more years, widening of the intercondylar notch, complete loss of the joint space, extensive eburnation and diffuse osteoporosis are seen. Despite the joint destruction, no osteophytes are present.

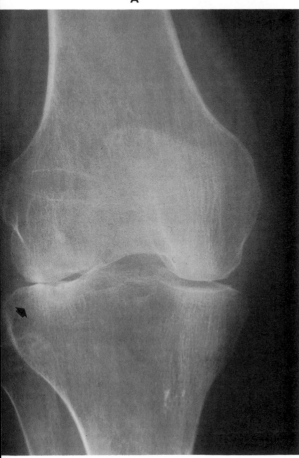

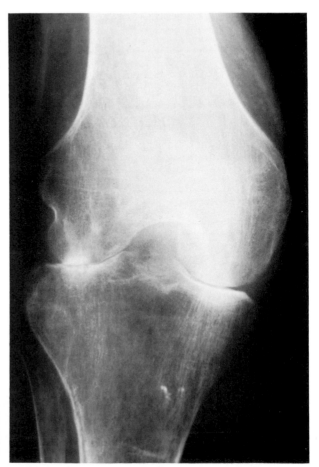

B

C

A

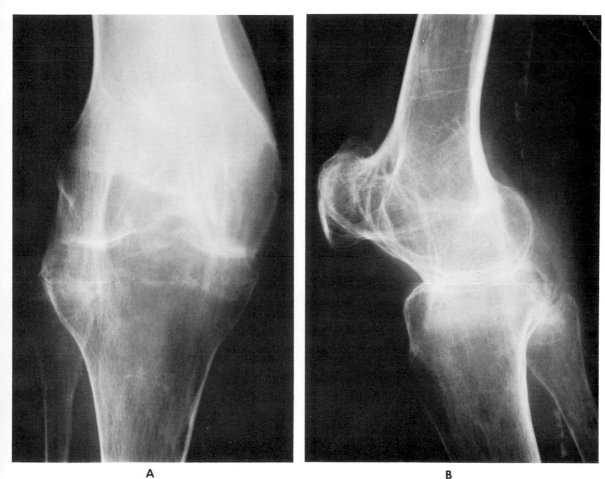

A   **B**

Figure 6–27. Juvenile rheumatoid arthritis.
The residua of the juvenile onset of rheumatoid arthritis may be bony ankylosis and severe osteoporosis, as in this example. The patella and tibia are united with the femur by continuous lines of trabeculae.

lines of stress, continuous arcs of bone are present, welding the three bones together.

Osteoarthritis

The pattern of osteoarthritis is distinctive enough that it is usually easily distinguished from the changes of inflammatory arthritides. It occurs in response to degeneration of cartilage and therefore develops along the lines of maximal stress of weight bearing or in areas subjected to trauma or poor nutrition. Because the periphery of the cartilage is most poorly nourished, osteophytes develop along the margins of the joints.

Degenerative changes in the cartilage precede the formation of osteophytes. Since the knee is a weight-bearing joint and therefore subject to undue stress and trauma, it is not surprising that mild degenerative changes are eventually present in the majority of knees. Figure 6–28 shows a specimen from the knee of a scrubwoman and illustrates splitting and fraying of the cartilage (arrows). A radiograph showed the typical hypertrophic changes of the adjacent bone that characterize osteoarthritis.

Trauma. A patient with a torn medial meniscus that was documented by arthrography has developed narrowing of the joint on the side of the injured cartilage (Fig. 6–29). The associated osteo-

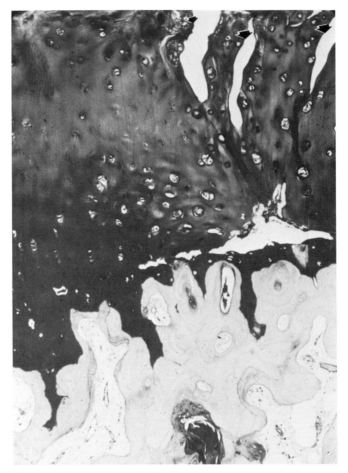

Figure 6–28. Degenerative changes of cartilage.
Splitting and fraying of the cartilage (arrows) leads to hypertrophic changes of the articular bone and the pattern of osteoarthritis. (Courtesy of The Arthritis Foundation.)

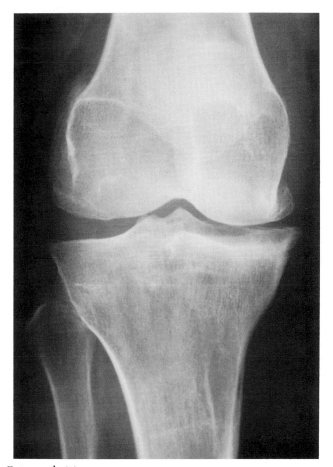

Figure 6–29. Osteoarthritis.

A medial meniscus tear initiated the series of events leading to degenerative changes in the cartilage and the subsequent radiographic finding of medial joint narrowing and prominent osteophytes.

phytes that have grown along the margins of the tibia and femur verify the destructive changes of the underlying cartilage.

Primary Osteoarthritis. A more advanced stage of osteoarthritis is present in a 70 year old woman (Fig. 6–30). The nonuniform narrowing of the joint and the pronounced development of osteophytes again characterize the findings of osteoarthritis and distinguish it from rheumatoid and psoriatic arthritis. Although such changes may be secondary to specific traumata, mild changes can occur as a result of aging alone. In a postmenopausal woman with no elicitable history of local injury, the possibility that these radiographic changes are a component of Kellgren's or erosive osteoarthritis is always a consideration,

since both conditions occasionally affect the large joints. Correlation with arthritic changes in the hands is important.

Osteoarthritis and Chondrocalcinosis. It must not be forgotten that degenerative changes of the cartilage result in the most common cause of chondrocalcinosis. Since pseudogout and hyperparathyroidism are associated with normal joint spaces and articular bones, osteoarthritis is easily distinguished from these two conditions. Figure 6–31 shows narrowing of the medial side of the joint and calcification in both menisci as well as small osteophytes on the narrowed side of the joint.

Ochronosis. Any process that results in degeneration of cartilage will initiate the changes of osteoarthritis. Ochronosis

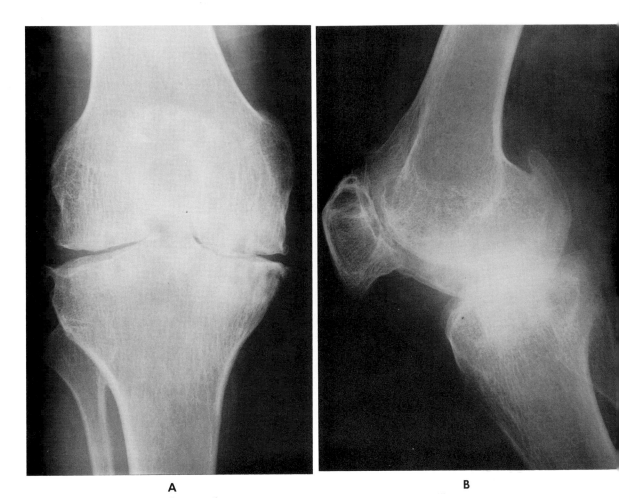

A

B

Figure 6–30. Osteoarthritis.

A. Non-uniform narrowing of the joint space, subchondral cysts and osteophytes are characteristic of osteoarthritis.

B. The lateral view illustrates narrowing of the patellofemoral joint space and prominent spurs along the posterior aspect of the femur.

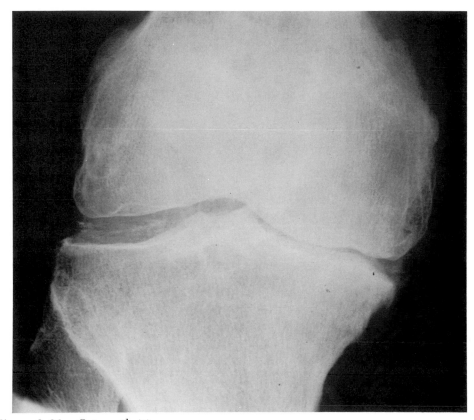

Figure 6–31. Osteoarthritis.
Non-uniform joint space narrowing and osteophytes distinguish this example of osteo-arthritis from rheumatoid arthritis. Extensive chondrocalcinosis, involving both menisci as well as the hyaline articular cartilage, indicates more advanced changes than the appearance of the articulating bones would imply.

is a hereditary disease in which an excess of homogentisic acid is present in the blood. This results in a precipitation of pigment in the soft tissues and cartilage. The deposition of abnormal pigment results in degeneration of cartilage, and patients with this disease have symptoms related to the superimposed osteoarthritis.

Typical changes of degenerative joint disease are seen in a patient with ochronosis (Fig. 6–32). There are numerous loose calcified bodies within the joint capsule. They represent either osteochondromatosis or fragments of articular bone. Although chondrocalcinosis is usually a prominent feature of ochronosis, it is not present in this knee.

Acromegaly. Overgrowth of cartilage and widening of the joint space are among the earliest radiographic signs of acromegaly. The same process that in-

creases the size of the cartilage results in its vulnerability and early senescence. The changes here are indistinguishable from the findings in any degenerative condition, with osteophytes forming in the areas of abnormal cartilage. In the weight-bearing joints of the hip and knee, these changes may occur early and more severely and should lead one to suspect an underlying systemic disease such as acromegaly.

These nonspecific changes can be seen in a film of the knee of a patient with acromegaly (Fig. 6–33), the same patient whose hand was seen in Chapter 4 (Fig. 4–32). There are medial joint space narrowing and marginal osteophytes similar to those in the patient with the torn medial meniscus (Fig. 6–26).

Neuropathic Joint. Although neuropathic joints are essentially a form of degenerative joint disease, there are sev-

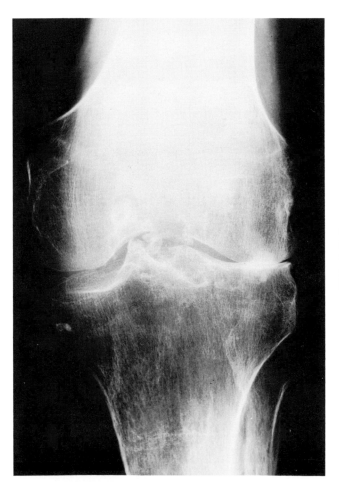

Figure 6–32. Ochronosis.
Joint narrowing, osteophytes and numerous ossified loose bodies are seen. Although chondrocalcinosis is usually a prominent feature of ochronosis, it is not evident at the time of this film.

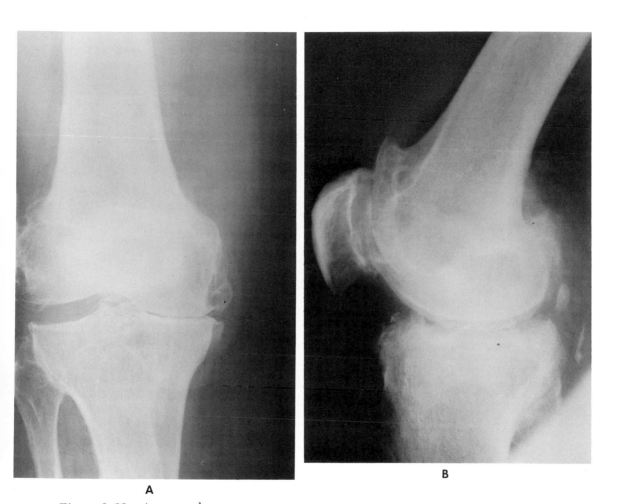

A

B

Figure 6–33. Acromegaly.
Degenerative joint disease follows the cartilage overgrowth and is characterized both by non-uniform narrowing of the joint and by osteophytes, as in this example (*A* and *B*).

eral features that make the radiographic picture distinctive. Frequently there is a massive chronic joint effusion, the result of complex factors including vasomotor instability. The effusion is typically non-inflammatory, thus distinguishing it from an infectious arthritis. Figure 6–34B shows marked distension of the joint capsule with obliteration of the normal muscle planes and anterior displacement of the patella. A film taken six months earlier (Fig. 6–34A) was normal.

Rapid destruction is a second hallmark of the neuropathic joint. Although taken only seven months after the previous film, Figure 6–34C shows proliferation of new bone and anterior subluxation of the tibia. There is no demineralization despite massive destructive changes. The final stage of a neuropathic joint is often associated with ectopic bone formation in the soft tissues.

The dependability of the radiographic signs as indicators of a neuropathic condition is reinforced by a second example of a Charcot joint (Fig. 6–35). Although the findings are less exaggerated than in the previous patient, the presence of ectopic bone in the soft tissue, the malalignment of the articular surfaces, the

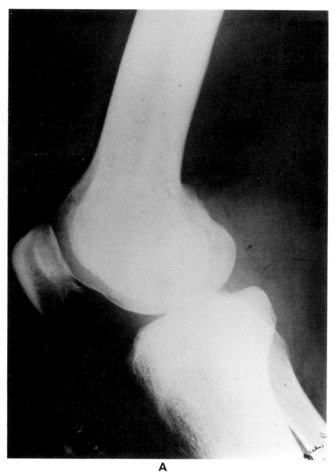

A

Figure 6–34.   Charcot joint.

A. The initial film appeared normal.

B. Six months later, however, massive effusion has displaced the patella anteriorly. Early fragmentation of the articular surface of bone is evident (arrow).

C. Seven months later, destruction of the joint space laterally and ectopic new bone within the soft tissues can be seen in addition to the joint effusion.

D. The knee nine years later is typical of the end stage of a Charcot joint.

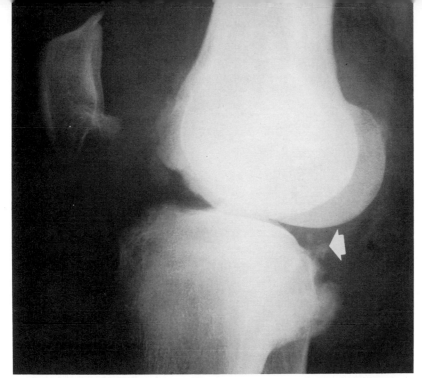

B

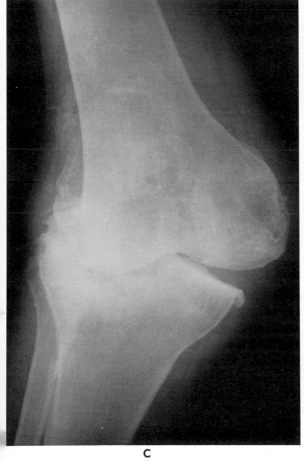

C

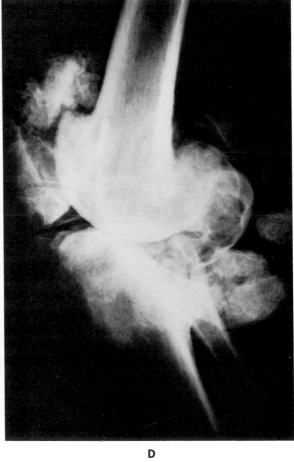

D

241

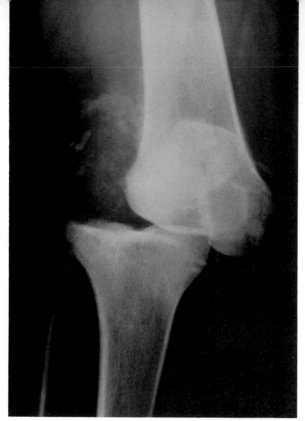

Figure 6–35. Charcot joint.
Subluxation, ectopic bone formation within the soft tissue and preservation of the bony mineralization characterize a neuropathic joint.

Figure 6–36. Charcot joint.
A sagittal section through the knee illustrates destructive changes similar to those seen in the preceding radiograph (Fig. 6–35), with subluxation and ectopic bone in the soft tissue (arrows). (Courtesy of The Arthritis Foundation.)

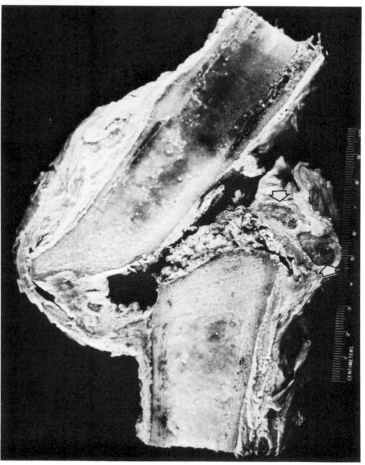

preservation of normal bony mineralization and the complete disruption of the joint space are classic findings and therefore allow an unequivocal diagnosis of neuropathic joint.

A sagittal section through the knee again demonstrates the hallmarks of a neuropathic joint (Fig. 6–36). Complete disruption of the joint with resorption of the ends of the articular bones and ectopic bone in the soft tissues are similar to findings in the preceding example.

SUGGESTED READINGS

Bocher, J., H. L. Mankin, R. N. Berk, et al. Prevalence of calcified meniscal cartilage in elderly persons. New Eng. J. Med. 272:1093 (1965).

Bohrer, S. P. Tuberculous synovitis with widening of the intercondylar notch of the distal femur. Brit. J. Radiol. 42:703 (1969).

Cassidy, T., G. L. Brody, and W. Martel. Monarticular juvenile rheumatoid arthritis, J. Pediat. 70:867 (1967).

Good, E., and R. Rapp, Chondrocalcinosis of the knee with gout and rheumatoid arthritis, New Eng. J. Med. 277:286 (1967).

Hall, A. P., and L. A. Healey. Infected synovial cysts arising as a complication of septic arthritis in a patient with rheumatoid arthritis. Arthritis Rheum. 11:579 (1968).

Harris, R. D., and H. L. Hecht, Suprapatellar effusions: A new diagnostic sign. Radiology 97:1 (1970).

Kiss, J., J. R. Martin, F. McConnell, and G. Wlodek. Angiographic and lymphangiographic examination of neuropathic knee joints. J. Canad. Ass. Radiol. 19:19 (1968).

Leach, R. E., T. Gregg, and F. J. Siber. Weight-bearing radiography in osteoarthritis of the knee. Radiology 97:265 (1970).

Palmer, D. G. Synovial cysts in rheumatoid disease. Ann. Int. Med. 70:61 (1969).

Perri, J. A., P. Rodman, and H. J. Mankin. Giant synovial cysts of the calf in patients with rheumatoid arthritis. J. Bone Joint Surg. (Amer.) 50A:709 (1968).

Pollock, S. F., J. M. Morris, and W. R. Murray. Coccidioidal synovitis of the knee. J. Bone Joint Surg. (Amer.) 49A:1397 (1967).

Taylor, A. R. Arthrography of the knee in rheumatoid arthritis. Brit. J. Radiol. 42:493 (1969).

EXERCISES

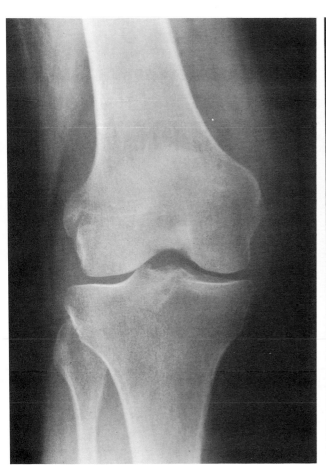

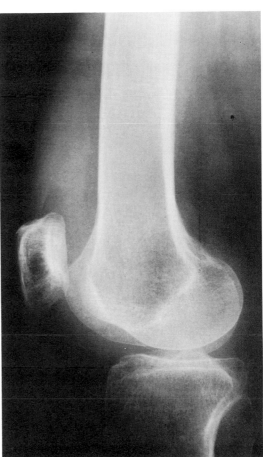

E6–1A.

E6–1B.

Exercise continued on following page.

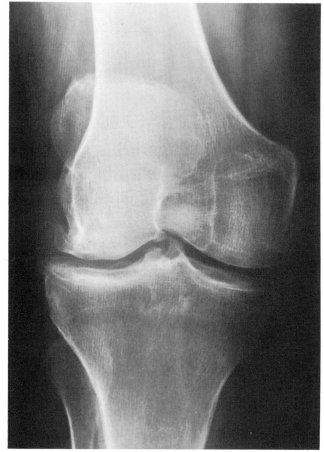

E6–1C.

E6–1. Although the changes hallmarking degenerative joint disease are generally considered to be those of the cartilage and bone, occasionally the synovium and capsule participate. The inflammatory synovitis may be marked and may precede visible radiographic changes in the bones, as in this example of a massive joint effusion of the knee (E6–1A and B). When this occurs it compounds the clinical confusion between osteoarthritis and rheumatoid arthritis. Since a joint effusion is so much more commonly seen in rheumatoid arthritis, the laboratory data are helpful: a negative latex fixation and a normal sedimentation rate.

Even more helpful are hand films when arthritis is present. This patient's hand was illustrated in Chapter 4, Figure 4–29. With such a classic distribution and characteristic type of joint destruction, there is no question that one is dealing with *primary generalized osteoarthritis.*

Eventually the development of nonuniform joint space narrowing and osteophytes make the distinction from rheumatoid arthritis in this knee much easier, as seen in E6–1C.

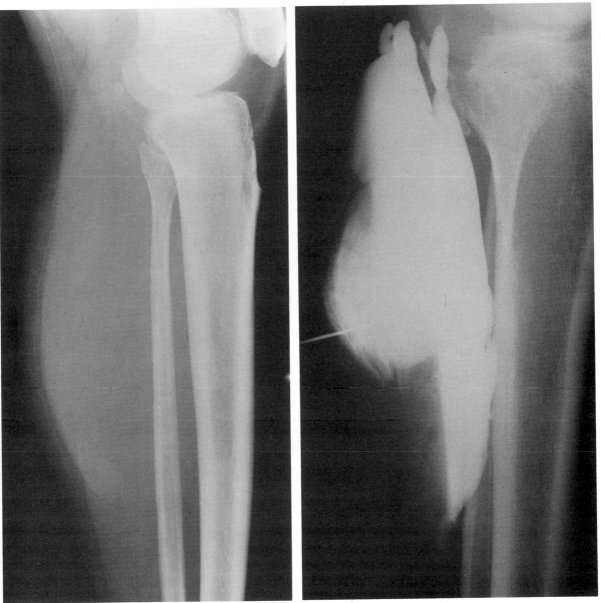

E6–2A.

E6–2B.
Exercise continued on following page.

E6–2. The abrupt onset of calf swelling and a positive Homan's sign most frequently indicate an underlying thrombophlebitis. In patients with *rheumatoid arthritis* and a chronic knee effusion, however, as in this case, an acute rupture of one of the popliteal bursae with extravasation of synovial fluid into the muscle exactly duplicates this clinical picture. Since patients with rheumatoid arthritis are treated not with anticoagulants but with rest, immobilization and at times intra-articular cortisone injections, the distinction between the two conditions is critical. Sudden disappearance of a knee effusion coincident with swelling of the calf is a common story.

This clinical situation calls for an emergency arthrogram to establish whether there is communication between the joint capsule and the calf mass. Although direct injection of contrast into the calf may be done, as in this patient, it frequently fails to show the connection with the joint capsule and only verifies the cystic nature of the mass. Even if contrast material is placed in the knee joint, weight bearing and walking may be necessary before the material makes its way into the synovial cyst, establishing the diagnosis.

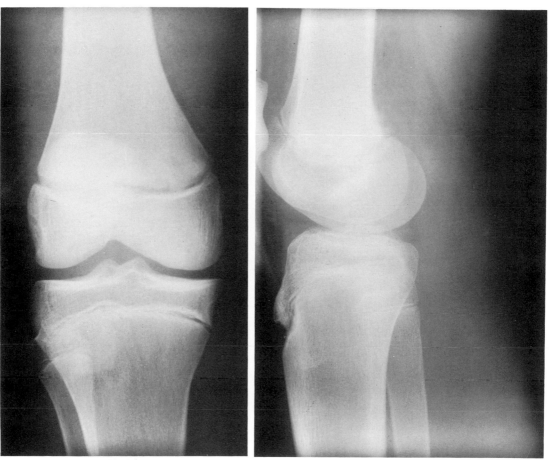

E6–3A.

E6–3B. One month later.
Exercise continued on following page.

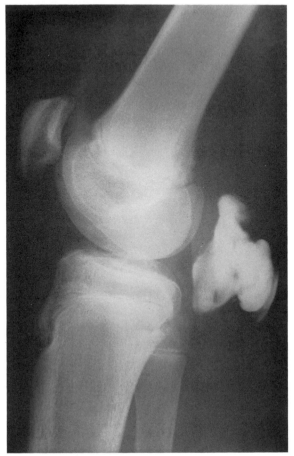

E6–3C.

E6–3. Although difficult to diagnose, horizontal fractures through the radiolucent cartilage can be suspected by the radiographic finding of widening and irregularity of the epiphyseal plate (E6–3A).

The epiphyseal fracture was missed initially in this teenage boy, and a film taken a month later because of persistent knee pain revealed the alarming findings of irregular cortical bone and periostitis along the distal femur and an associated popliteal mass (E6–3B). The initial gloom that this combination of findings provoked was immediately dispelled when the earlier fracture through the epiphyseal plate was recognized, and thoughts of osteosarcoma quickly were forgotten. An arthrogram (E6–3C) documented the cystic nature of the mass and established it as a traumatic *Baker's cyst* communicating with the joint capsule.

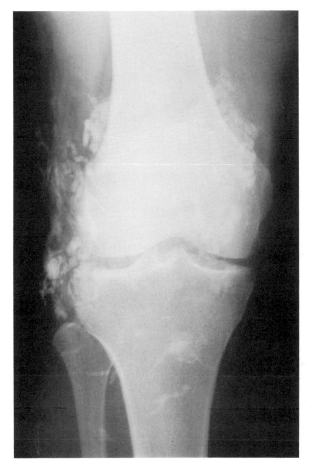

E6–4.

E6–4. Because progressive systemic sclerosis may present with a symmetrical polyarthritis and the joint fluid may be similar to that in rheumatoid arthritis, radiographic findings are essential in separating the two entities. Extensive subcutaneous deposits of calcium and a normal joint, as seen in this patient, should always suggest the diagnosis of the former entity when a connective tissue disorder is suspected.

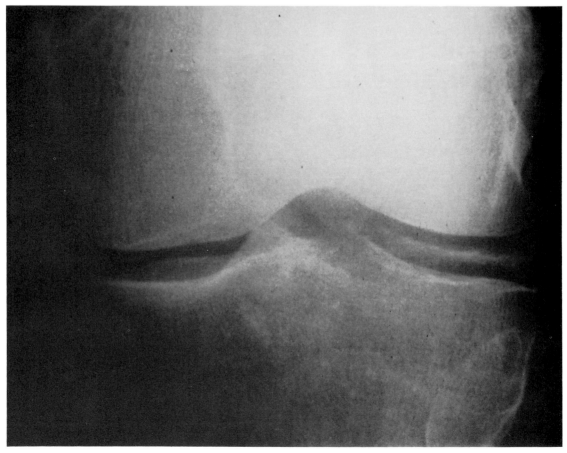

E6–5.

E6–5. What gout is to the great toe, *pseudogout* is to the knee.

Like gout, pseudogout is a crystal-induced arthritis, and an acute attack may mimic the clinical picture of gout. It occurs most frequently in the knee, and the presence of calcified cartilage is a helpful clue to the proper diagnosis. Neither the radiographic picture nor the presence of calcium pyrophosphate crystals in the joint aspirate excludes such other diagnostic possibilities as hyperparathyroidism and hemochromatosis, since these too may have chondrocalcinosis, calcium pyrophosphate crystals and intact articular bones, and even attacks of acute arthritis. The diagnosis of idiopathic chondrocalcinosis or pseudogout is therefore one of exclusion, and is established only by the process of elimination.

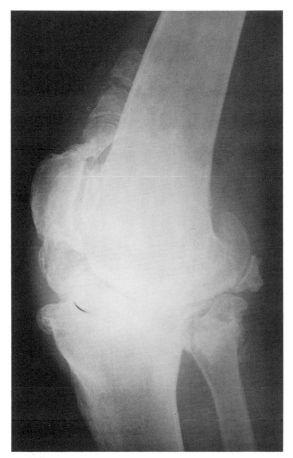

E6–6.

E6–6. "The excesses of our youth are drafts upon our old age, payable with interest, about 30 years after date."*

Tabes dorsalis extracts its payment 10 to 20 years after the primary syphilitic in-fection, and posterior column involve-ment of the spinal cord not infrequently leads to paresis and a neuropathic arthri-tis of the joints of the lower extremity. This single picture summarizes the radio-graphic findings in a *Charcot knee:* disor-ganization of the joint, exaggerated os-teophytes and ectopic bone within the soft tissues.

*Charles Caleb Colton

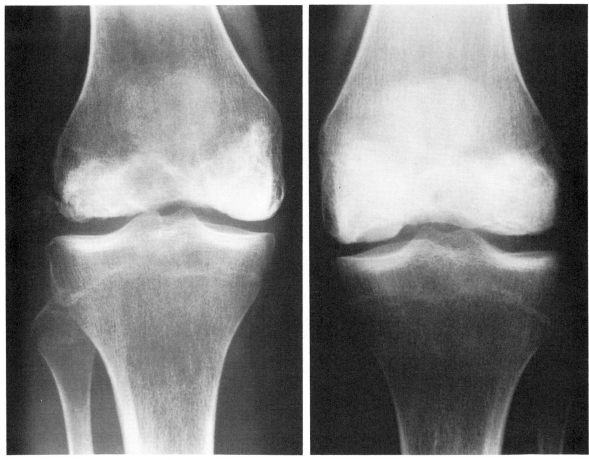

E6–7A.

E6–7B.
Illustration continued on opposite page.

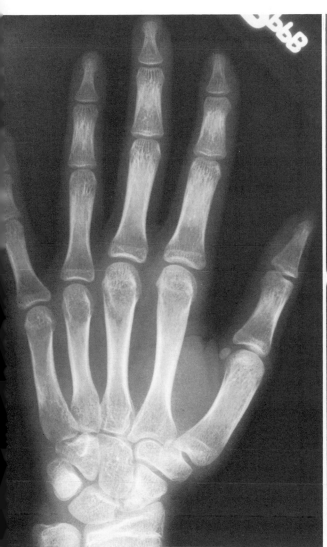

E6–7C.

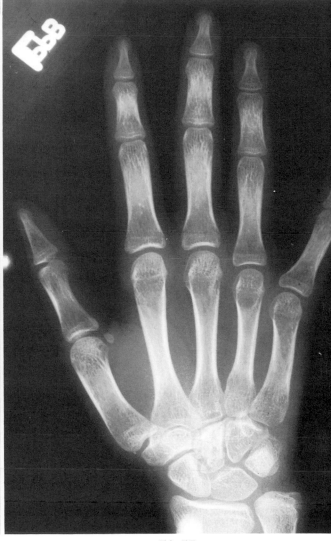

E6–7D.

E6–7. When extensive alteration in bone texture is confined to the epiphysis there are few likely causes other than chronic infection and avascular necrosis. A rare case of reticulum cell sarcoma or osteosarcoma may look similar, but multicentric disease, as in this 22 year old woman, virtually excludes these possibilities.

Tapering of the soft tissue around the distal phalanges and bone destruction of the tip of the index finger of the right hand (E6–7C) suggest the diagnosis of *Raynaud's phenomenon*. High doses of adrenocorticosteroids have caused diffuse bony demineralization in addition to *avascular necrosis* of both distal femoral epiphyses.

Two additional unusual sites of steroid-induced avascular necrosis are illustrated by the films of the hands. The proximal half of the navicular bone on the right hand (E6–7C) and the capitate bone on the left (E6–7D) have a mottled, sclerotic appearance with marked loss of volume of the bone, identical to the changes in the femoral epiphyses.

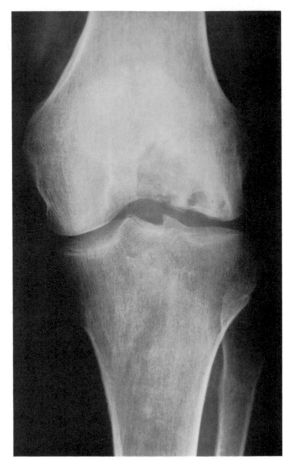

E6–8.

E6–8. Because in this case the radiographic abnormality is limited to the epiphysis, the diagnostic possibilities are similar to those in the preceding example. Destruction of the central portion of the distal femoral epiphysis appears as a large, radiolucent, excavated area, and breaks in the cortical margin suggest crumbling of the bone due to its structurally weakened condition. This patient had well-documented sarcoidosis and massive hepatosplenomegaly from granulomatous involvement. Because of the rarity of sarcoid granulomas of bones,

other than those of the hand and feet, extensive attempts were made to document a more likely cause of the knee changes. However, neither tuberculosis nor any other infectious agent could be implicated, and biopsy of the femoral epiphysis as well as the synovium of the knee joint revealed noncaseating granulomas consistent with *sarcoidosis.*

Since this example doubles the world's literature on such cases, sarcoidosis should be the last consideration in the differential diagnosis of a destructive arthritis of the large joints.

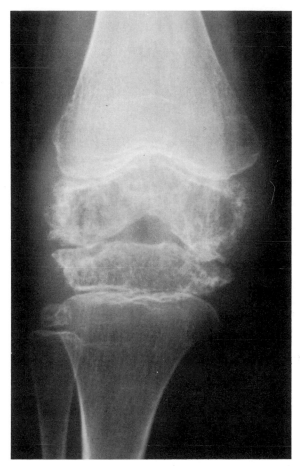

E6–9.

E6–9. A distended joint capsule, combined with overgrowth and erosions of the epiphyses, is as likely to reflect hemophilia as *juvenile rheumatoid arthritis,* but the two conditions are easily distinguished clinically.

The horizontal bandlike area of rarefaction in the femoral metaphysis can be diagnostically unnerving, as it is not uncommonly seen in patients with leukemia. Since a quarter of children with juvenile rheumatoid arthritis have lymphadenopathy and splenomegaly, and leucocytosis is frequent, the diagnosis of leukemia is often a serious consideration. Recognition of the radiolucent line as a nonspecific reflection of altered bone metabolism and awareness of its occurrence in juvenile rheumatoid arthritis as well as leukemia are essential in correctly assessing the clinical problem.

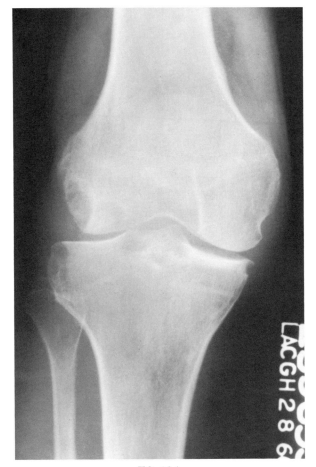

E6–10A.

Exercise continued on opposite page.

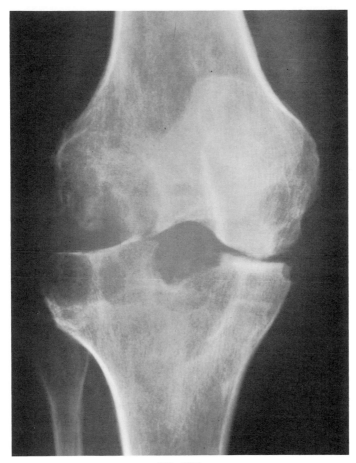

E6–10B.

E6–10. A film of this horse-trainer's knee during hospitalization for an unrelated problem revealed marginal erosions of the femoral and tibial condyles (E6–10A). A hasty departure before diagnosis and treatment, however, allowed an interval of two years to pass before the patient hobbled back, this time because of the knee.

With the advent of antibiotics it is rare to see *tuberculous arthritis* following its natural course. This patient offers an opportunity to study the progressive destructive changes of a chronic granulomatous infection unaltered by medication.

Whenever marginal erosions are seen, two categories of disease must be considered: those associated with synovial hypertrophy, and those associated with para-articular erosions contiguous to subcutaneous masses (such as gout and lipodermatoarthritis). Patients in both groups give a chronic history of joint problems. Either type of disease may cause total destruction of the joint space and large scooped-out erosions of bone. Only laboratory evidence obtained by biopsy distinguishes among the multiplicity of causes.

Chapter 7

THE HIP

ANATOMY

The anatomy of the hip is relatively uncomplicated. The acetabular cavity is formed by the union of the inferior portion of the ilium and superior ends of the pubic and ischial bones. The femoral head fits snugly into this large spherical joint cavity, forming a ball and socket type of articulation. A synovium-lined capsule encases the entire femoral head and attaches to the neck. Within the capsule there is no periosteum. Hence the radiographic sign of periosteal new bone which signifies an inflammatory process will only be seen along the distal femoral neck. The articular cartilage covers the epiphysis and extends along the femoral neck to the point of capsular attachment.

Water soluble contrast material was injected into the hip joint of a child and delineates the extent of the capsule and outlines the articular cartilage (Fig. 7–1).

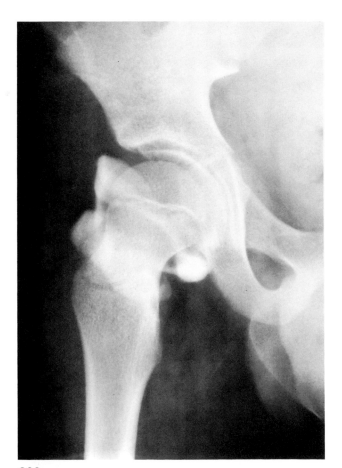

Figure 7–1. Normal arthrogram. Contrast material demonstrates the narrow limits of the joint capsule and the width of the articular cartilage (appearing as the radiolucent crescent between the femoral head and the contrast material).

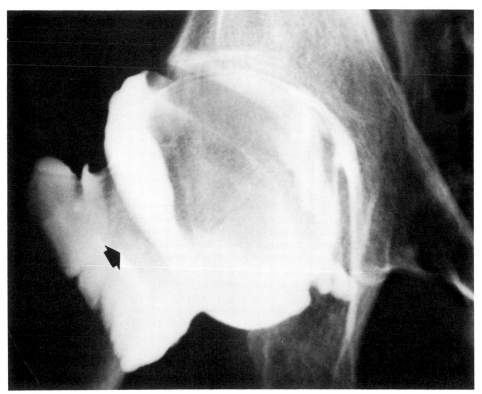

Figure 7–2. Adult hip.
The extent of the joint capsule and its limited distensibility is demonstrated by an arthrogram in an adult. The width of the articular cartilage is noticeably narrower than the child's. The radiolucent collar (arrow) is caused by a thickening of the capsule, the zonae orbicularis, and is normal.

The lower extent of the capsule is well defined, and its oblique attachment is illustrated by the disparity between the anterior and posterior margins of the contrast material superimposed on the femoral neck. The articular cartilages of the acetabulum and femoral head and neck cast a radiolucent shadow between the bones and the contrast-filled capsule. The small size of the capsule and its lack of distensibility are obvious from this study; it differs dramatically from the joint capsule of the knee.

An arthrogram of an adult (Fig. 7–2) demarcates a very similar appearing joint space. The striking difference in the width of the articular cartilage between the child and the adult is apparent when one compares the dimensions of the radiolucent crescent above the femoral head.

SOFT TISSUE ABNORMALITIES

Joint Effusion

Joint effusions of the hip are extremely difficult to diagnose clinically. They are just as difficult to see radiographically. Detection of abnormal quantities of fluid in other joints of the body is easy because the fluid deforms the contour of the extremity. The location of the hip deep to the thigh muscles and its relative nondistensibility precludes these radiographic findings. However, despite these anatomic hurdles, there are three very different radiographic signs that indicate the presence of fluid.

DISLOCATION OF THE FEMORAL HEAD
Occasionally an effusion may be large enough to displace the femoral head from

the acetabular cavity. This occurs in children rather than adults because of the shallow acetabulum and the surrounding structures which hold the femoral head less firmly in place. Because it occurs in childhood, dislocation secondary to a joint effusion is seen most commonly associated with juvenile rheumatoid arthritis and infectious arthritides.

Tuberculous Arthritis. A patient with tuberculosis initially presented with a dislocated hip (Fig. 7–3A). The femoral head is laterally displaced because of the fluid in the joint capsule. After treatment was begun the effusion subsided and the hip returned to its normal position (Fig. 7–3B). A large lytic area of the metaphysis can be seen in addition to the joint fluid on the first film but is better defined on the later frogleg view. The sharp borders are typical of a granulomatous process. A joint effusion and epiphyseal irregularity in combination with an intraosseous destructive lesion indicates an osteomyelitis as well as an arthritis. Figure 7–3C illustrates the residual deformity and undermodelling of the acetabular cavity 22 years later. Since the acetabulum develops in response to the forces of weight bearing, the presence of

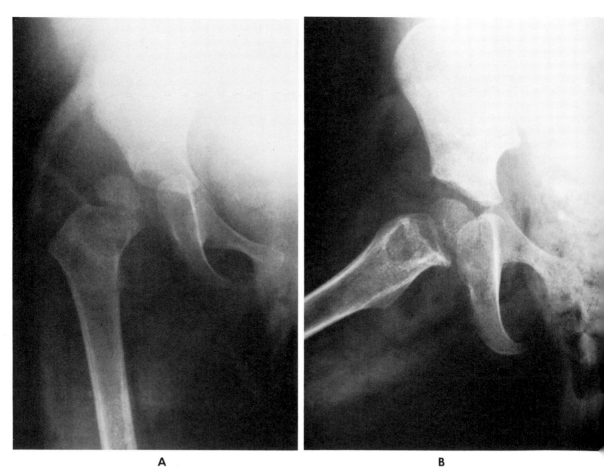

A B

Figure 7–3. Tuberculous arthritis.

A. Effusions may be massive enough to displace the hip from the acetabular cavity. A large radiolucent defect in the metaphysis indicates granulomatous involvement of the bone in addition to inflammation of the joint space.

B. The metaphyseal defect with its well-defined sclerotic border is better defined on the frogleg view.

Illustration continued on opposite page.

a dislocation and disuse in the formative period resulted in this hip deformity.

VACUUM EFFECT

In order to detect small effusions, attempts have been made to utilize the phenomenon of the "vacuum effect," which occurs when a sudden negative pressure is created in a normal joint. If there is no inflammatory process, manual traction of the femur results in a negative pressure within the capsule. Gas is released that will appear as a radiolucent crescent between the articular cartilages. This does not occur in a joint that contains abnormal amounts of fluid.

Infectious Arthritis. A vacuum may be created on a routine examination by the slight amount of traction that results from positioning a hip in external rotation for the frogleg view. Figure 7–4A illustrates the black crescent of gas between the articular cartilages in a normal hip. An infectious process was present in the opposite hip, despite its normal appearance on a film of the pelvis (Fig. 7–4B). The absence of gas in the joint on the left is not diagnostic of the presence of abnormal amounts of fluid, however. It may represent only an inadequate amount of traction to create a significant decrease in pressure. In fact, inability to produce a vacuum in an inflamed joint may be secondary to spasm and splinting on the part of the patient. Adequate traction can only be assumed if the femoral head is separated at least two millimeters from the acetabulum. Since this example is a routine frogleg view rather than a specific traction manuever, the absence of a vacuum effect on the left only supports

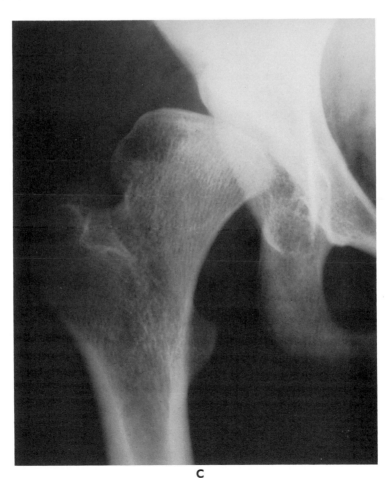

C

Figure 7–3. Continued.
C. Twenty-two years later, residual deformity of the femoral head and the acetabular cavity reflect the dislocation and disuse during the formative period of acetabular development.

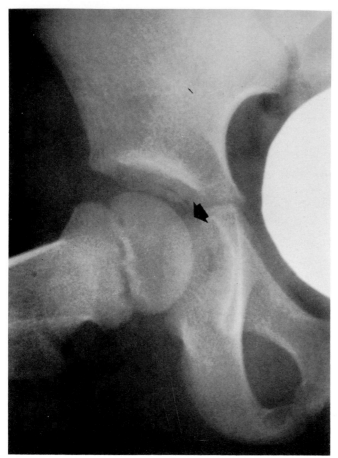

A

Figure 7–4. Infectious arthritis.

A. The vacuum created by sudden negative pressure within the capsule appears as a thin black line between the articular cartilages of the hip (arrow) and occurs only in joints without an excess of fluid.

B. The opposite hip failed to exhibit a vacuum, supporting the clinical diagnosis of an infectious arthritis and joint effusion.

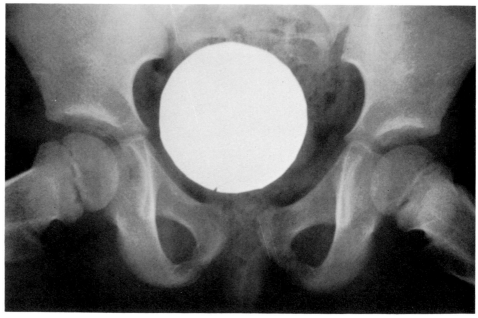

B

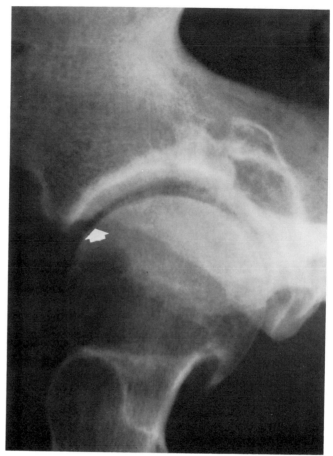

Figure 7–5. Vacuum phenomenon.

Degenerative changes of the femoral head and the acetabular cavity followed an episode of trauma. The radiolucent line paralleling the femoral head indicates a normal amount of joint fluid but delineates marginal loss of cartilage as its shadow approximates the superior margin of the femoral head.

the clinical suspicion of an inflammatory arthritis.

A second example of the vacuum effect is present in a radiograph of an adult patient, again a routine frogleg view (Fig. 7–5). The femoral head and acetabulum are deformed from old trauma and secondary degenerative joint disease. The radiolucent crescent of gas between the articular cartilages of the acetabulum and femoral head indicates the absence of excess joint fluid and demarcates the width of the cartilage, revealing its loss along the superior margin of the femoral head (arrow).

DEMINERALIZATION

Disappearance of the sharp white subchondral line of bone of the femoral head indicates an inflammatory process in the joint capsule. It is a sign of demineralization and is secondary to hyperemia. Since infections and inflammatory processes are accompanied by effusions, this radiographic finding signals an otherwise undetectable joint effusion.

Pyogenic Arthritis. Figure 7–6 is a radiographic example of an infectious arthritis. There has been extensive demineralization of the femoral head, resulting in a fuzzy, poorly defined outline and apparent widening of the joint space. The demineralization reflects the synovitis, and by inference a joint effusion can be suspected *without* any *soft tissue signs*.

Soft Tissue Calcifications

The presence of periarticular soft tissue calcification of the hip is nonspecific and may reflect many underlying processes, including a connective tissue disorder, hypercalcemia, old trauma or dys-

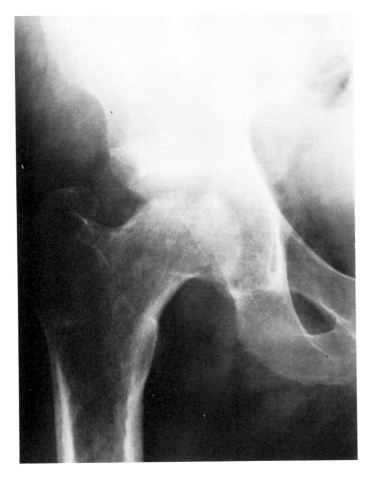

Figure 7–6. Pyogenic infection.

Extensive demineralization has obliterated the normal sharp cortical margin of the femoral head, giving it a fuzzy appearance.

trophic calcification secondary to infection or bleeding.

CALCIFICATION IN MUSCLE

Dermatomyositis. The characteristic picture of calcification within muscle is demonstrated in Figure 7–7. With two views of the thigh taken at a 90 degree angle to each other, the abnormal calcium is localized deep to the subcutaneous tissues. Extensive calcification is present in striated muscle of an eight year old girl with dermatomyositis. It is similar in location and appearance to the calcification that occurs in myositis ossificans following trauma and intramuscular bleeding.

SUBCUTANEOUS CALCIFICATION

Progressive Systemic Sclerosis. The distinction between the amorphous appearance of the calcification in a young patient with scleroderma (Fig. 7–8A) and the muscular calcification of derma-

tomyositis is made by contrasting the appearance and location of the deposits. The subcutaneous nature of the calcium is suggested by its peripheral location lateral to the greater trochanter. The isolated finding of subcutaneous calcification in the absence of inflammatory joint disease is a nonspecific finding. When a patient has clinical evidence of a connective tissue disorder, however, the most likely disease is scleroderma.

There is an additional important finding on the film which, although subtle, denotes a serious complication in this patient. A slight irregularity of the margin of the femoral epiphysis can be seen in the AP (anteroposterior) view. When the femur is externally rotated into a frogleg position (Fig. 7–8B), the slight amount of traction *exaggerates* the separation of the cortical margin. The tiny radiolucent line which parallels the cortex (arrow) and the

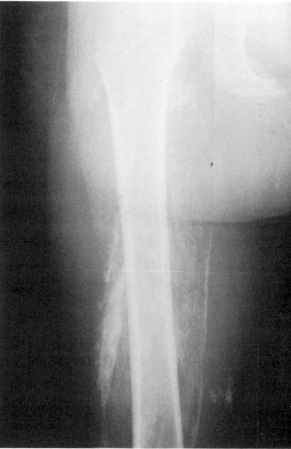

A

Figure 7–7. Dermatomyositis.
Two views of the thigh establish the extensive calcification deep to the subcutaneous tissues and within the muscles (*A* and *B*).

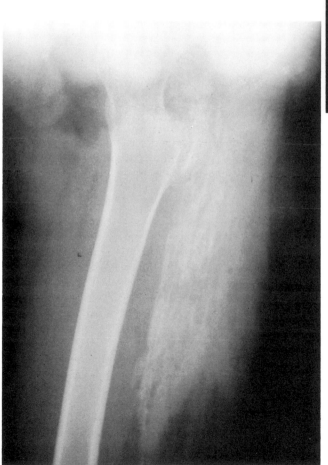

B

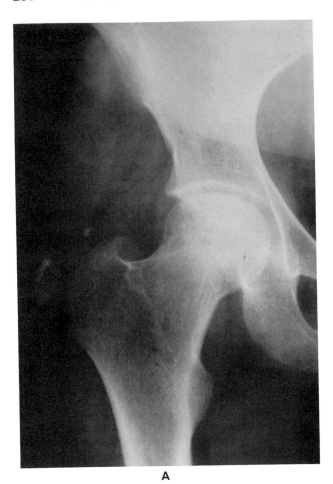

A

Figure 7–8. Progressive systemic sclerosis.

A. Amorphous calcification adjacent to the greater trochanter is deposited in the subcutaneous tissues. On the AP view the femoral head appears normal.

B. The frogleg view causes traction on the hip, separating the cortex from the underlying necrotic bone and illustrating the earliest radiographic sign of avascular necrosis. The thin black radiolucent line beneath the cortex and the breaks in the cortical margin are apparent only on this view (arrow).

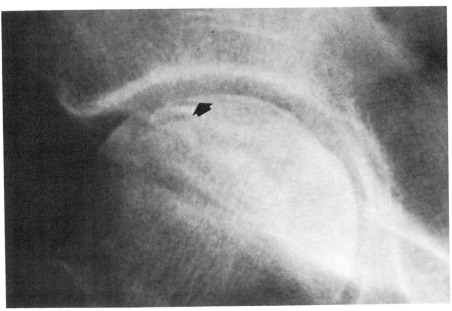

B

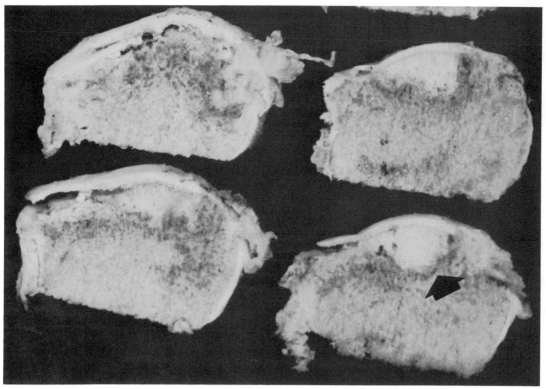

Figure 7–9. Avascular necrosis.
Serial sections through a resected femoral head illustrate the separation of cortex from subchondral bone and the mottled texture of the femoral head. The white sclerotic new bone (arrow) indicates healing within the gray areas of necrosis. (Courtesy of The Arthritis Foundation.)

unobtrusive break in the arc of the cortical outline are the earliest signs of *avascular necrosis.* Although these are minor findings, their importance is obvious. They are caused by crumbling of the necrotic bone beneath the cortical margin.

Avascular necrosis is not infrequently seen in patients who have been placed on long-term adrenocorticosteroid therapy; it is a complication that must be looked for in this vulnerable group of patients. Multiple sections through the femoral head illustrate the separation of cortex from subchondral bone in a patient with avascular necrosis (Fig. 7–9). In addition to the radiolucent line beneath the cortex and the gray areas of necrotic bone throughout the femoral head, the sclerotic new bone indicates healing (arrow).

CHONDROCALCINOSIS
Articular cartilage may calcify in any of

the conditions which result in its degeneration. In addition, deposition of calcium pyrophosphate crystals in the cartilage of patients with gout, pseudogout and hyperparathyroidism will cause a radiodense shadow.

The radiographic appearance of chondrocalcinosis in the hip is that of a sharp, thin, curvilinear arc of calcium which parallels the contour of the femoral head or the acetabular cavity. It should not be confused with the sharp shadow cast by the acetabular rim.

Hyperparathyroidism. The radiographic appearance in a patient with hyperparathyroidism is illustrated in Figure 7–10. The calcified cartilage is usually best seen peripherally, as in this example (arrow), since its thin shadow centrally often is obscured by the superimposed acetabulum. Extensive calcification of the femoral artery is an addi-

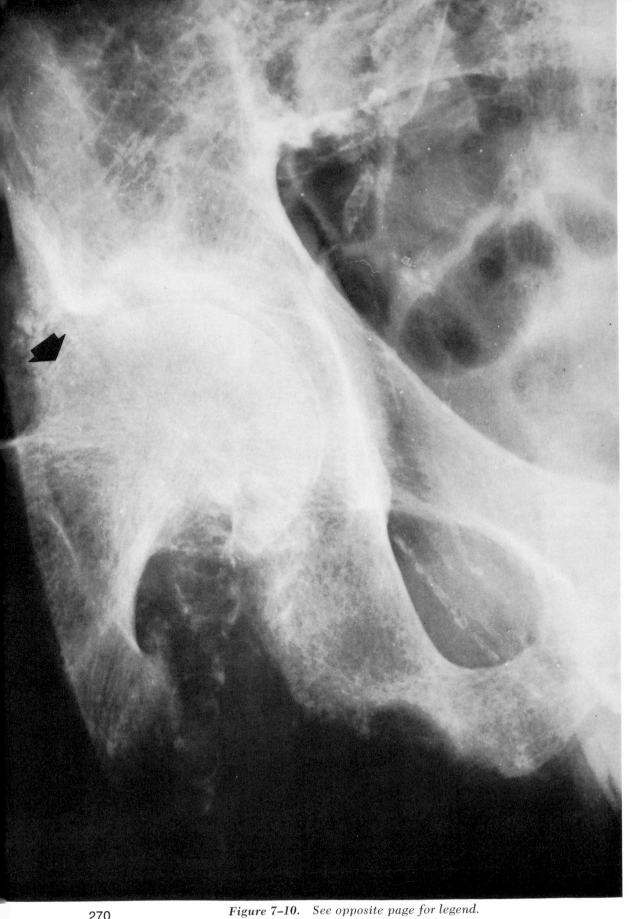

270   **Figure 7-10.** *See opposite page for legend.*

tional complication of hypercalcemia. Although chondrocalcinosis and vascular calcification could as easily suggest diabetes as hyperparathyroidism, there is one additional radiographic abnormality that allows a specific diagnosis of hyperparathyroidism from this single film. The large shallow erosion that has altered the inferior margin of the ischium reflects the exaggerated osteoclastic activity of hyperparathyroidism. Wherever major muscles attach (in this case, the adductor magnus), the process is accelerated and a scalloped defect advertises the metabolic abnormality.

ALIGNMENT ABNORMALITIES

The most common malalignment seen in the hip is an abnormal angle between the shaft of the femur and its neck. Normally this angle is between 120 and 130 degrees. An increase in the angle above 130 degrees is called a valgus deformity; a decrease below 120 degrees is a varus deformity. These are frequently related to congenital defects or underlying disease conditions which result in bone softening, such as osteomalacia or Paget's disease. Since these changes are confined to the femur rather than reflecting primary joint disease, they will not be considered in this monograph.

When there are abnormalities in the relationship of the femur to the acetabulum, in traumatic dislocations, permanent sequelae may result. These abnormalities of alignment are easily detected radiographically as well as clinically.

Posterior Dislocation. The most common type of dislocation is one where the femoral head is displaced posteriorly, superiorly and laterally (Fig. 7–11A). Often, as in this case, the lip of the acetabulum is fractured (arrow). A blow to a flexed hip such as occurs in an automobile accident causes this type of dislocation. A film nine months later shows restoration of the normal anatomic relationship (Fig. 7–11B). However, there are marked changes in the appearance of the femoral head. Instead of a homogeneous appearance of the bone, there is a large radiolucent defect surrounded by ill-defined sclerotic borders. This nonuniform appearance is a later stage of avascular necrosis than the one previously seen in the patient with scleroderma. The sclerosis represents formation of new bone around the necrotic fragments. With posterior dislocations, the superior retinacular vessels which provide the main blood supply to the femoral head are often damaged. Not infrequently, avascular necrosis follows this type of trauma if the blood supply from the ligamentum teres or the inferior retinacular vessels is inadequate.

Anterior Dislocation. It is much less common to see an anterior dislocation. When it occurs, the femoral head is displaced inferiorly, anteriorly and medially and is superimposed on the obturator foramen. Since pelvic films are taken in the supine position, the anteriorly dislocated head is farther from the film than the normally positioned hip, and its shadow is magnified. Figure 7–12 is an example of an anterior dislocation; it demonstrates how easily the two types of dislocations can be differentiated.

ABNORMAL BONE MINERALIZATION

Changes of bone mineralization are manifested in the hip in the same manner as in other regions of the body. An inflammatory process within the joint capsule is reflected in the bone early by

---

Figure 7–10. Hyperparathyroidism.

Chondrocalcinosis, vascular calcification and subperiosteal resorption are the hallmarks of hyperparathyroidism. The thin arc of calcified cartilage is best seen superior to the femoral head (arrow). The large, shallow, scalloped defect of the ischium represents exaggerated osteoclastic activity at the attachment of the adductor magnus.

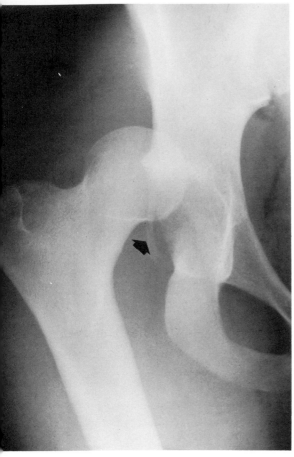

A

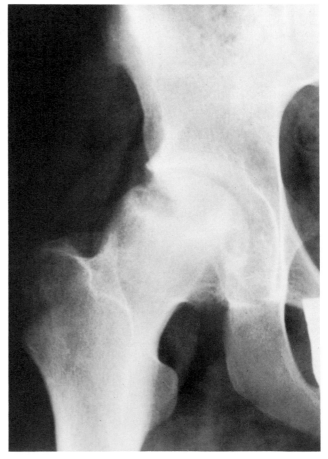

B

Figure 7–11. Posterior dislocation of the hip.

A. In a posterior dislocation, the femoral head is superior and lateral to the acetabulum. Frequently, as in this example, the acetabular rim is fractured (arrow).

B. Following reduction, the normal relationship of the head to the acetabular cavity can be seen. However, disruption of the blood supply during the episode of dislocation has resulted in avascular necrosis. The femoral head is deformed, and large radiolucent areas within it represent necrotic bone.

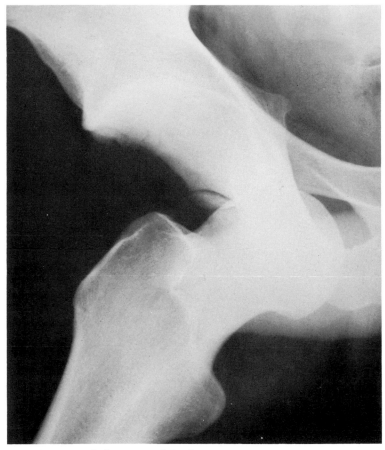

Figure 7–12.   Anterior dislocation of the hip.
Anterior dislocation of the femoral head has resulted in superimposition of its shadow medially over the obturator foramen. Its appearance is easily distinguished from that of a posterior dislocation.

the loss of the sharp cortical margin that normally defines the epiphysis. This radiographic appearance was illustrated earlier in the chapter as a subtle sign of joint fluid. Generalized osteoporosis of the femur is seen as thinning of the cortex and loss of trabeculae in the spongiosa and implies a problem *not limited* to the joint.

Nonspecific Synovitis.   The indistinct, out-of-focus appearance of the epiphyseal border of the femur is striking in Figure 7–13A. This patient had acute hip pain that was diagnosed as nonspecific synovitis by needle aspiration of fluid and biopsy of the synovium. The subtle alteration in bone mineralization is more apparent when compared to a film of the same hip taken six months later (Fig. 7–13B). With quiescence of the inflamma-

tory process, the bone has remineralized and the sharp cortical margin has returned.

Tuberculous Arthritis Secondary to a Psoas Abscess.   Any inflammatory process may result in identical subtle alterations in the mineralization of the femoral head. Tuberculous arthritis of the hip was suspected in a patient with a psoas abscess by this chance finding on a diagnostic study of his kidneys (Fig. 7–14). Loss of the sharp defining margin of cortical bone (arrows) indicated an inflammatory process; this was confirmed by needle aspiration. An arthrogram demonstrated the communication between the joint capsule and the psoas abscess. Not uncommonly, an abscess will dissect down the psoas muscle to its point of attachment on the lesser tro-

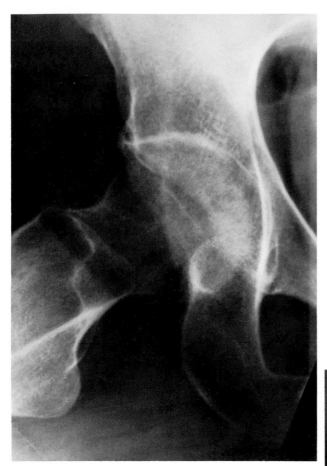

A

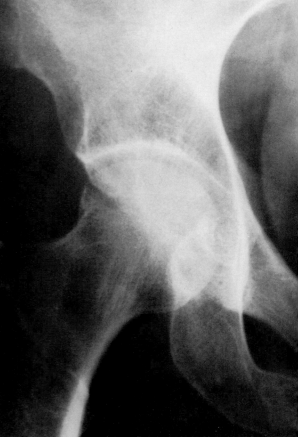

B

Figure 7–13. Nonspecific synovitis.

A. Demineralization of the femoral head secondary to a non-infectious synovitis has resulted in resorption of calcium and loss of the sharp defining cortical margin of the femoral head.

B. Six months later, quiescence of the inflammatory process has resulted in restoration of the subchondral line.

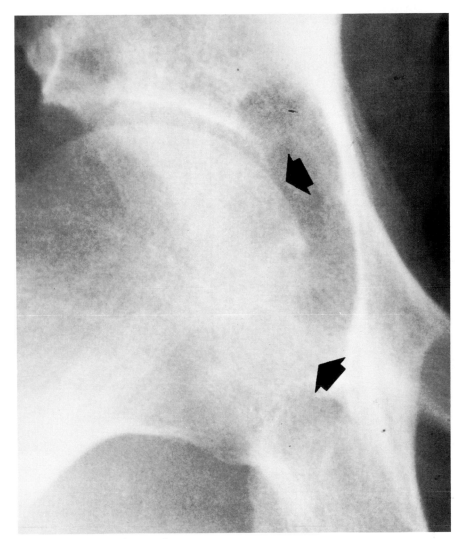

Figure 7–14. Tuberculous arthritis.

Extension of the abscess to the area of psoas muscle insertion on the lesser trochanter and subsequent dissection into the hip joint itself have caused inflammatory changes of the femoral head and destruction of the articular cartilage. Joint narrowing can be seen medially, and adjacent to it the indistinct cortical margin with its accompanying demineralization of the medial portion of the femoral head is apparent (arrows).

chanter and the adjacent hip joint becomes a vulnerable site for its extension, as in this case.

Tuberculous Arthritis Secondary to Osteomyelitis. A series of films shows the development of osteoporosis in the femur secondary to an inflammatory arthritis. Figure 7–15A demonstrates a well-defined radiolucent defect in the acetabulum caused by a localized focus of tuberculosis. The joint is uninvolved, and the femur is normally mineralized with fine, sharp white trabeculae. There is a well-defined homogeneous thick cortex along the shaft of the femur. The shallow indentation of the femoral head (arrow) is not an erosion but demarcates

the attachment of the ligamentum teres.

A film taken one year later (Fig. 7–15B) illustrates the changes following the development of a tuberculous arthritis. The once well-circumscribed destructive lesion in the acetabulum is now more diffuse, and multiple lytic areas are present which have broken through the cortex. The joint space is markedly narrowed, indicating dissolution of the articular cartilage. The change in bone mineralization is dramatic. The loss of trabeculae has resulted in a mottled appearance of the entire femur. The femoral head and neck appear gray, as does the lesser trochanter; this is particularly obvious when compared to the density of the normally

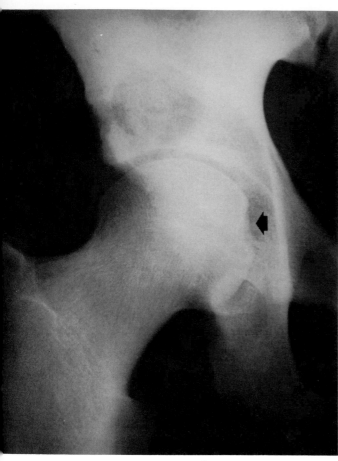

A

Figure 7–15. Tuberculous arthritis.

A. A focus of osteomyelitis is seen as a circular radiolucency in the superior acetabulum. The saucerlike indentation of the femoral head (arrow) indicates the site of attachment of the ligamentum teres and is not an erosion.

B. A tuberculous arthritis occurred when the bone infection broke into the joint. Destruction of articular cartilage has resulted in diffuse joint narrowing. Generalized demineralization of the femur is due to disuse as well as inflammation of the joint.

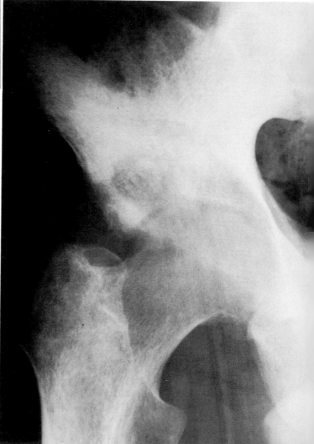

B

mineralized iliac wing. The cortex here is thin compared to that seen in the initial film. Such diffuse demineralization, not confined to the juxta-articular area, when it is associated with a primary arthritis of the hip, is usually a sign of disuse osteoporosis.

ABNORMALITIES OF THE CARTILAGE SPACE

Bony Ankylosis

Complete obliteration of the joint space and bony ankylosis may result from any inflammatory process and is most frequently seen in association with the rheumatoid diseases, particularly juvenile rheumatoid arthritis. An infection, however, may also result in fusion of the hip.

Juvenile Rheumatoid Arthritis. Figure 7–16 illustrates complete bony union of the acetabulum to the femoral head, with continuous lines of new bone bridging the joint space. Also seen are severe osteoporosis of all of the bones and deformity of the pelvis due to the abnormal medial position of the femoral head. The acetabular cavity has been remodeled to accommodate the protruding femur.

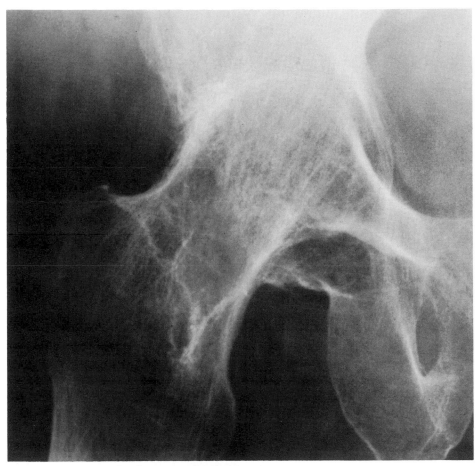

Figure 7–16. Juvenile rheumatoid arthritis.
The presence of bony ankylosis is most frequently associated with the juvenile onset of rheumatoid arthritis. Remodeling of the acetabulum and a mild protrusio acetabuli can be seen, as well as diffuse bony demineralization.

Cartilage Destruction

In contrast to other regions of the body, diagnosis of the primary cause of hip joint abnormalities from the radiographic appearance alone is extremely difficult. Unlike the hand, which has relatively nonspecific changes early in the course of the disease and develops the features of a specific arthritis later, changes in the hip from any disease are most typical early in their course, before superimposed avascular necrosis or osteoarthritis complicates the picture. It is essential to be aware of the point in time at which the film of the hip was taken in relation to the course of the patient's disease in order to accurately interpret the radiographic finding.

As an example, the changes of rheumatoid arthritis may be altered by a secondary avascular necrosis of the femoral head. Likewise, deformity of the femoral head epiphysis from avascular necrosis results in abnormal forces of weight bearing. What begins as destruction limited to the femoral head eventually develops a superimposed degenerative arthritis with subsequent alteration of both the cartilage space and the acetabulum. In unraveling a diagnostic dilemma in the hip, the most helpful radiographic aid is a series of films revealing the sequence of pathophysiologic events.

UNIFORM CARTILAGE LOSS

Uniform destruction of the articular cartilage characterizes the rheumatoid diseases (rheumatoid arthritis, psoriatic arthritis and ankylosing spondylitis) and is followed by cystic erosion of the articular bones and superimposed degenerative changes. A sagittal section through a hip destroyed by rheumatoid arthritis shows complete absence of cartilage (Fig. 7–17). Despite the absence of cartilage, the smooth round contour of

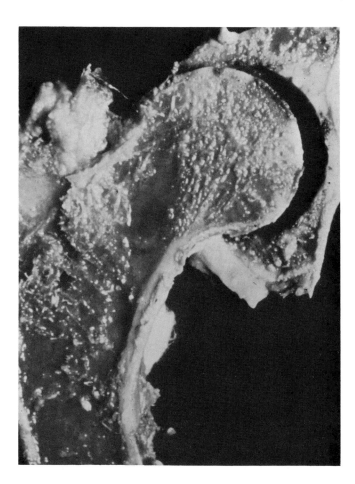

Figure 7–17. Rheumatoid arthritis.

A sagittal section through the hip joint of a patient with long-standing rheumatoid arthritis illustrates the typical pattern of destruction: uniform loss of articular cartilage of both the femoral head and the acetabulum. The apparent widening of the joint space is an artifact from positioning of the specimen for photography. Loss of cartilage resulted in uniform narrowing of the joint space. (Courtesy of Roger Terry, M.D.)

the femoral head and the acetabulum attest to the absence of erosions. The wide separation between the two bones is an artifact of positioning the hip section for the photograph. A film prior to surgical resection showed the uniform joint space narrowing that one would anticipate from such uniform destruction of cartilage.

Psoriatic Arthritis. Sequential films taken over a long period are helpful in analyzing the progression of changes that occur in response to an arthritis. Rheumatoid arthritis, psoriatic arthritis and ankylosing spondylitis may cause identical changes in the hip. A series of four films taken at two year intervals shows the progressive changes that have occurred in a patient with psoriatic arthritis. The articular cartilage has been destroyed in a uniform manner, causing a symmetrical narrowing of the joint space.

The initial study shows a normal joint with sharply defined articulating bones (Fig. 7–18A). Uniform narrowing has occurred in a two year period (Fig. 7–18B) and is identical in appearance to the preceding pathologic specimen of rheumatoid arthritis. There is also a striking change in the mineralization. Alternating lucent and sclerotic areas indicate erosions of the femoral head. Their contiguity with the joint space is not apparent, as the erosions are viewed en face and the shadows of the acetabulum and femoral head are superimposed on each other. Although this mottling is similar to the radiographic appearance of avascular necrosis, an inflammatory arthritis is easily distinguished from a primary pathologic process of the femoral head by the simultaneous loss of the joint space.

With further narrowing of the joint space, there are pressure changes on the acetabulum and remodeling of bone around the medially displaced femoral head. Figure 7–18C shows actual protrusion of the head of the femur into the pelvis. This phenomenon is called by several names: protrusio acetabuli, Otto pelvis, arthrokatadysis. Protrusion of the femoral head results in limitation of motion as well as pelvic dystocia in the child-bearing female. A final film (Fig. 7–18D) demonstrates the severe displacement that can occur as an end stage of any severely destructive arthritis. Bone has been laid down around the head to form a new acetabular cavity, and the remodeled femoral head demonstrates severe loss of volume and distortion of the normal spherical configuration.

Throughout this series of films there is progressive demineralization of bone. It is significant that despite the severe changes in the hip over this six year period, only minimal signs of a superimposed osteoarthritis are seen. Despite alterations in the biomechanics with abnormal stresses of weight bearing, very little stimulus to new bone formation is present in rheumatoid and psoriatic arthritis; osteophytes are small or, as in this example, not present even though the joint is destroyed.

Rheumatoid Arthritis. A second series of films shows a different pattern of changes in a rheumatoid disease.

The initial film demonstrates uniform narrowing of the joint space identical to that in the patient with psoriatic arthritis (Fig. 7–19A). Extensive erosions are seen in both the acetabulum and the femoral head. In addition, there are prominent osteophytes along the lateral aspect of the acetabulum and the inferior acetabular lip. Since the film of the opposite hip shows similar osteophytes but no other abnormalities, it suggests that the patient's rheumatoid arthritis of the right hip is superimposed on an underlying osteoarthritis. A film of the same hip a year later (Fig. 7–19B) shows large cystic erosions of both the acetabulum and the femoral head. There is further progression of the joint space narrowing. Examination yet another year later (Fig. 7–19C) again demonstrates progressive changes and, in addition, a large subchondral cyst in the mid-acetabulum (arrow). At this advanced stage it is impossible to know whether the severely deformed femoral head is a result of synovial proliferation with erosions or secondary avascular necrosis.

The osteophytes which were present on the initial film are absent on the final examination. It is interesting to speculate on a possible pathophysiologic mechanism to explain the relative lack of os-

Text continued on page 284.

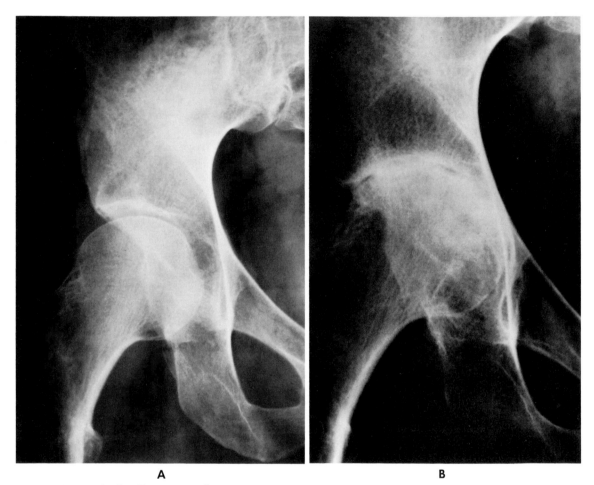

A   **B**

Figure 7–18. Psoriatic arthritis.

A. The pathologic changes of psoriatic arthritis are identical to rheumatoid arthritis when it involves the hip. The initial film illustrates a normal hip joint.

B. Two years later, uniform narrowing of the joint indicates extensive cartilage destruction. Irregularities of the femoral head are secondary to erosive changes.

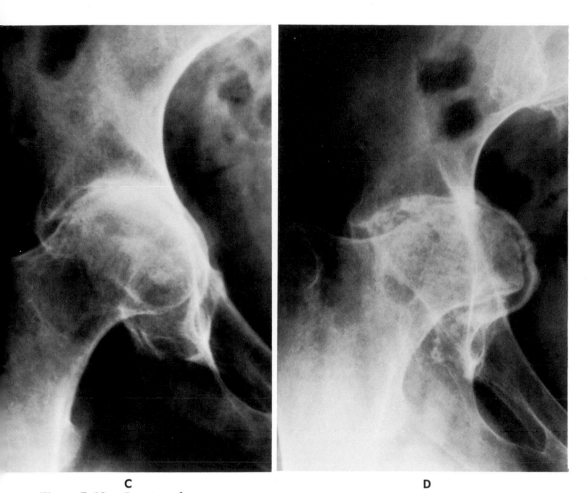

C **D**

Figure 7–18. Continued.
C. Further narrowing and remodeling of the acetabular cavity have resulted in a mild protrusio acetabuli, or Otto pelvis.
D. The final film shows marked loss of volume of the femoral head, severe protrusio and diffuse osteoporosis. Despite the severe changes of the hip joint, a superimposed osteoarthritis is not apparent.

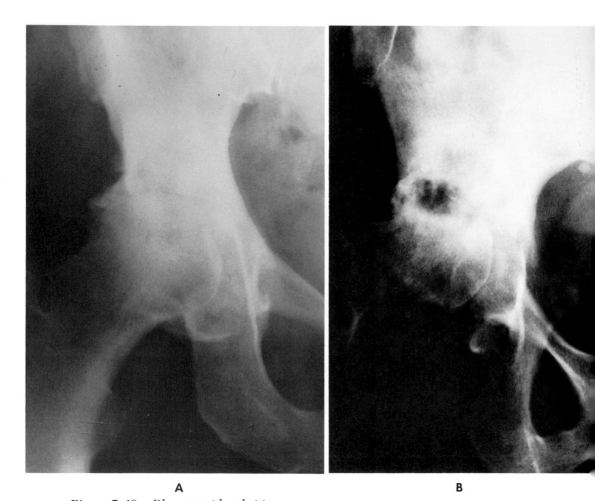

A **B**

Figure 7–19. Rheumatoid arthritis.

A. Superimposed on an osteoarthritis are the changes of rheumatoid arthritis, with uniform narrowing of the hip joint and subchondral cysts of the acetabulum.

B. A year later, progressive destruction of the femoral head and acetabulum can be seen.

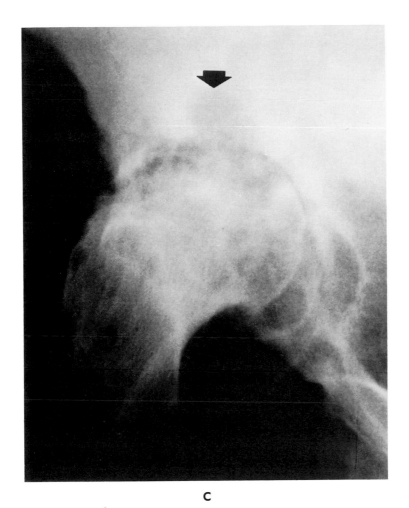

C

Figure 7–19.   Continued.
C. A large subchondral cyst has developed in the acetabulum over the intervening year (arrow). At this stage, the appearance of the femoral head may be due to either extensive erosions or a superimposed avascular necrosis.

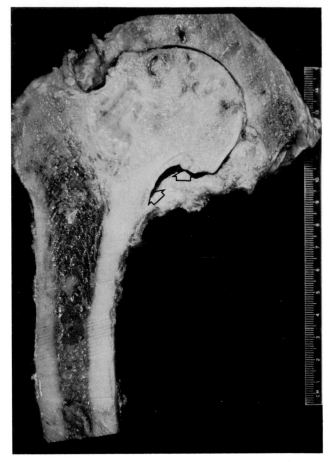

Figure 7–20. Osteoarthritis.
A sagittal section through the hip illustrates the prominent osteophytes along the superior and inferior margins of the acetabulum and the increased bone of the adjacent borders of the femoral head. In addition, buttressing of the femoral neck can be seen as a thickening of the cortex along the inferior border (arrows). Severe loss of cartilage is present in this example, and only a tiny remnant of articular cartilage remains along the medial femoral head. Except for the presence of prominent osteophytes, the joint changes are similar to rheumatoid arthritis. (Courtesy of Roger Terry, M.D.)

teophytes in association with rheumatoid arthritis. The series of films in this patient suggests that they too are involved in the inflammatory destructive process and have been obliterated or eroded simultaneously with the erosions of the other bony structures.

NON-UNIFORM CARTILAGE LOSS

Degenerative joint disease, in contrast to rheumatoid arthritis and its variants, causes loss of cartilage and narrows the joint space in areas of major lines of force (Fig. 7–20). Remnants of articular cartilage are found along the medial femoral head and acetabulum. The remainder has degenerated, leaving a narrowed joint space. New bone is laid down along the rim of the acetabulum at the outer margin of the femoral head, altering its spherical shape. Frequently, buttressing of the inferior femoral neck occurs, and a solid thick layer of appositional new bone can be seen (arrows).

Degenerative Joint Disease. The difference between the patterns of change in rheumatoid diseases and in degenerative joint disease is illustrated by a series of films which show the asymmetric loss of cartilage at the weight-bearing areas and the early development of osteophytes.

The initial film (Fig. 7–21A) shows normal bone mineralization, an intact acetabular cavity and a round femoral head. Years later (Fig. 7–21B) there is narrowing of the joint space superiorly along the line of the weight-bearing forces. In addition, osteophytes have developed and eburnation has occurred along the periphery of the acetabulum; the superior margin of the femoral head has become deformed in a fashion characteristic of degenerative joint disease. As seen in the preceding pathologic specimen (Fig. 7–20), buttressing of the femur has occurred and new bone widens the inferior cortical margin of the femoral neck. The mottled appearance of the femoral head is similar to that in Figure 7–19B and may indicate subcortical cysts or necrotic bone from a superimposed avascular necrosis. The final film (Fig. 7–21C) demonstrates loss of the femoral head and remodeling of the acetabular cavity with projection of the femoral neck into the pelvis. The dramatic loss of bone suggests that avascular necrosis may have been a major contributor to the radiographic findings on the previous film.

Figure 7–22 illustrates an uncomplicated case of degenerative joint disease and emphasizes the features that distinguish osteoarthritis from rheumatoid diseases. The joint narrowing is asymmetric and involves the superior portion of the joint in the direct line of stress, leaving the medial side of the joint intact. In addition, osteophytes or spurs along the acetabular rim are prominent components of the pathologic change. Small subchondral cysts may be seen in either condition and are not helpful in differentiating one arthritis from another.

The microscopic appearance of subchondral cysts in osteoarthritis is illustrated in Figure 7–23. The femoral head was resected because of pain and severe limitation of motion. Total loss of articular cartilage is apparent, in addition to multiple cysts. The increase in number of trabeculae around the cysts and in the subchondral bone is the equivalent of the radiologic finding of eburnation or sclerosis.

The cartilage degenerates where it is most poorly nourished (peripherally) or where it has received the greatest amount of trauma (along the lines of weight bearing), and hence the joint narrowing is very nonuniform in contrast to that seen in rheumatoid arthritis. Any cause for cartilage degeneration will result in clinical and radiographic pictures of degenerative joint disease. Such degeneration is commonly seen on routine films that include the hip and therefore appears to be an inevitable accompaniment of aging. Congenital or systemic diseases which alter the femoral epiphyses or the articular cartilage will also eventually lead to osteoarthritis. Because these diseases often are expressed at birth or have an onset in youth, degenerative change in an unusually young patient should always make one suspect as a cause a specific underlying disease process or a history of localized trauma to the hip.

Hemophilia. The destructive changes that occur in the cartilage and articular bones from multiple episodes of bleeding in patients with hemophilia may mimic juvenile rheumatoid arthritis. However, in the weight-bearing joint, degenerative changes may overshadow the changes of the primary arthritis.

Gross specimens from a normal and a hemophilic joint (the humeral rather than femoral head) graphically illustrate the pathologic changes leading to the radiographic findings (Fig. 7–24). Multiple episodes of bleeding into the right joint have discolored the tissues and evoked a synovial response. The surface of the bone is extensively eroded, and the joint capsule is thickened and pigmented.

Figure 7–25 shows severe hip disease in a young patient. Associated with the loss of cartilage superiorly are localized cystic changes of both the acetabulum and the femoral head. Although cystic changes may accompany osteoarthritis, as seen in the preceding section, their extensive size in this patient suggests an origin of either synovial proliferation or intraosseous bleeding.

Ochronosis. Deposition of pigment within the cartilage in patients with the hereditary condition of ochronosis results in early senescence and subsequent degenerative joint disease. Since the homogentisic acid pigment is deposited

Text continued on page 291.

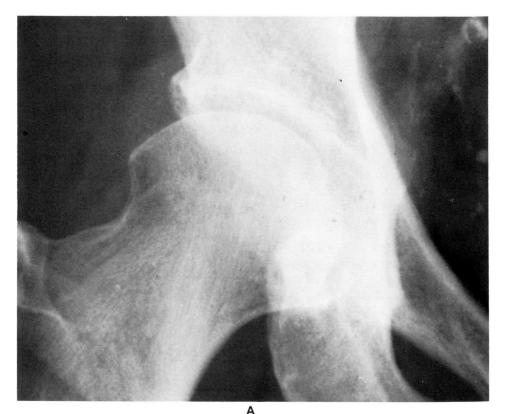

Figure 7–21. Osteoarthritis.
A. Initially the hip joint appeared normal.

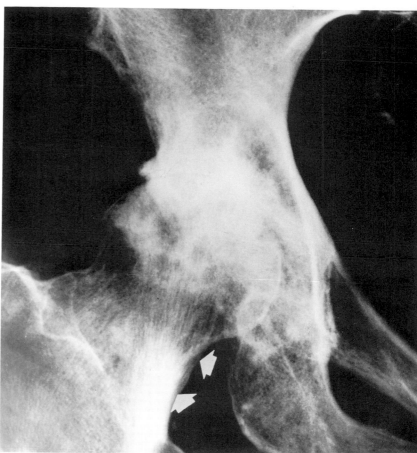

B

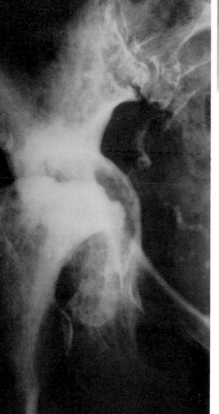

C

Figure 7-21. Continued.

B. Three years later the typical changes of osteoarthritis have developed: narrowing of the joint space (more severe along the superior aspect of the femoral head), prominent osteophytes of the superior acetabular lip, cystic erosions of the articulating bones and eburnation in the areas of weight-bearing stress. In addition, buttressing of the femur is commonly seen; here, a thick layer of new bone has been laid down along the inferior margin of the neck (arrows).

C. Five years later, an end stage arthritis is evident. The severe loss of bone and remodeling of the acetabular cavity suggest a superimposed avascular necrosis on the underlying degenerative joint disease. The wide femoral neck and thick cortex indicate the amount of new bone that has been produced along the inferior neck during the time interval.

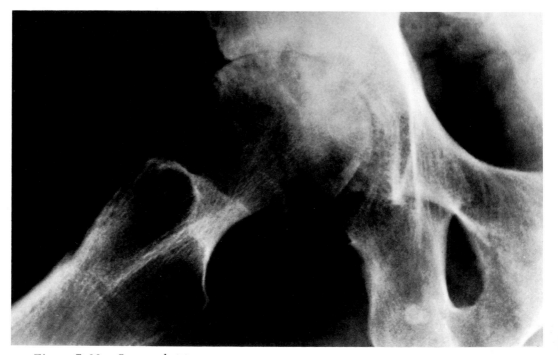

Figure 7–22. Osteoarthritis.
Early changes of degenerative arthritis can be similar to those of rheumatoid arthritis, and only the presence of osteophytes and the non-uniform cartilage loss help to differentiate the two conditions. In this example, the joint space narrowing is characteristically greatest in the line of weight bearing, at the superior aspect of the joint. Although prominent osteophytes are present along the superior and inferior acetabular lips, they are not clearly seen in the reproduction.

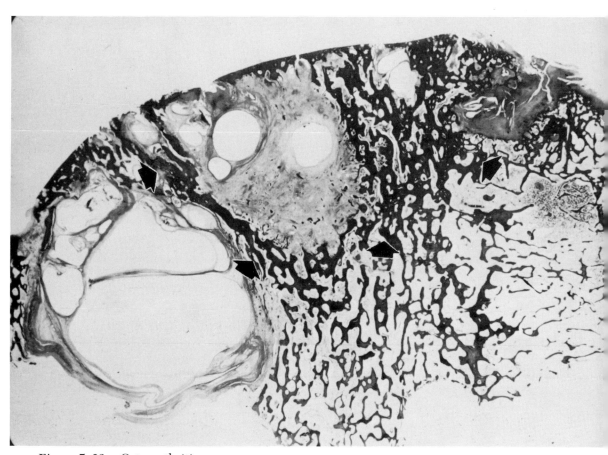

Figure 7–23. Osteoarthritis.
　　A section from the articulating margin of a femoral head shows several subchondral cysts in a patient with typical degenerative joint disease. Increased thickness and number of trabeculae (arrows) surround the cysts; the appearance on a radiograph is that of eburnation. (Courtesy of The Arthritis Foundation.)

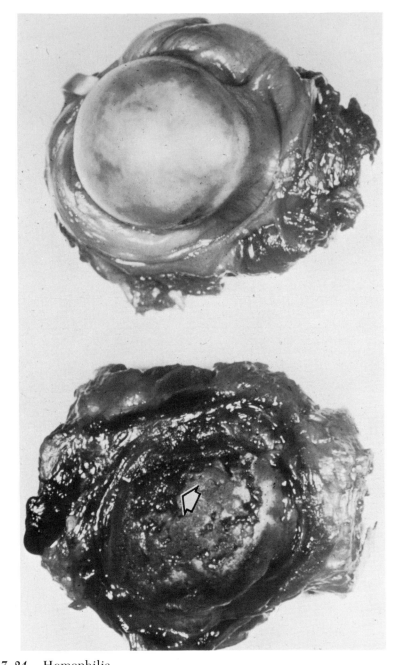

Figure 7-24. Hemophilia.
Comparison of a humeral head involved by a hemophilic arthritis with an uninvolved specimen dramatizes the destructive changes. Irregular loss of cartilage and subsequent erosions of the denuded articular surface are apparent as irregularities over the convexity of the affected humeral head (arrow). Multiple episodes of hemarthrosis have caused hypertrophied synovium and excessive deposition of pigment in the capsule. (Courtesy of The Arthritis Foundation.)

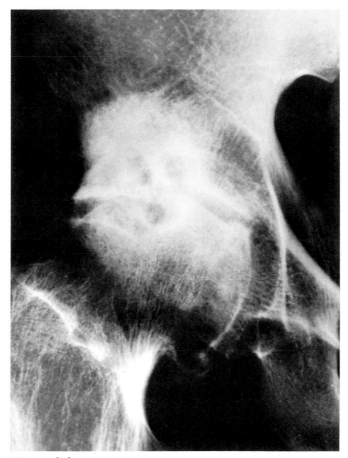

Figure 7–25. Hemophilia.
In the weight-bearing joints, the changes of hemophilia are those of a severe osteoarthritis. Loss of cartilage at the weight-bearing surfaces, large subchondral cysts of both the acetabulum and the femoral head and eburnation are the radiographic stigmata of osteoarthritis. The thick white cortex of the inferior femoral neck indicates buttressing in the typical location.

throughout the cartilage, it is not surprising that the joint narrowing is much more uniform than in other conditions associated with osteoarthritis (Fig. 7–26). Chondrocalcinosis is universal in patients with this disease and in this example can be seen along the inferior aspect of the joint. Because of the uniform narrowing, the destructive changes mimic the pathologic findings in rheumatoid arthritis. In our experience, however, the chondrocalcinosis that accompanies rheumatoid arthritis appears only in fibrocartilage; this contrasts with the hyaline cartilage calcification that is present in this joint.

Neuropathic Arthritis. The destructive changes that occur in the hip from a neuropathic condition are similar to such changes in the ankle and the elbow. They are characterized by disorganization of the joint and the production of ectopic new bone.

Figure 7–27 shows all these findings in a patient with syphilis and a Charcot hip. There are fragmentation of the superior acetabular lip and extensive new bone in the medial soft tissues. The femoral head has been resorbed, with subsequent widening of the joint space.

Figure 7–28 is an even more flagrant example of the exaggerated changes that can be seen with a neuropathic joint. The remodeling of both the acetabular cavity

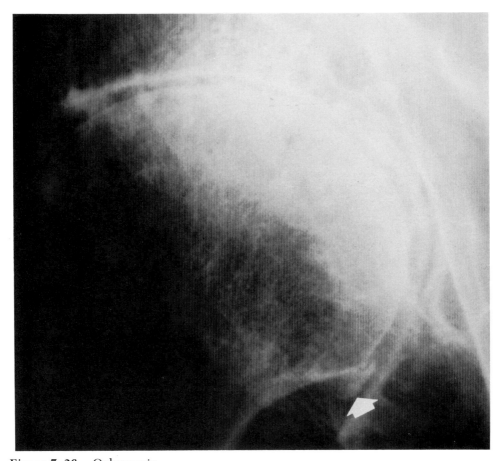

Figure 7–26. Ochronosis.
Any cause of cartilage destruction leads to degenerative joint disease. When it is uniform, as is often the case in ochronosis, the symmetrical joint destruction mimics the changes of rheumatoid arthritis. Chondrocalcinosis (arrow) is evident.

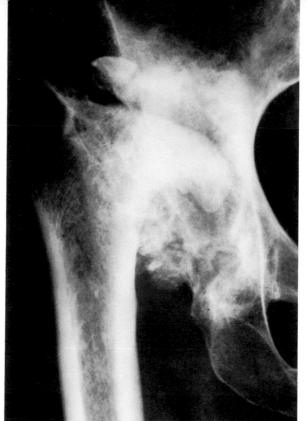

Figure 7–27. Charcot joint.
Whenever complete disorganization of a joint is accompanied by ectopic new bone in the para-articular soft tissues, the diagnosis of a Charcot joint should be made. Preservation of normal bony mineralization is an additional important radiographic sign.

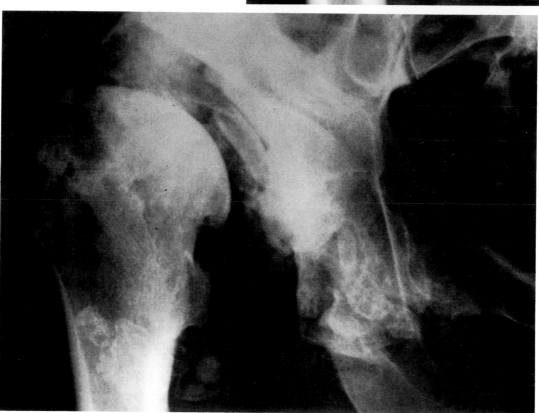

Figure 7–28. Charcot joint.
Lateral subluxation of the femoral head and excessive new bone within the acetabular cavity as well as the soft tissues have developed in a patient with tertiary syphilis.

and the femoral head have resulted in a laterally displaced hip. The medial joint space is widened and prominent fragments of ectopic bone are present, as in the preceding example.

SUGGESTED READINGS

Chung, S. M. K., and E. L. Ralston. Necrosis of the femoral head associated with sickle cell anemia and its genetic variants. J. Bone Joint Surg. (Amer.) 51A:33 (1969).

Glick, E. N. A radiological comparison of the hip joint in rheumatoid arthritis and ankylosing spondylitis. Proc. Roy. Soc. Med. 59:1229 (1966).

Golding, J. S. R., J. E. MacIver, and L. N. Went. The bone changes in sickle cell anaemia and its genetic variants. J. Bone Joint Surg. (Brit.) 41B:711 (1959).

Hurwitz, D., and H. Roth. Sickle cell-thalassemia presenting as arthritis of the hip. Arthritis Rheum. 13:422 (1970).

Madle, S. H., and L. M. Freeman. Avascular necrosis of bone in Cushing's syndrome. Radiology 83:1069 (1964).

Martel, W., and A. K. Poznanski. The effect of traction on the hip in osteonecrosis. Radiology 94:505 (1970).

Martel, W., and A. K. Poznanski. The value of traction during roentgenography of the hip. Radiology 94:497 (1970).

Martel, W., and B. H. Sitterley. Roentgenologic manifestations of osteonecrosis. Amer. J. Roentgen. 106:509 (1969).

McCollum, D. E., R. S. Mathews, and M. T. O'Neil. Aseptic necrosis of the femoral head: Associated diseases and evaluation of treatment. Southern Med. J. 63:241 (1970).

Miller, T., and R. A. Ristifo. Steroid arthropathy. Radiology 94:509 (1970).

Rosen, R. A. Transistory demineralization of the femoral head, Radiology 94:509(1970).

Samuelson, C., J. R. Ward, and D. Albo. Rheumatoid synovial cyst of the hip. Arthritis Rheum. 14:105 (1971).

Sevitt, S., and R. G. Thompson. The distribution and anastomosis of arteries supplying the head and neck of the femur. J. Bone Joint Surg. (Brit.) 47B:560 (1965).

Swezy, R. L., Transient osteoporosis of the hip, foot, and knee. Arthritis Rheum. 13:858 (1970).

Velayos, E. , E., J. D. Leidholt, C. J. Smyth, and R. Priest. Arthropathy associated with steroid therapy. Ann. Int. Med. 64:759 (1966).

Wilde, A., H. J. Mankin, and G. P. Rodman. Avascular necrosis of the femoral head in scleroderma. Arthritis Rheum. 13:445 (1970).

Yaghmai, I., and P. Mirbod. Tumoral calcinosis. Amer. J. Roentgen. 111:573 (1971).

EXERCISES

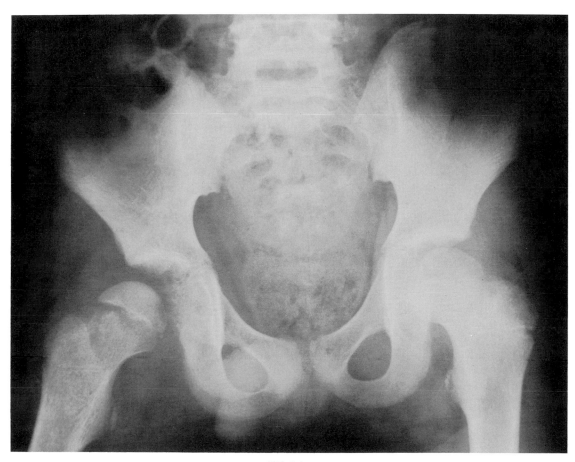

E7–1A.

Exercise continued on following page.

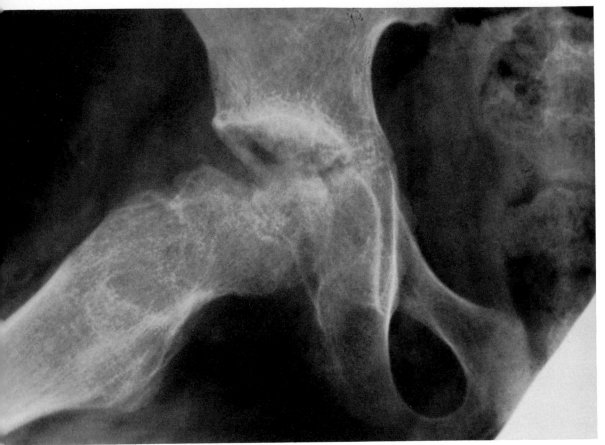

E7–1B. Five months later.

E7–1. Monoarticular arthritis must always suggest a bacterial infection first since early recognition and treatment are critical in preserving the joint cartilage and articular surfaces of bone. In a child, pain is frequently referred to the knee, and radiographs of both hip and knee must be obtained to avoid missing the true site of disease.

In the younger age groups, a joint effusion of the hip may present as a dislocation since the fluid easily displaces the femoral head from the acetabular cavity. The widened space between the right acetabulum and femoral head, as well as the interrupted Shenton's line, signify a hip subluxation in this patient (E7–1A).

Spread of infection from the joint capsule to bone may also occur in *pyogenic arthritis*. Its entry is at the vulnerable point where capsule attaches to bone; this complication is likewise seen more frequently in children than in adults. Five months later, despite therapy, irreversible destruction of this patient's joint space and femur has occurred (E7–1B).

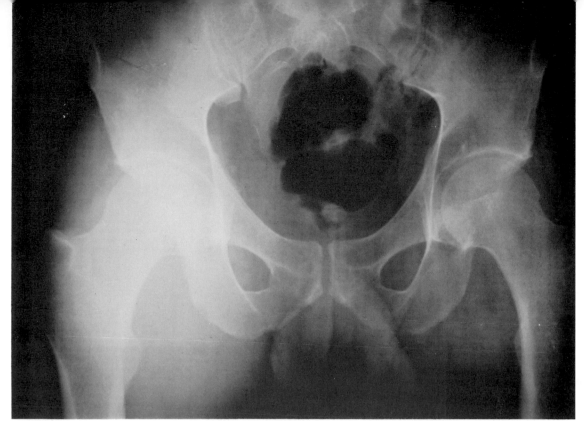

E7–2A.

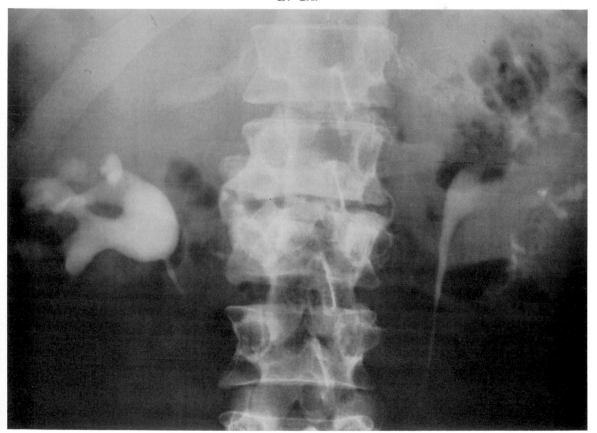

E7–2B.   *Exercise continued on following page.*

297

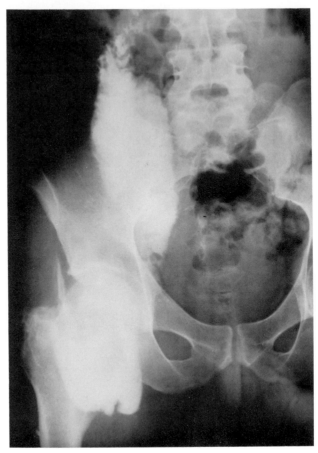

E7–2C.

E7–2. Massive soft tissue swelling of the right thigh, seen radiographically as an increase in density as well as mass, is so nonspecific a finding that anything from hematoma to synovial sarcoma is in the realm of possibility. The film from the intravenous urogram (E7–2*B*), however, provides two critical clues that enable a specific diagnosis to be made with such assurance that one hardly needs help from the bacteriologist. Dilatation of the pelvis and calyces of the right kidney suggests obstruction at the ureteropelvic junction, and similar changes localized to the upper collecting structures of the left kidney imply an additional site of stenosis involving the superior infundibulum. Tuberculosis characteristically affects the points of normal narrowing in the urinary tract causing fibrosis and subse-quent obstruction of the proximal collecting structures. Ureteropelvic junction or infundibular stenosis with subsequent hydronephrosis, as in this example, typifies renal *tuberculosis.*

The lumbar spine offers additional evidence for the presence of this granulomatous infection. Narrowing of the intervertebral space between the first and second lumbar vertebrae, with irregularity of the bony end plates and reparative new bone, indicates an additional site of tuberculous infection and explains the soft tissue shadow of the hip. A psoas abscess, originating from the slips of muscle to the infected vertebrae and dissecting down to the attachment on the lesser trochanter, was shown by injecting contrast and documenting the extent of the abscess cavity (E7–2*C*).

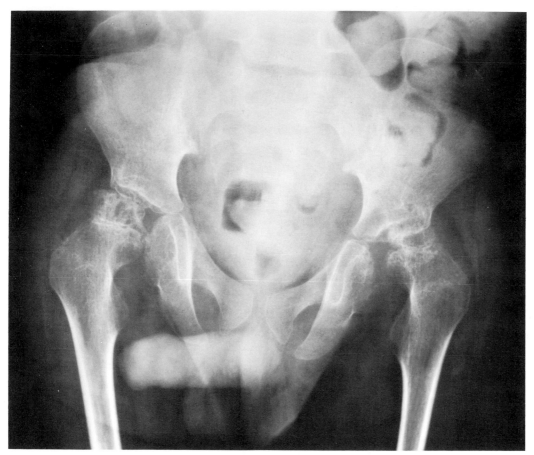

E7–3.

E7–3. Hip involvement is common in the polyarticular form of *juvenile rheumatoid arthritis,* some series suggesting as high an incidence as 64 per cent. The radiographic picture is the opposite from what one sees in adult rheumatoid arthritis. Instead of joint narrowing and protrusion of the femoral head into the pelvis, the femur may remain laterally displaced. The actively growing bones of the pelvis often remodel an acetabular cavity around the oversized epiphysis, suggesting restoration of a joint and minimizing the actual degree of destruction, as in this child's right hip.

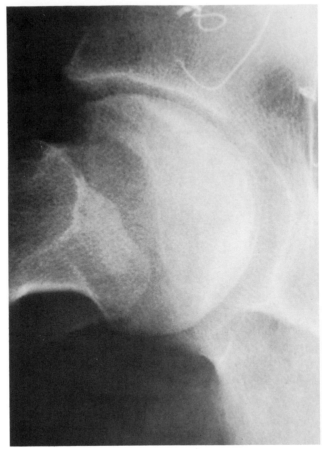

E7–4.

E7–4. The earliest sign of *avascular necrosis* is the radiolucent line paralleling the cortical margin of the femoral epiphysis. It must be searched for in patients with a predilection for this complication, and frogleg views of the hip are essential for its early detection. Patients on adrenocorticosteroids who begin to complain of hip pain must be repeatedly examined if the initial films appear normal.

The metallic sutures overlying the ilium in this example mark the surgical incision for a renal transplant, and the avascular necrosis reflects one of the many ominous complications in this group of patients.

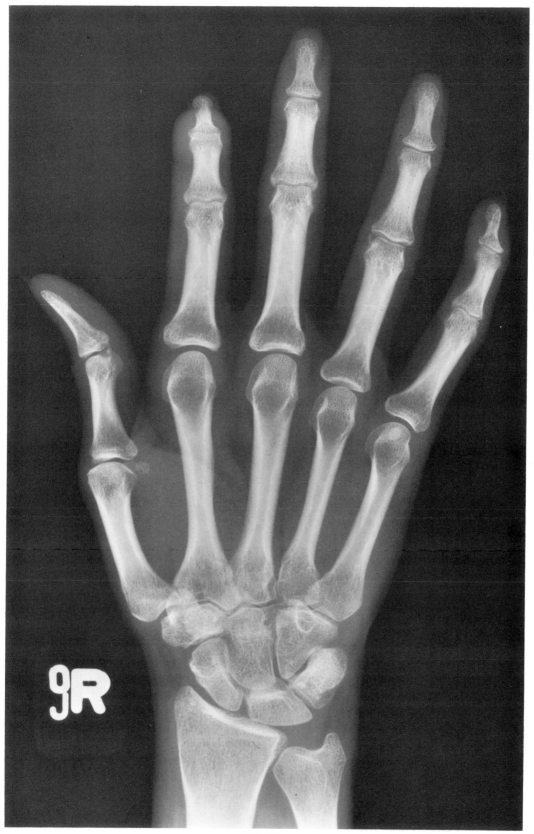

E7–5A.   *Exercise continued on following page.*

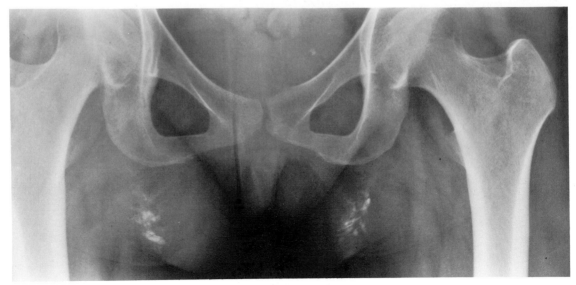

E7–5B.

E7–5. Bilateral calcific deposits beneath the ischial bones may reflect nothing more than a localized ischial bursitis or myositis ossificans from local trauma, but it may also mirror a systemic abnormality. The connective tissue disorders are common causes of extensive dystrophic calcification and must always be of prime consideration in the list of diagnostic possibilities.

Atrophy of the soft tissues of the tips of the fingers (E7–5A), gangrene with ulceration (as seen in the index finger) and juxta-articular demineralization of all the joints of the hand are so typical of the complex of radiographic findings in Raynaud's phenomenon that the diagnosis of a connective tissue disorder is almost certain. This patient had a typical "butterfly rash" and positive tests for lupus erythematosus (L.E. cells). In addition, lung, heart and esophageal changes developed. Although subcutaneous calcification is most common in *progressive systemic sclerosis* and is rare in *systemic lupus erythematosus,* it occasionally occurs. Patients with this combination of findings, however, frequently have elements of both diseases and cannot be pigeonholed into a single category.

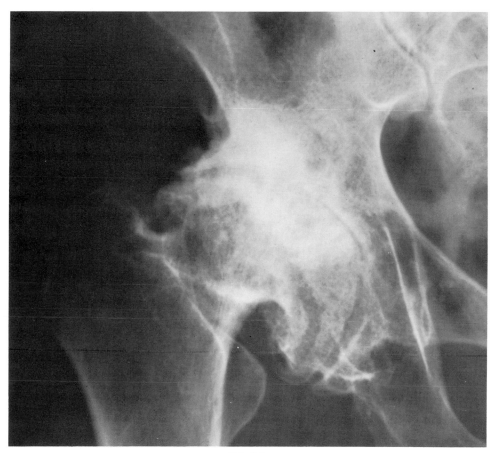

E7-6A.

Exercise continued on following page.

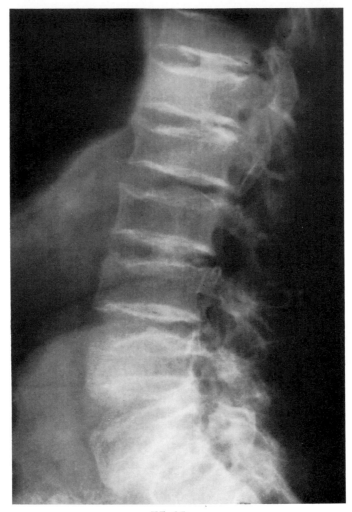

E7–6B.

E7–6. Severe degenerative joint disease, characterized by irregular joint narrowing, eburnation and osteophytes, is not uncommon in the weight-bearing joints of the hip and the knee. Although crippling to the patient, it is somewhat mundane as a choice for a textbook exercise.

Whenever the femoral head is as misshapen and flattened as in this example, however, the suspicion of an underlying epiphyseal disorder must be considered: an earlier episode of avascular necrosis or a slipped capital femoral epiphysis, for example—or, as in this case, a generalized epiphyseal dysplasia. A specific diagnosis from the joint film alone is impossible. The universal vertebra plana, seen on the lateral view of the lumbar spine, clinches the diagnosis of *Morquio's disease* (E7–6B).

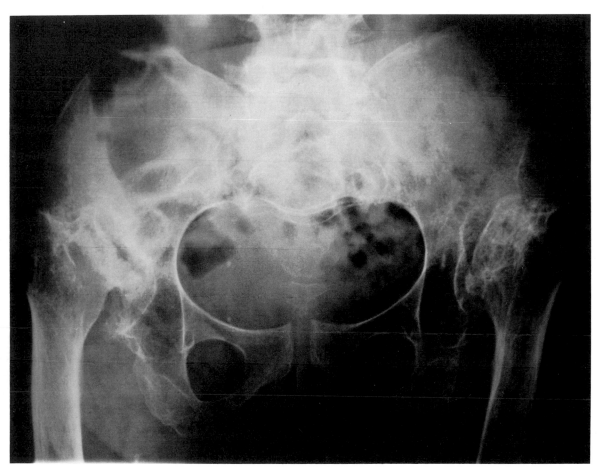

E7–7A. *Exercise continued on following page.*

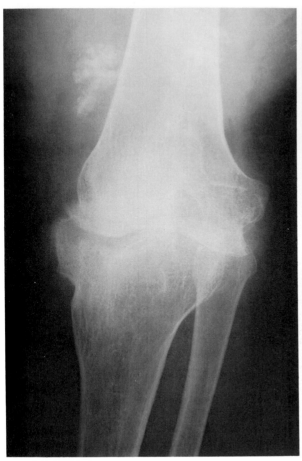

E7–7B.

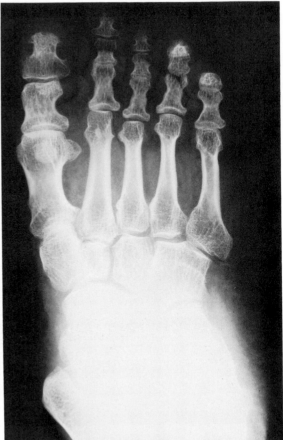

E7–7C.

E7–7. *Dysplasia epiphysealis multiplex* is frequently familial. It affects the epiphyses, resulting in degenerative changes of the weight-bearing joints in young adults in a similar fashion to Morquio's disease. The severe hip derangement might just as easily be secondary to the residua of congenital dislocated hip or Legg-Calvé-Perthes disease. Thus it is important to establish the distribution of the arthritis. Its presence in the knees excludes diseases limited to the hip joint. The knee in this condition characteristically has a flat intercondylar notch in addition to the changes of degenerative joint disease (E7–*B*). Morquio's disease and spondyloepiphyseal dysplasia tarda are easily distinguished from dysplasia epiphysealis multiplex on a lateral spine projection, normal in the latter entity and diffusely abnormal in the other two conditions.

A hand or foot film is also helpful in establishing the diagnosis, as the carpal and tarsal bones are hypoplastic and the tubular bones are short and square; this is classically manifested in E7–7*C*.

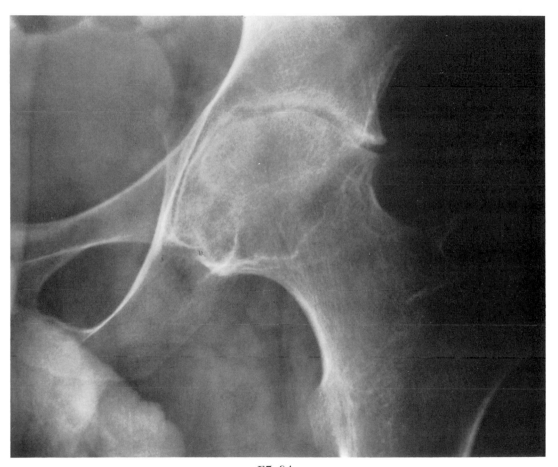

E7–8A.

Exercise continued on following page.

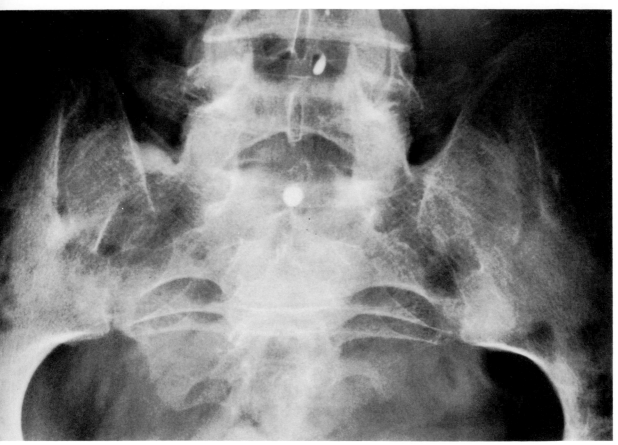

E7–8B.

E7–8. Even though a straight AP view of normal sacroiliac joints may result in a mistaken impression of arthritis, no semblance of a joint can be deciphered in the lower third of the joints seen in this example. Oblique views verified inflammatory destruction of these synovial joints and substantiated the suspicion of *spondylitis.* The hip seems at first glance to have suffered the changes of rheumatoid arthritis, with uniform joint space narrowing. About 50 per cent of patients with *ankylosing spondylitis* will develop symptoms of peripheral joint involvement; the shoulders and hips are the areas most frequently affected. Half of *these patients* will progress to chronic changes that can be seen radiographi-cally. Since the pathologic changes in ankylosing spondylitis begin with osteitis and progress to fibrosis and new bone formation, it is not surprising that ultimately a distinction may be made between the two entities.

Absence of proliferative bone characterizes the inflammatory joint disease of rheumatoid arthritis, but in ankylosing spondylitis, a collar or rim of new bone may form around the femoral head and acetabulum as the osteitis heals, enlarging and deforming their contours. This tendency is suggested by the illustration: the superior acetabular lip is prominent, and the femoral head, instead of being round, has a wedgelike wing of new bone along the superior margin.

Chapter 8

THE ELBOW

ANATOMY

The elbow joint is composed of three bones: the humerus, the radius and the ulna. The humero-ulnar articulation permits hingelike motion only (flexion and extension) and restricts lateral movement. The radio-ulnar articulation allows pronation and supination. The joint capsule attaches to the articulating ends of the three bones, and while it would appear to enclose a relatively small space and contain a limited synovial membrane, the extension of the synovium is rather vast. It is reflected upward along with the joint capsule and covers the anterior and posterior fossae of the humerus before attaching to the epiphysis. An arthrogram obtained by injecting contrast material into the joint capsule demonstrates the extent of these upward reflections (Fig. 8-1).

Between the synovial membrane and the capsule are three fat pads which fill the fossae of the distal humerus. The posterior fat pad is the largest and is pressed into the olecranon groove by the triceps tendon. Because of its recessed position it is hidden on a film of a normal elbow. Two smaller anterior fat pads lie in the coronoid and radial fossae. On a lateral film they are superimposed upon each other and appear as a single triangular radiolucency just above the humeral epicondyle. There is a large bursa posterior to the olecranon; like the prepatellar bursa in the knee, it does not communicate with the joint space.

ABNORMALITIES OF SOFT TISSUE

Abnormalities of the soft tissue of the elbow fall into the same categories as other regions of the body previously discussed. Therefore, soft tissue swelling and wasting as well as localized lumps and calcific deposits must be searched for. In addition, the peculiar anatomy of the elbow provides soft tissue signs of effusion unique to this joint and invaluable as a diagnostic aid to the clinician.

SUBCUTANEOUS NODULES

Palpable masses around the elbow are most frequently rheumatoid nodules or gouty tophi, although these may be simulated by infectious processes and other inflammatory nodules. There are specific characteristics that are revealed on films which may distinguish these pathologic processes from one another despite their similar clinical appearances.

Rheumatoid Arthritis. Rheumatoid nodules occur in approximately 25 per cent of patients with rheumatoid arthritis. They develop in the para-articular subcutaneous tissue and in the elbow are seen adjacent to the olecranon process and along the proximal extensor surface of the forearm. The frequency of this location attests to the likelihood that repetitive pressure phenomena or microtraumata, contributing to a localized vasculitis, underlie the pathology of rheumatoid nodules.

The nodules are usually discrete, well-circumscribed, painless masses which occasionally grow to a diameter of several centimeters. Rarely they are multicentric. Although movable, they are not encapsulated and hence blend into the surrounding tissue. When they are subperiosteal rather than subcutaneous, they are fixed to palpation and may rarely cause pressure erosions of the underlying bony cortex.

Figure 8–2 illustrates the two common sites of soft tissue changes in patients with rheumatoid arthritis: the outline of

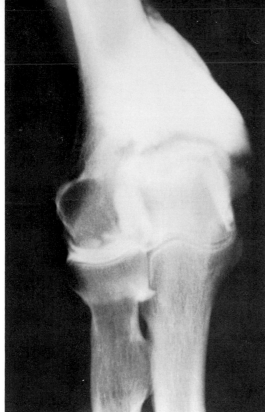

Figure 8–1. Normal elbow arthrogram. Contrast material outlines the extent of the joint capsule, demonstrating its downward reflection over the head of the radius and its extensive upward reflection enclosing the radial and coronoid fossae anteriorly and the olecranon groove posteriorly.

A

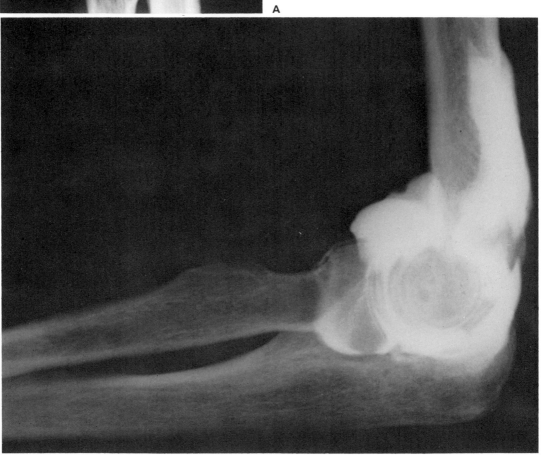

B

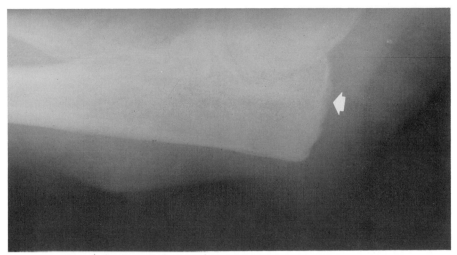

Figure 8–2.   Rheumatoid Nodules
The typical location and appearance of rheumatoid nodules can be seen as discrete masses adjacent to the olecranon process and along the proximal extensor surface of the forearm. Irregularity of the bone (arrow) attests to the inflammatory bursitis.

the elbow is distorted by a mass in the olecranon bursa, and a rheumatoid nodule is present along the extensor surface of the forearm. The irregular rough posterior margin of the olecranon process (arrow) indicates an associated bursitis with its accompanying erosions of the adjacent bone.

Gout.   There are three helpful signs that differentiate a gouty tophus from a rheumatoid nodule. (1) The nodules are rarely as discrete or distinct from the surrounding soft tissues as rheumatoid nodules. (2) Where sufficient calcium urate is present, the increased density of the tophus delineates it from the adjacent soft tissue, whereas, radiographically a rheumatoid nodule is always of water density. (3) Tophi often produce adjacent bony erosion and stimulate new bone formation, and so the contiguity of a sharply marginated erosion with a soft tissue mass typifies the picture of gout. *Rheumatoid nodules,* on the other hand, rarely produce contiguous erosions. Bone destruction is limited to the synovium-lined capsule and bursa and therefore is not associated with an adjacent soft tissue nodule. In long-standing gout the destructive lesions are not limited to the para-articular area but also involve the joint itself, and therefore look similar to rheumatoid arthritis. In this situation, the most revealing radiographic sign of gout is an increased density of the associated nodules from their calcium content. Since gout and rheumatoid arthritis rarely coexist, the usefulness of these two criteria — calcium within the mass and an erosion that is contiguous with it — becomes apparent in distinguishing the two diseases.

Two of the three signs of a gouty tophus are seen in Figure 8–3. The nonhomogeneity of the mass that fills and distends the olecranon bursa indicates the presence of calcium urate. The erosion of the olecranon is sharply circumscribed and is associated with new bone proliferation. A radiolucent defect adjacent to the erosion suggests a tophus within the bone itself (arrow). The subchondral extension of pannus in rheumatoid arthritis may result in an identical finding; therefore, the presence of this cystic bony lesion is not helpful in separating the two entities.

Figure 8–4 shows all of the characteristic signs of chronic tophaceous gout: (1) A poorly circumscribed mass distorts the soft tissues and extends along the posterior humerus, filling the olecranon bursa and widening the subcutaneous tissues of the extensor surface of the forearm. (2)

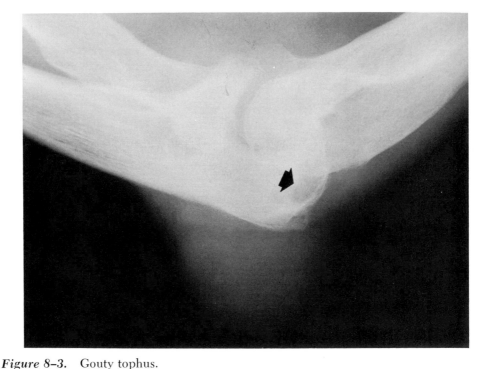

Figure 8–3. Gouty tophus.

Massive distention of the olecranon bursa with a density slightly more than the surrounding soft tissues indicates the presence of calcium within a gouty tophus. Erosion of the posterior olecranon as seen here is a frequent finding in chronic tophaceous gout when the olecranon bursa is involved. A radiolucent defect within the olecranon reflects an intraosseous tophus (arrow).

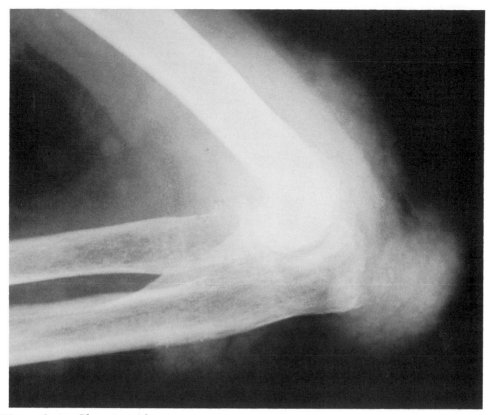

Figure 8–4. Chronic tophaceous gout.
Tophi are less well circumscribed than rheumatoid nodules; they often contain calcium; and they are frequently associated with adjacent bony erosions. All of these distinguishing characteristics can be seen in this patient with a history of gout since the age of 18.

The nonhomogeneous increased density of the nodular mass indicates the presence of calcium. (3) The erosion of the posterior olecranon is contiguous with the tophus.

Capsular Distention

The joint capsule is lined by a thin synovial membrane. Between it and the capsule wall lie the three fat pads that fill the radial, coronoid and olecranon fossae. These radiolucent structures demarcate the extent of the capsule that would otherwise fade imperceptibly into the surrounding shadows of the water-density muscles and tendons. As the capsule distends with fluid, the two anterior fat pads are elevated out of their fossae. The posterior fat pad, normally obscured by the lateral projections of the posterior humerus, is also pushed out of its groove and thus becomes visible. The fat pads therefore provide a valuable sign by which capsular distention may be detected.

Proliferation of the synovium or the presence of blood within the joint space has precisely the same effect on the fat pads as does distention with synovial fluid. The "fat pad" sign resulting from a hemarthrosis is well recognized by orthopedic surgeons, who rely on it as a clue to what might otherwise be an undetected fracture of the elbow. It is less frequently recognized in association with inflammatory arthritides because fat becomes edematous when inflamed, and its radiolucent shadow is obliterated.

Trauma. Without the telltale sign of the fat pads, the lateral projection of an elbow gives no clue to the major trauma that has been inflicted on it (Fig. 8–5A).

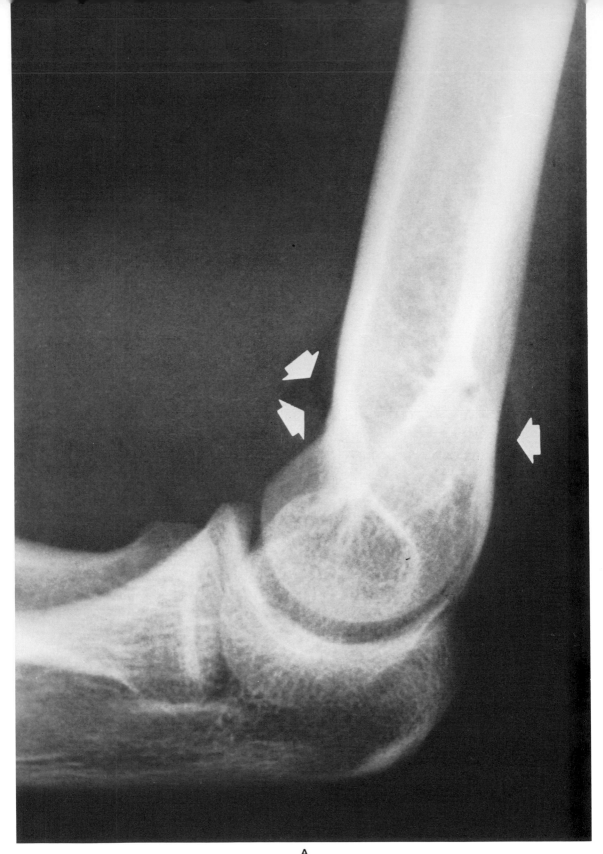

A

Figure 8–5. See legend on opposite page.

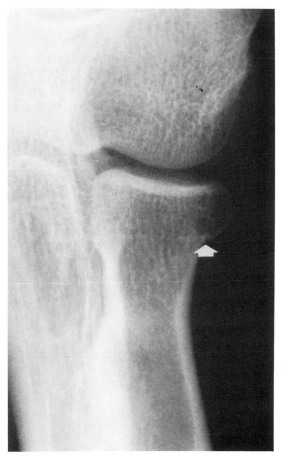

B

Figure 8–5. The fat pad sign in trauma.
A. Elevation of the anterior fat pads out of their radial and coronoid fossae and displacement of the posterior fat pad from the olecranon groove indicate abnormal distention of the joint capsule (arrows).
B. Two weeks following trauma, the vertical hairline fracture of the radial head is visible (arrow).

However, the posterior fat pad is visible, and the triangular anterior pads have been lifted out of their fossae by the accumulation of blood within the joint capsule. The hairline vertical fracture of the radial head is revealed on a film taken two weeks after the trauma (Fig. 8–5B, arrow), when enough demineralization has taken place to delineate it.

The head of the radius is a notoriously difficult area in which to discover a fresh fracture. The consistent value of the fat pad sign in revealing the extent of trauma suggests this as the location of a fracture if none other can be found in an adult.

As in this case, films obtained after demineralization has occurred generally reveal the fracture line. In children, the supracondylar area of the humerus is the most frequent location of an occult elbow fracture, and the abnormally situated fat pads may confirm a suspicion of extensive trauma. These nondisplaced fractures would remain unsuspected were it not for the useful fat pad sign.

Rheumatoid Arthritis. Elevation of the fat pads is frequently seen in rheumatoid arthritis when it involves the elbow and may result from an early effusion or from a later synovial proliferation.

The fat pad sign, in conjunction with demineralization of the juxta-articular bones, indicates radiographically the presence of an inflamed joint. This is seen in a patient with rheumatoid arthritis (Fig. 8–6). The irregularity of the posterior olecranon implicates the bursa as an additional site of involvement by this arthritis.

A second example of rheumatoid arthritis demonstrates the change in the position of the fat pads following the onset of acute inflammatory involvement of the elbow. The intial film (Fig. 8–7A) shows the anterior fat pads snug in their fossae and does not show the posterior fat pad. A later film (Fig. 8–7B) demonstrates elevation of the anterior fat pads and sig-nals the presence of a flare up of the arthritis. During the interval since the first film the inflammatory involvement of the olecranon bursa has left a permanent mark on the olecranon, an irregular erosion altering its posterior border.

Pyogenic Arthritis. Infection is less likely than trauma or rheumatoid arthritis to produce a positive fat pad sign because early edema renders these structures indistinguishable from the surrounding water-density soft tissues. Occasionally, early in the course of a pyarthrosis the fat pads will not be obliterated, and the presence of an effusion may be easily discernible.

A 15 year old girl with gonococcal arthritis (Fig. 8–8) had such pronounced

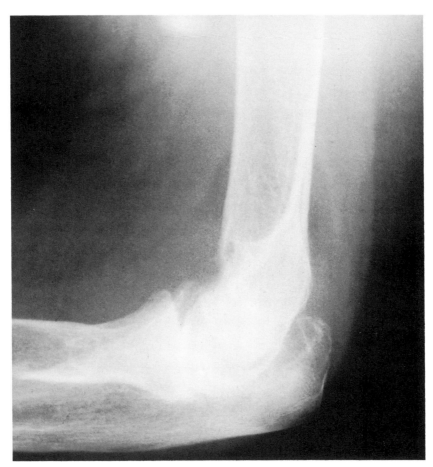

Figure 8–6. Rheumatoid arthritis.
Elevation of the anterior and posterior fat pads due to capsular distention is commonly seen in rheumatoid arthritis. Narrowing of the joint space attests to the chronicity of the involvement.

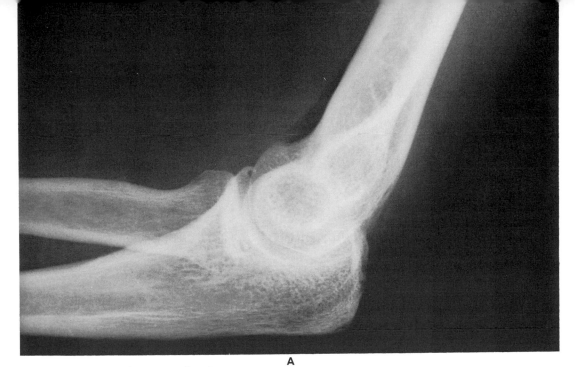

A

Figure 8–7. Rheumatoid arthritis.

A. The normal appearance of the fat pads on a lateral view is illustrated.

B. Onset of inflammation has caused a joint effusion, lifting the anterior fat pads from their fossae. Involvement of the olecranon bursa has resulted in a shallow erosion of the posterior olecranon.

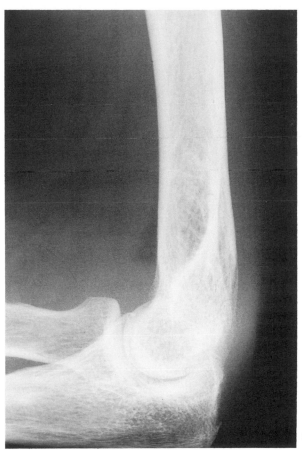

B

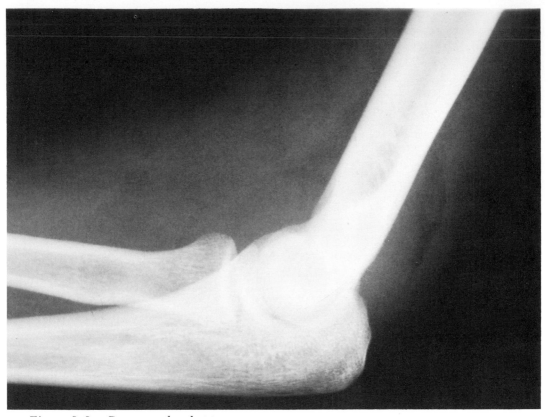

Figure 8–8. Gonococcal arthritis.
A massive joint effusion has displaced the anterior fat pads upward and the posterior fat pad away from the margin of the humerus.

capsular distension that the posterior fat pad was not only visible but was actually elevated upward! Arthrocentesis demonstrated a serous effusion with no detectable organisms by gram stain or culture. Serous pyarthroses occur in certain phases of gonococcal arthritis, and the organism responsible is notoriously difficult to culture.

Soft Tissue Calcification

The type and location of soft tissue calcification of the elbow is similar to that of the knee, and its presence has the same diagnostic usefulness in separating the arthritides. It is necessary, as in the other regions of the body, to determine first which anatomic structure is calcified. Only then does its significance become apparent.

Subcutaneous calcification

Progressive Systemic Sclerosis. The presence of dystrophic calcification in the subcutaneous tissues and the absence of associated joint destruction characterize the radiographic picture of scleroderma (Fig. 8–9). The anatomic position of the calcium is easily assessed because of its superficial location just under the skin. Clinically, this shallow location allows the white calcium deposits to be visible through the skin, and they mimic the appearance of gouty tophi. Radiographically, the absence of an associated noncalcified component to the mass easily distinguishes the two conditions.

Calcinosis Circumscripta. An unusual example of a subcutaneous calcification is included for two reasons. It demonstrates the anatomic location of the olecranon bursa, and it also cautions against assuming that amorphous calcifications bespeak an underlying connective tissue disorder (Fig. 8–10). Thorough evaluation of this patient for scleroderma and systemic lupus erythematosus was undertaken because of the radiographic findings, but evidence for

318

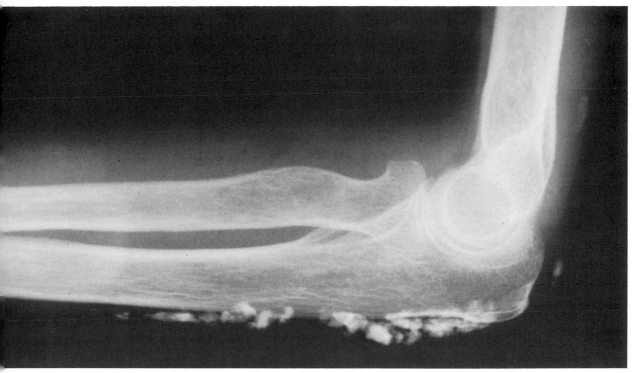

Figure 8–9. Progressive systemic sclerosis.
The subcutaneous location of calcium deposits is characteristic of scleroderma. The elbow is a frequent site of involvement.

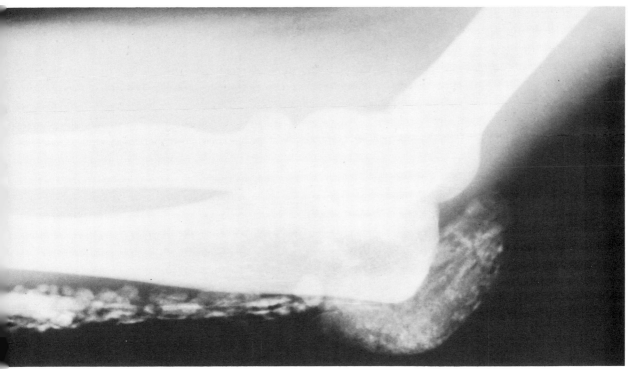

Figure 8–10. Calcinosis circumscripta.
Massive deposits of calcium along the extensor surface of the forearm and within the olecranon bursa were an isolated abnormality in this patient. Although the appearance and location were identical to scleroderma, there was no evidence of any systemic disease.

both of these diseases was unsubstantiated. The condition was thus given the descriptive label calcinosis circumscripta. Similar involvement of multiple areas of the body in the absence of any systemic disorder is appropriately labeled calcinosis universalis. The appearance of the abnormal subcutaneous calcific deposits is sufficiently suggestive of progressive systemic sclerosis that clinical evaluation should be undertaken when it is seen on a film.

CALCIFICATION OF MUSCLE

Dermatomyositis. The radiographic appearance of calcification in dermatomyositis is easily distinguished from that of scleroderma by its presence in the muscles, deep to the subcutaneous layers (Fig. 8–11). Soft tissue wasting accompanies the severe calcification in this patient, and the abnormal alignment of the bones is attributable to severe contractures. Osteoporosis accompanies the muscular changes and is caused partly by disuse and partly by chronic adrenocorticosteroid administration.

CALCIFICATION OF TOPHI

Gout. Although the severe joint destruction and fat pad elevation might be that of a patient with rheumatoid arthritis, the soft tissue changes seen in Figure 8–12A are far out of proportion to those found in this disease: they are typical of severe tophaceous gout. Even the olecranon erosion has the overhanging edge, typifying the proliferative osseous changes produced in gouty arthritis.

Three years later, the irregular, nonuniform destruction of the joint and the deposition of calcium within the soft tissue mass further distinguish this picture from that of rheumatoid arthritis (Fig. 8–12B). The tophus within the olecranon bursa has disappeared in the interim, leaving only the bony erosion as a permanent sign of previous involvement.

CALCIFICATION OF NERVES

Leprosy. This example of soft tissue calcification is included not because it demonstrates the presence of arthritis but because its localization outlines an anatomic structure not previously demon-

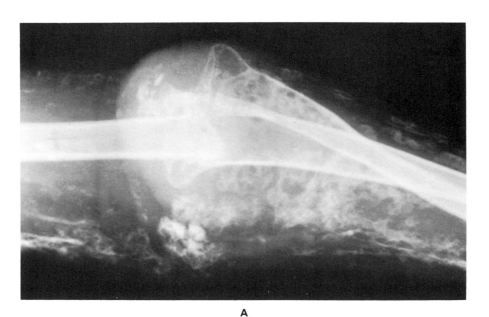

A

Figure 8–11. Dermatomyositis.

A. Extensive calcification of the soft tissues, diffuse osteoporosis, and subluxation of the forearm on the humerus illustrate the end stage of the juvenile onset of dermatomyositis.

B. A lateral view localizes the major portion of calcium within the muscles, deep to the subcutaneous tissue.

strated. The amorphous calcification within the soft tissues follows the path of the ulnar nerve and its branches (Fig. 8–13). The metallic markers with their radiopaque adhesive tape covers were placed at the extremes of a palpable mass in the arm of this 27 year old student from Thailand. In addition to a "lump" in his arm, this patient also complained of cutaneous anesthesia of his fourth and fifth fingers and a saucerlike skin lesion on his forearm with an anesthetic center. Although calcification of a nerve is rare, localized nerve abscesses may develop in tuberculous leprosy, and resultant dystrophic calcification has been reported as an unusual accompaniment of this disease.

Although similar in location and course, the *hollow, tubular* configuration of vascular calcification is easily distinguished from the solidly calcified nerve, as is seen in Figure 8–14.

CALCIFICATION WITHIN THE CAPSULE

Trauma. The elbow may develop peri-articular calcification in the muscles, tendon and capsule following repeated bouts of trauma. It is a hazard of tennis players, golfers and pitchers; and Little Leaguers are advised not to throw curve balls to avoid the sequelae of a traumatic arthritis following avulsion of the medial epicondyle. Loose bodies may form within the joint capsule (osteochondromatosis) or from fragments of bone that separate from the epiphysis (e.g., in osteochondrosis dissecans or avulsion fractures).

Calcification is present adjacent to the

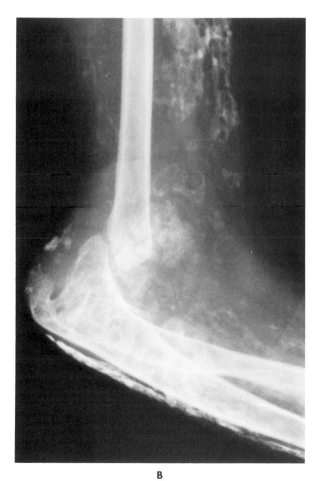

B

Figure 8–11. Continued.

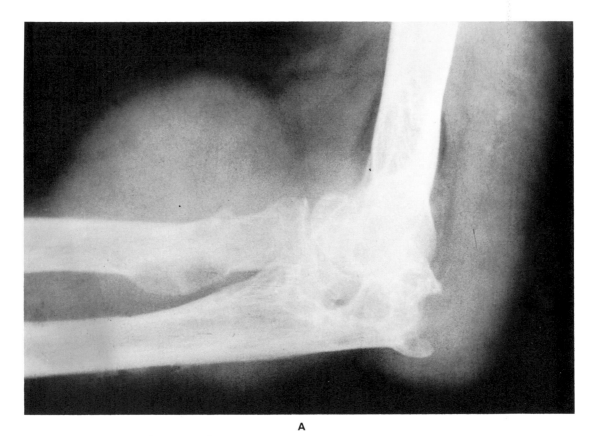

A

Figure 8–12. Chronic tophaceous gout.

A. In addition to grotesque distortion of the soft tissues by tophi, distention of the capsule is signaled by the fat pad sign. Involvement of the olecranon bursa is apparent from the soft tissue distention as well as the adjacent olecranon erosion with the typical overhanging edge.

B. Three years later severe destructive changes of the joint are seen. Multiple erosions demarcated by bony sclerosis have caused the articular ends of the bones to have a mottled appearance. The tophus within the olecranon bursa has disappeared, leaving only the telltale bone erosion. Extensive deposition of calcium within the remaining tophi has occurred, giving the soft tissues the characteristic appearance of long-standing gout.

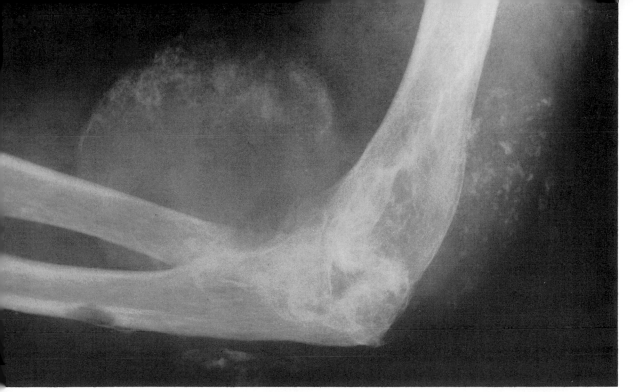

Figure 8–12. Continued.   **B**

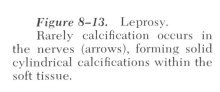

Figure 8–13. Leprosy.
Rarely calcification occurs in the nerves (arrows), forming solid cylindrical calcifications within the soft tissue.

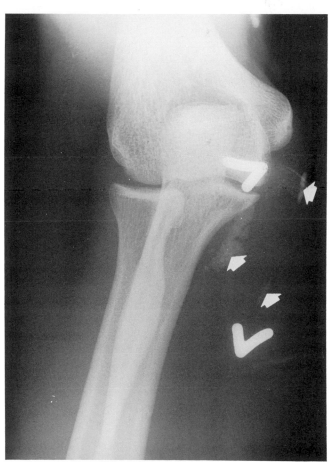

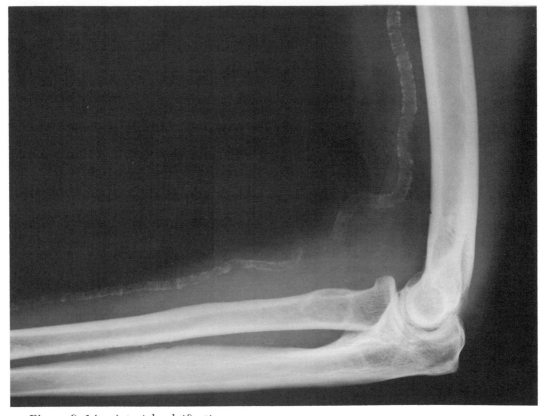

Figure 8–14. Arterial calcification.
The hollow tubular configuration of vascular calcification is easily distinguished from the solid collections within nerves.

radial head in the region of the capsule (Fig. 8–15A). Its structured appearance indicates the formation of trabeculae and cortex, and hence it is more appropriately designated ossification. This bony structure is more clearly seen on the anterior view (Fig. 8–15B), where it simulates a deformed radial head. The loose body lies above the lateral epicondyle (arrow). The joint space is narrowed asymmetrically along the radial side. Osteoarthritis of the elbow, unlike the hand, is rare, and is always secondary to trauma.

CALCIFICATION OF CARTILAGE

Hyperparathyroidism. The hyaline cartilage that covers the articular ends of the bones may become calcified in any condition that results in the deposition of calcium pyrophosphate crystals (see section in Chapter 1 on chondrocalcinosis). When such deposition occurs in the elbow, it is most commonly associated with hyperparathyroidism or pseudogout, and in both diseases the joint itself is normal.

Extensive calcification of the cartilage is seen in a patient with hyperparathyroidism (Fig. 8–16A). Its thin sharp line parallels the lateral condyle of the humerus and the edge of the radial head on the lateral view. On the anterior view (Fig. 8–16B), the calcification outlines the entire margin of the humerus and the coronoid process of the ulna.

Figure 8–15. Traumatic arthritis.

A. A large soft tissue ossification is seen adjacent to the radial head.

B. Asymmetric joint space narrowing is typical of degenerative joint disease and is evident on the side of the soft tissue ossifications, between the radius and distal humerus. A loose body is present superior to the lateral epicondyle (arrow).

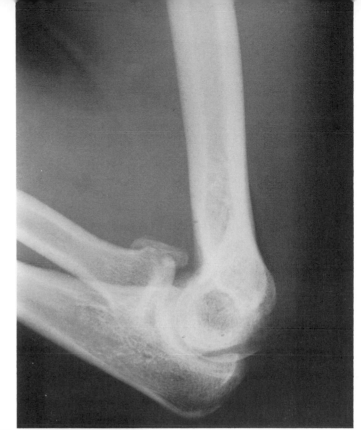

A

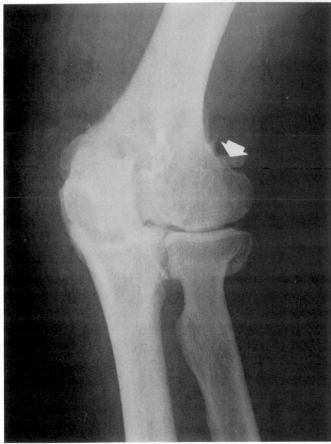

B

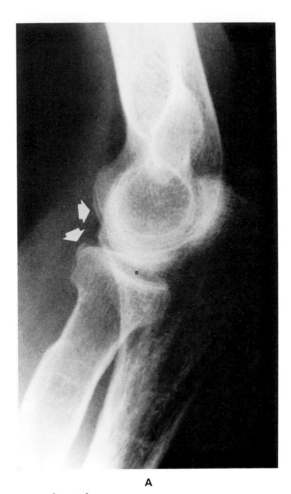

A

Figure 8–16. Hyperparathyroidism.
Extensive chondrocalcinosis outlines the hyaline articular cartilage of the humerus, radius and ulna (arrows).

Illustration continued on opposite page.

ABNORMALITIES OF ALIGNMENT

Normally the forearm makes an angle of approximately 170 degrees with the humerus, deviating slightly laterally. Medial deviation (cubitus varus) and lateral deviation (cubitus valgus) of the forearm may result from a variety of conditions. Trauma, connective tissue diseases, infections and neuropathic diseases are the most common culprits.

Dislocation may also occur at the elbow joint. The forearm is generally displaced posteriorly and, therefore, on a lateral projection the humerus is seen to lie anterior to the ulna.

Traumatic Dislocation. Traumatic dislocations, frequently from a fall on the outstretched arm, result in the typical deformity seen in Figure 8–17A. Considerable damage to the joint capsule, ligaments and tendons must occur to allow this degree of dislocation.

A film taken six weeks after the injury shows complete restoration of the normal bony relationships following closed reduction (Fig. 8–17B). The development of calcification in the soft tissues is related to the trauma. These calcified tissues are not dissimilar in appearance to

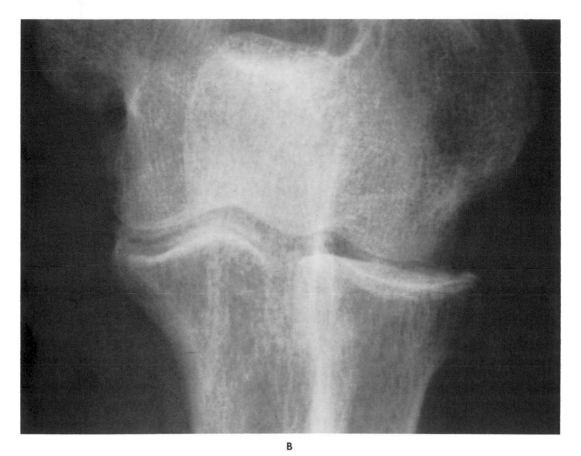

B

Figure 8–16. Continued.
As so often occurs in hyperparathyroidism associated with calcified cartilage, the bony mineralization appears normal and does not reveal the abnormal calcium metabolism (*A* and *B*).

those seen in osteochondromatosis of the knee (see Figure 6–12) and differ significantly from the amorphous calcifications occurring in scleroderma and dermatomyositis. The presence of trabeculae in these soft tissue masses indicates their bony nature. In the muscles, ossification secondary to hemorrhage is called myositis ossificans. Technically this term refers to a rare genetic disease characterized by microdactyly and progressive ossification of fibrous structures related to muscle (fibrodysplasia ossificans progressiva). In popular usage, it describes ossification within muscle from any cause.

Monteggia Fracture. Figure 8–18 demonstrates the difference between a forearm dislocation and a dislocation of the radius alone. In the latter, the olecranon is in a normal position and the radial head has been displaced anteriorly. The cause of this dislocation is a fracture through the ulna with overriding of the two fragments and subsequent foreshortening of the bone. Since the radius and ulna span an equal distance from the elbow to the wrist, without a concomitant fracture of the radius there must be a dislocation for this bone to fit the foreshortened space. The combination of a primary ulnar fracture with a radial dislocation is called a Monteggia fracture. Awareness of this entity is important because often the elbow is not included on a film of the forearm, and detection of the dislocation is precluded. Failure to cor-

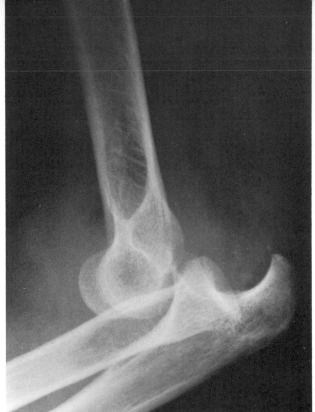

Figure 8–17. Traumatic elbow dislocation.

A. Dislocation of the elbow results in posterior displacement of both bones of the forearm.

B. A film six weeks later shows large ectopic deposits of bone. The appearance of myositis ossificans may rapidly follow an injury, as in this case. Normal restoration of the elbow joint can be seen, although a small bony fragment adjacent to the posterior olecranon suggests a chip fracture.

A

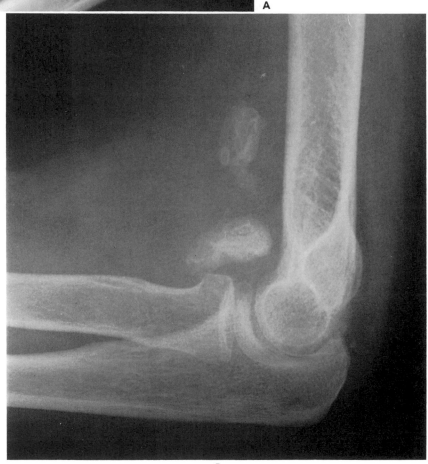

B

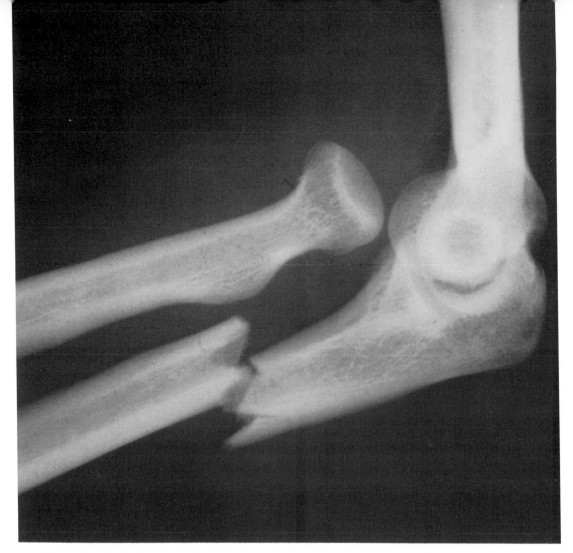

Figure 8–18. Monteggia fracture.

A fracture through the ulna is always accompanied by either fracture or dislocation of the radius when there is significant foreshortening of the forearm. The radial head is separated from the capitellum. The combination of ulnar fracture and radial head dislocation is termed a Monteggia fracture.

rect the malalignment results in permanent deformity and secondary osteoarthritis.

ABNORMALITIES OF MINERALIZATION

In general, the same signs of demineralization are looked for in the elbow as in the other regions of the body, but caution must be taken not to misread signs of osteoporosis or osteomalacia in a normal patient when interpreting this joint. The sparsity of trabeculae in the proximal radius and the coarsened appearance of the spongiosa of the distal humerus are normal and do not signal a metabolic abnormality.

Pyogenic Arthritis. A second example of gonococcal arthritis in the elbow of a young girl (Fig. 8–19A) differs from that shown in Figure 8–8 in three ways. There is loss of the sharp white defining margin of the distal humerus and the coronoid process of the ulna. The joint space is irregularly narrowed. In addition, there is periosteal new bone along the distal humerus and proximal radius, beginning at the point of capsular attachment (arrow). As in the previous example of gonococcal arthritis, there is elevation of the anterior fat pads and visualization of the posterior fat pad, indicating the presence of a joint effusion (Fig. 8–19B). The fact that the fat pads are still of radiolucent density and have not been visually obliterated by edema is unusual in an infectious arthritis, but re-

emphasizes the fact that a positive "fat pad sign" may be seen in any condition that results in distention of the joint capsule.

Arthrocentesis verified the presence of pyogenic fluid, accounting for the acute demineralization and periosteal new bone so characteristic of bacterial infection. There is considerable evidence of cartilage destruction as seen by the joint space narrowing, despite the fact that this film was taken only one week after the onset of symptoms. It dramatizes the necessity for early diagnosis and treatment of pyogenic infection to preserve a functioning joint.

Coccidioidomycosis. A second ex-

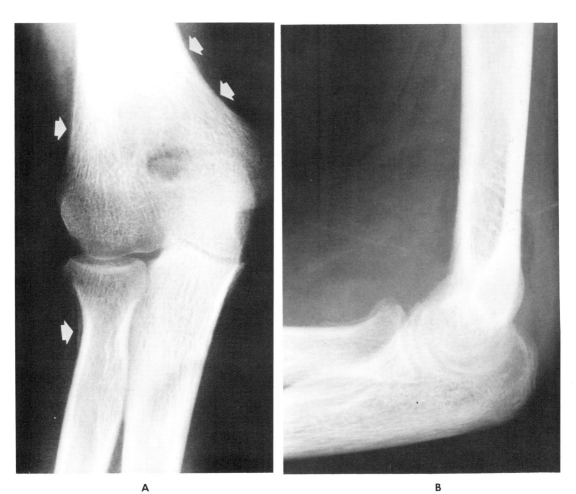

A   B

Figure 8–19. Gonococcal arthritis.

A. Joint space narrowing, loss of the sharp cortical margin and periosteal new bone (arrows) suggest an inflammatory arthritis.

B. Distention of the joint capsule by an effusion is demonstrated by the positive fat pad sign.

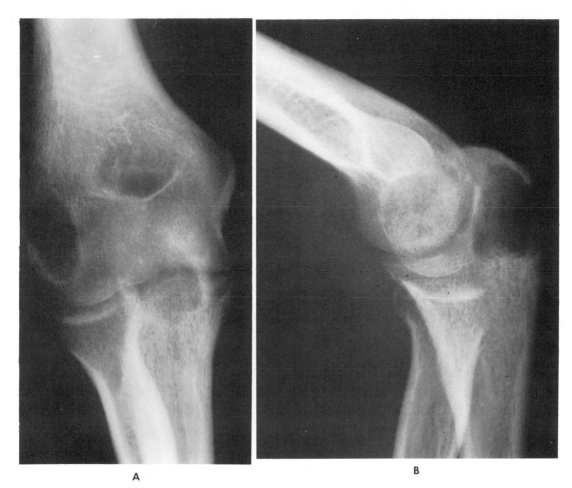

A   B

Figure 8–20. Coccidioidomycosis osteomyelitis.
Λ. A large, well-circumscribed intraosseous granuloma is present in the distal humerus.
B. A second granuloma, in the olecranon, is better seen on the lateral view. Demineralization of the articular bones indicates an arthritis as well as an osteomyelitis. Only minimal joint space narrowing is seen, typical of the slow destructive changes of granulomatous infections.

ample of juxta-articular demineralization is seen in a patient with disseminated coccidioidomycosis involving both bone and joint (Fig. 8–20). These films were taken three years after the diagnosis of pulmonary infection was made and treatment with amphotericin B instituted; the patient died soon after. The fuzzy, out-of-focus appearance of the ends of the bones indicates demineralization and loss of trabeculae. Despite the long history of joint involvement, the cartilage space is only minimally narrowed. This is characteristic of granulomatous infections. The well-circumscribed holes in the olecranon and lateral epicondyle of the hu-

merus define the *intra-osseous granulomas,* and their appearance is typical of this low-grade infection.

ABNORMALITIES OF CARTILAGE SPACE

Cartilage Destruction

Any disease process that causes low-grade inflammation and synovitis with synovial proliferation will result in a progression of changes beginning with destruction of the cartilage and marginal

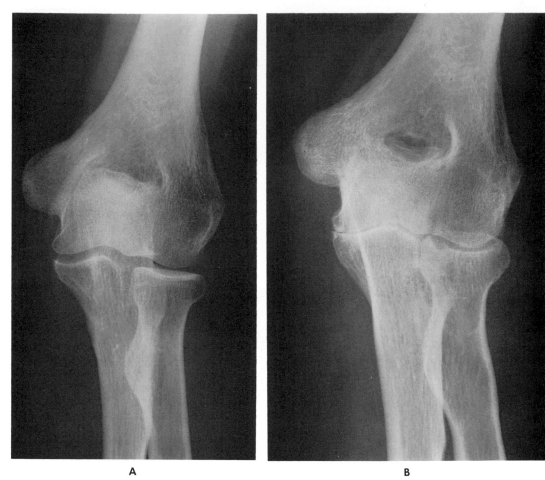

A   **B**

Figure 8–21. Rheumatoid arthritis.
A and B. Two films of the same elbow demonstrate the development of uniform joint space narrowing. The thin flange of bone along the radial side of the humerus should not be confused with periostitis.

erosion of the underlying bone. Subsequently, the entire joint space may be destroyed, and extensive changes of the denuded articulating bones may occur. Therefore, tuberculosis, coccidioidomycosis, blastomycosis, rheumatoid arthritis and hemophilia may produce identical radiographic abnormalities, and only correlation with history and laboratory data will permit correct diagnosis. The following series of patients with rheumatoid arthritis has been chosen to demonstrate the progressive changes that may occur in the joint space of an elbow.

Rheumatoid Arthritis. The earliest evidence of inflammatory involvement of the elbow is the presence of an effusion

and juxta-articular demineralization. In rheumatoid arthritis, cartilage tends to be destroyed uniformly, and narrowing of the entire joint results. Two films demonstrate the progression of changes that are so typical of this disease (Fig. 8–21A and B). A lateral view taken simultaneously with the later study (Fig. 8–21C) shows how difficult it is to detect narrowing in this projection. The fat pad sign is readily seen on the lateral view, however, and indicates the extent of capsular distention.

Identical findings are present in this patient's opposite elbow: uniform narrowing of the joint space and elevation of the anterior fat pad (Fig. 8–22). Symmetrical involvement of joints is typical of

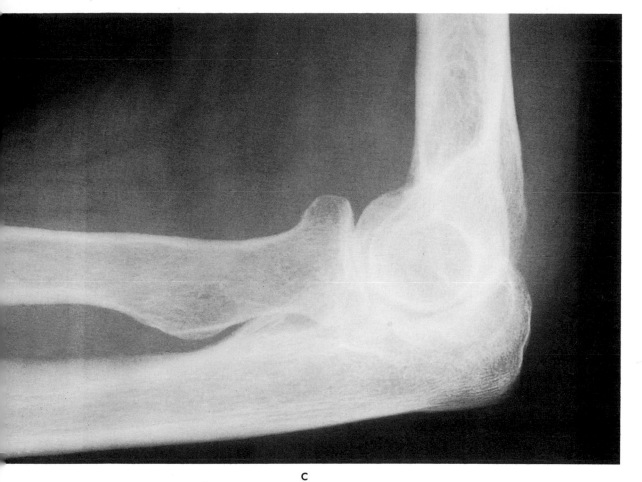

C

Figure 8–21. Continued.
    C. Joint narrowing is difficult to detect on a lateral view of the elbow. A fat pad sign indicates distention of the joint capsule.

rheumatoid arthritis and extremely un-usual in the other conditions causing joint destruction (e.g. infection), a helpful fact in pinpointing a precise diagnosis.

As the synovium erodes the margins of the bones, irregularity in the cortex de-velops (Fig. 8–23). When this is com-bined with bony demineralization, as in this patient with rheumatoid arthritis, the sharp white cortical outline disappears.

Erosions and subchondral cysts may be the most prominent findings in rheuma-toid arthritis, and cartilage destruction may be less dramatic, as in Figure 8–24. However, where this is the case it is wise to consider such other diagnostic possi-bilities as tuberculosis and the fungal in-fections. The large cystic erosion of the ulna (Fig. 8–24B, arrow) indicates the ex-tent of synovial proliferation and illus-trates the mechanism by which severe destruction of a joint occurs.

The end result of a destructive arthritis in the elbow may be such extensive ero-sions and bone resorption that widening of the joint space and subluxation occur. At this stage, all of the arthritides may look identical, and no distinguishing fea-tures are present to implicate a specific disease. Figure 8–25 is an example of these changes in a patient with rheuma-toid arthritis. Identical radiographs, how-ever, have been seen in tuberculosis, blastomycosis and coccidioidomycosis.

Coccidioidomycosis. To demonstrate the similarity of changes that may be seen in all of the inflammatory arthri-tides, coccidioidomycosis of the elbow

Text continued on page 337.

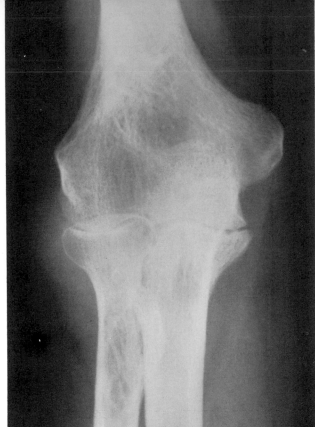

Figure 8-22. Rheumatoid arthritis.

A. Uniform narrowing of the joint space and absence of secondary degenerative changes are characteristic of the pathologic alterations of rheumatoid arthritis.

B. The fat pad sign is frequently seen in rheumatoid arthritis. Elevation of the anterior fat pads can be seen as a sail-like shadow.

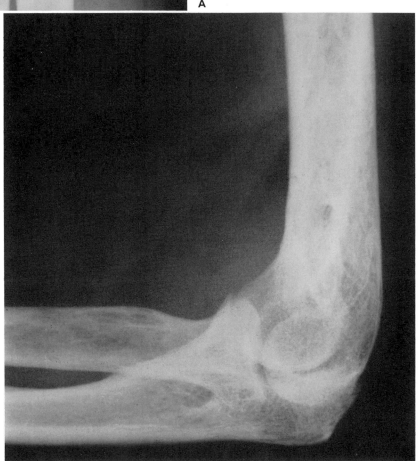

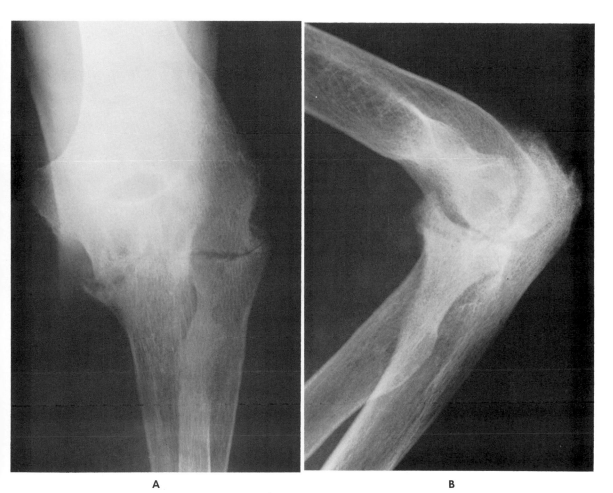

A   B

Figure 8-23. Rheumatoid arthritis.
Synovial proliferation has caused destruction of the cartilage and the articular bone, leaving in its wake a narrowed joint with irregular margins of bone.

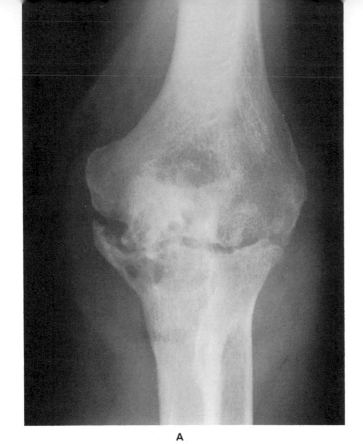

A

Figure 8–24. Rheumatoid arthritis.

A. Bony erosions and subchondral cysts may sometimes be a more prominent feature than cartilage destruction. Other causes of synovial proliferation, such as granulomatous diseases and hemophilia, must in such cases be considered as diagnostic possibilities.

B. A large radiolucency completely surrounded by bone is present in the ulna (arrow); it represents a subchondral cyst.

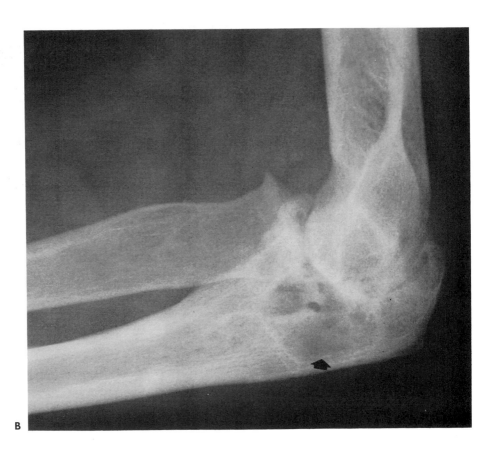

B

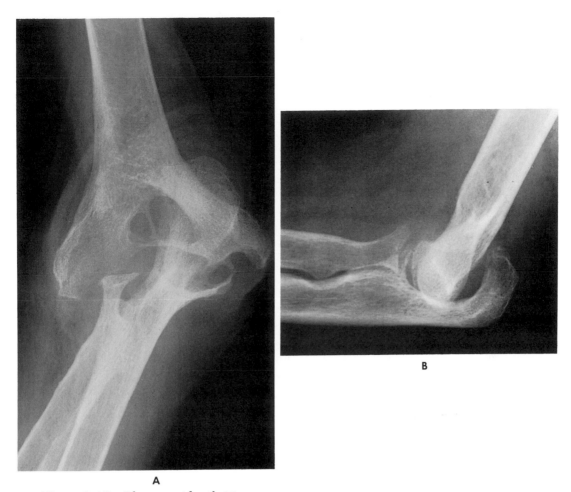

Figure 8-25. Rheumatoid arthritis.
The end stage of any inflammatory arthritis may be identical to this picture. Huge erosions of the articular ends of the bones have resulted in a markedly deformed elbow.

joint in an elderly Chinese man is illustrated (Fig. 8-26). The joint widening is caused by the erosions which most severely involve the coronoid process of the ulna. Granulomatous changes of the synovium distort the soft tissues. The olecranon bursa is also involved, and irregularity of the underlying bone is apparent. The prominent flange of bone along the lateral aspect of the humerus (Fig. 8-26A) is exaggerated because of the underlying bony demineralization and does not represent periosteal new bone.

Hemophilia. Repeated episodes of intra-articular bleeding cause proliferation of synovium and erosions of the bones in a similar manner to the previously illustrated diseases.

A young patient with hemophilia illustrates these changes (Fig. 8-27). Cartilage narrowing and erosions of the articular surfaces are identical to those seen in the examples of rheumatoid arthritis. The large cystic area in the radius may be the result of either synovial proliferation beneath the cortex or intra-osseous bleeding.

Ankylosis

Any destructive inflammatory process can cause total obliteration of the joint

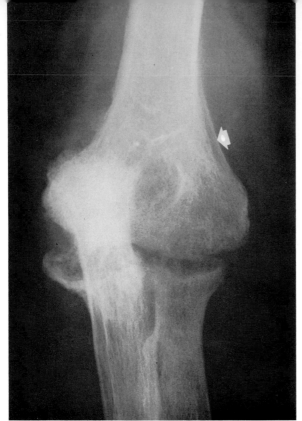

Figure 8–26. Coccidioidomycosis. Chronic granulomatous infection has resulted in synovial hypertrophy with marked distention of the soft tissues. Widening of the joint space and erosion and resorption of the articular bones are similar to the changes of rheumatoid arthritis. The normal flange of bone (arrow) is exaggerated because of the diffuse osteoporosis.

A

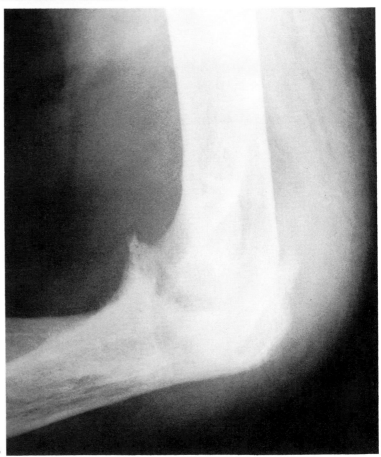

B

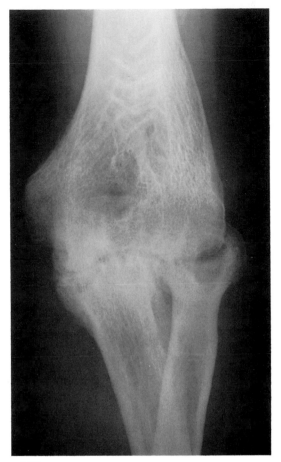

Figure 8–27. Hemophilia.
Destruction of articular cartilage with joint narrowing and erosion is similar to the pathologic changes of rheumatoid arthritis. The large cystic lesion in the radial head may represent either a subchondral cyst secondary to synovial proliferation or an intraosseous hemorrhage.

space and fusion with loss of mobility. Most commonly loss of function is from *fibrous ankylosis*; however, bony ankylosis may occasionally occur. When it occurs in a connective tissue disorder, it is most commonly associated with juvenile rheumatoid arthritis, but occasionally it is seen in the adult onset of this disease.

Juvenile Rheumatoid Arthritis. Continuous lines of trabeculae bridge the adjacent bones in the elbow of a patient with juvenile rheumatoid arthritis (Fig. 8–28). Despite total destruction of the joint, the bones are not deformed by erosions. Although it is rare, extensive erosion may occur in juvenile rheumatoid ar-

thritis. It is more common, however, to see growth disturbances alter the normal contour of the bones. The thick cartilage in the joint space of children seems to protect the articular bone from the proliferating synovium, and erosions are less common than in the adult onset of rheumatoid arthritis.

Joint Destruction and Ectopic New Bone

Neuropathic Joint. The presence of new bone in the elbow along with severe destructive joint changes is most common in the neuropathic joint. In the

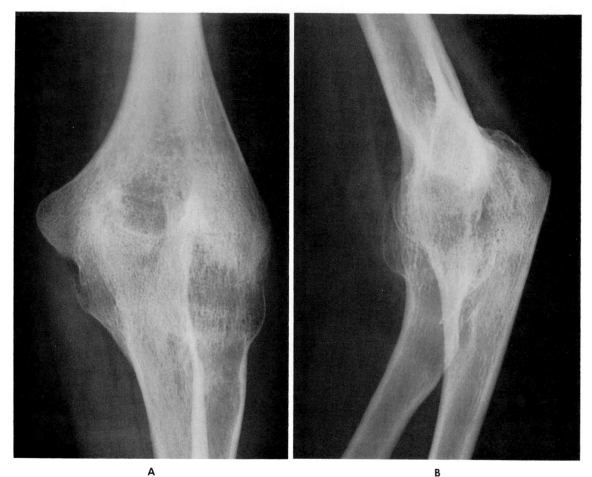

A   **B**

Figure 8–28.   Juvenile rheumatoid arthritis.
A. Bony ankylosis of the radius, ulna and humerus are apparent by the continuous lines of trabeculae and the absent cartilaginous space.
B. A slight flexion deformity distorts the appearance of the bones on the AP view but is better viewed on the lateral projection.

elbow, this is usually associated with syringomyelia. It is interesting that the characteristic changes of a neuropathic joint that occur in the weight-bearing regions of the body are also seen in the non-weight-bearing elbow. The etiologic roles of lack of proprioception and consequent abnormal stress, leading to disorganization of the joint and production of new bone within the capsule and soft tissues, must therefore be questioned, since these mechanisms are not as predominant in the elbow. The primary insult, no matter how minor, appears to initiate an unrelenting series of responses and, regardless of subsequent trauma, results in a completely disorganized joint.

Neuropathic disease of the elbow is seen in a patient with syringomyelia (Fig. 8–29A and B). There is total disorganization of the joint with subluxation of the radial head and massive new bone formation both in the soft tissues and along the articulating margins of the joint (ectopic ossification). Despite severe destructive changes the bony mineralization is normal. This is characteristic of a neuropathic arthropathy.

Figure 8–29. Charcot joint.
There is total disorganization of the joint, with subluxation of the radial head and massive new bone formation in the soft tissues and along the articulating margins of the joint. The mineralization is normal.

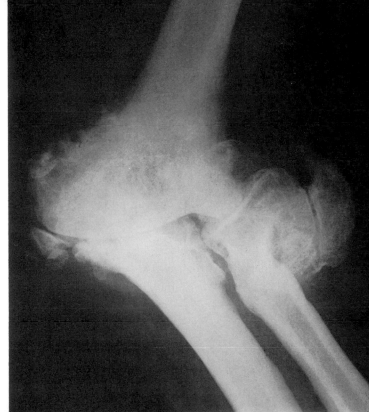

A

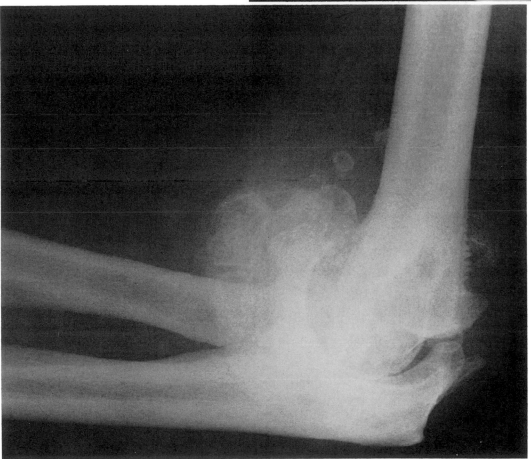

B

SUGGESTED READINGS

Brogdon, B. G., and N. E. Crow. Little Leaguer's elbow. Amer. J. Roentgen. 83:671 (1960).

Holmes, K. K., G. W. Counts, and H. N. Beaty. Disseminated gonococcal infection. Ann. Int. Med. 74:979 (1971).

Wood, K. A. Omer, and M. T. Shaw. Haemophilic arthropathy. A combined radiological and clinical study. Brit. J. Radiol. 42:498 (1969).

EXERCISES

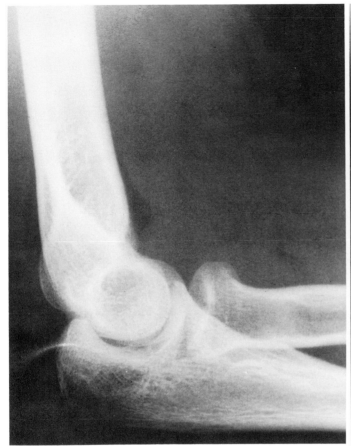

E8–1A.

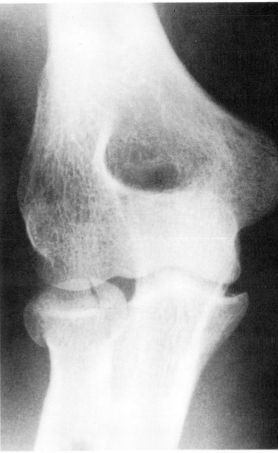

E8–1B.

E8–1. "The smallest hair throws its shadow."*

The reliability of the fat pad sign as an indicator of capsular distention is illustrated by this example. The only abnor-

---

*Goethe

mality on the lateral view is the appearance of the posterior fat pad (normally hidden) and elevation of the anterior pads from their radial and coronoid fossae. The AP view reveals the source of the trouble: a hemarthrosis from a *fractured radial head.*

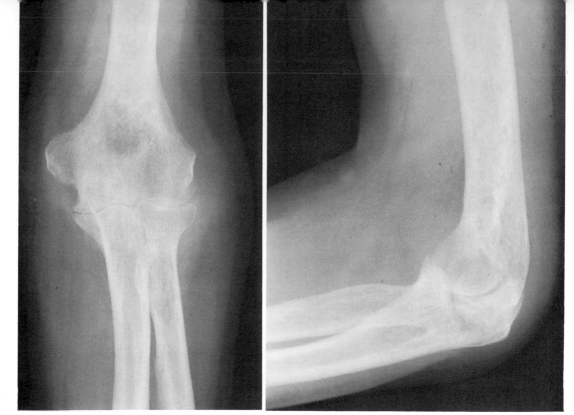

E8–2A. *E8–2B.*

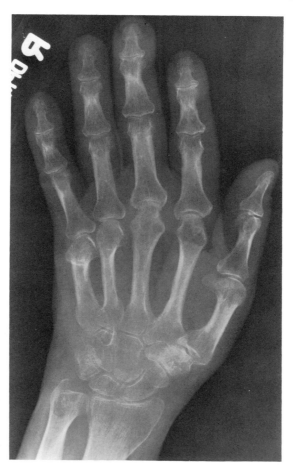

E8–2C.

344

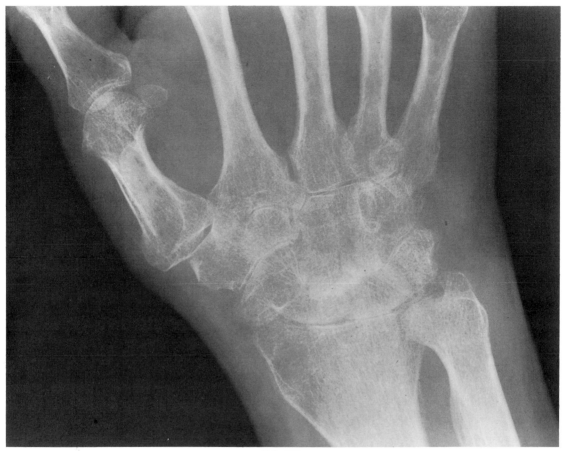

E8–2D.

E8–2. Uniform narrowing of the joint space is a dependable sign of *rheumatoid arthritis*, and when it occurs in any joint, this disease should be the primary consideration.

A film of the hand is often a helpful adjunct in verifying which arthritis one is dealing with, as the changes there tend to be more classic, unaltered by superimposed degenerative joint disease. The finding of narrowed metacarpophalangeal joints reflecting far advanced destruction is not uncommon in patients with rheumatoid arthritis and can be seen in this man's right hand (E8–2C). His left wrist illustrates involvement of all three joint spaces of the carpus (E8–2D). The distribution and pattern of destruction is so typical of rheumatoid arthritis that it is difficult to conceive of another diagnostic possibility other than a rheumatoid variant. Calcification of the fibrocartilage of the wrist occasionally is associated with rheumatoid arthritis and is present in this patient.

Although ulnar styloid erosion has often been touted as an important diagnostic criterion in the radiologic changes of rheumatoid arthritis, it frequently occurs adjacent to a tophus in gout, and as can be seen by this example, the ulnar styloid is the only area spared in this severely arthritic wrist.

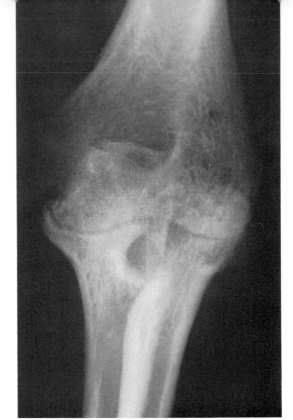

E8–3A.

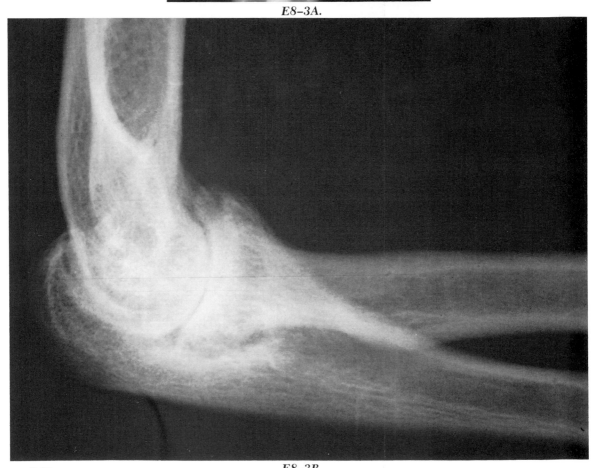

E8–3B.

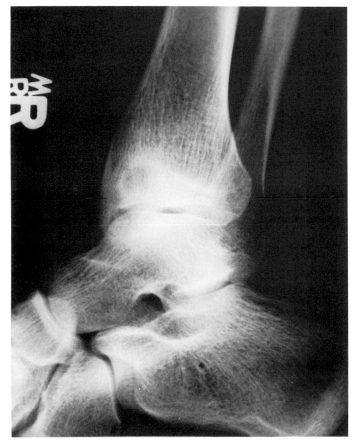

E8–3C.

E8–3. There is only one finding to distinguish this elbow from the preceding picture of rheumatoid arthritis: overgrowth of the coronoid process and the radial epiphysis. This finding suggests that the arthritis began in childhood, and the likeliest considerations to cause uniform destruction of the joint are juvenile rheumatoid arthritis and hemophilia.

The only other joint involved was this man's ankle (E8–3C). Narrowing of the tibiotalar joint and a subchondral cyst within the distal tibial epiphysis could as easily be from a patient with juvenile rheumatoid arthritis, but knowledge of this patient's long history of bleeding problems quickly established the diagnosis of *hemophilia*.

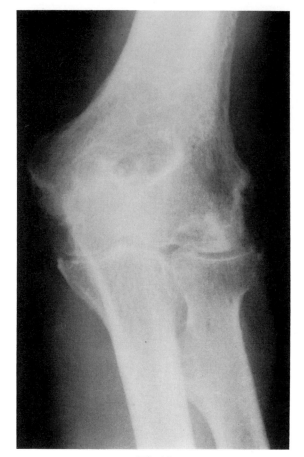

E8–4A.

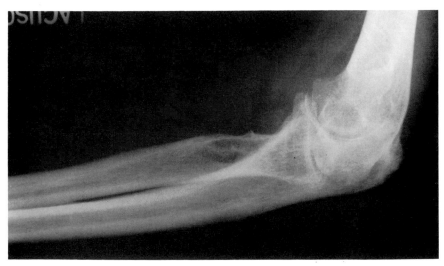

E8–4B.

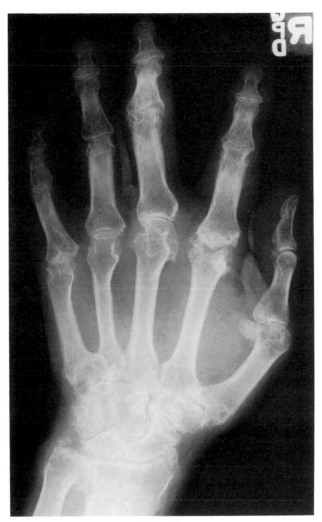

E8–4C.

E8–4. Unlike the two preceding exercises, the joint space in this example is normal in width, and the destruction is confined to the para-articular region. Sclerotic-based erosions deform all four margins of articulating bone and are typical of the proliferative bony changes of *gout.* Erosions similar in appearance may accompany a chronic granulomatous infection, and the determination of whether the patient has a monoarticular or polyarticular arthritis weights the judgment between an infectious and a metabolic problem.

The *distribution* of gouty arthritis of the joints in the hand may be identical to rheumatoid arthritis, and for this reason confusion as to the diagnosis may arise (E8–4C). The carpus and the metacar-pophalangeal joints may be involved, the ulnar styloid process eroded and the radioulnar joint destroyed. For this reason, the character of the erosions and the appearance of the joint spaces become critical. In this example, multiple joints demonstrate para-articular erosions but, if examined closely, frequently exhibit sclerotic bases, as at the fifth metacarpophalangeal joint and the base of the fifth metacarpal bone. Despite extensive involvement of the wrist, the intercarpal joint space is normal (except in the area of the eroded lesser multangular bone). Preservation of the cartilage in the presence of an extensive erosive arthritis should always make one suspicious that he is dealing not with rheumatoid arthritis but, in fact, with gout.

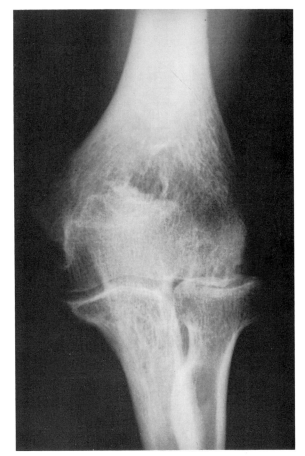

E8–5A.

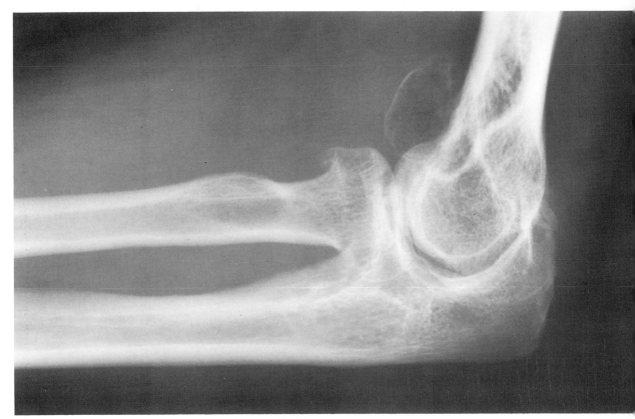

E8–5B.

E8–5. An unexplained radial palsy initiated the films of the elbow, and only after the large bony mass adjacent to the anterior humeral fossae was revealed by the lateral view was the history of a previous radial head fracture elicited from the patient.

Even without the history of earlier trauma, the appearance of the joint is that of an osteoarthritis, with asymmetric narrowing of the cartilage space and small osteophytes along the margin of articular bone signaling the underlying destroyed cartilage. It is so uncommon for the changes of *degenerative joint disease* to be seen in the non-weight-bearing elbow joint that previous trauma must always be suspected. The hemarthrosis that accompanied the radial head fracture must have resulted in a myositis ossificans and a unique cause of nerve entrapment.

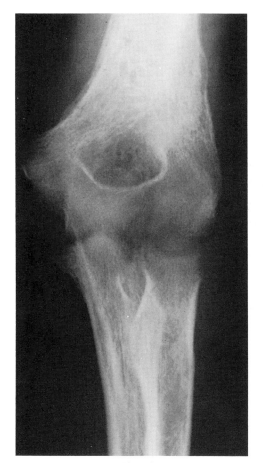

E8–6A.

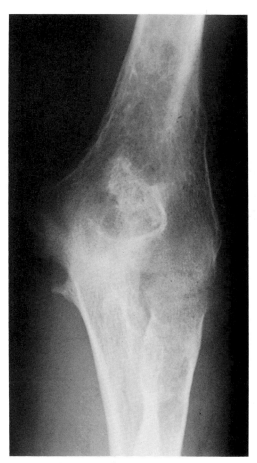

E8–6B. After synovectomy.

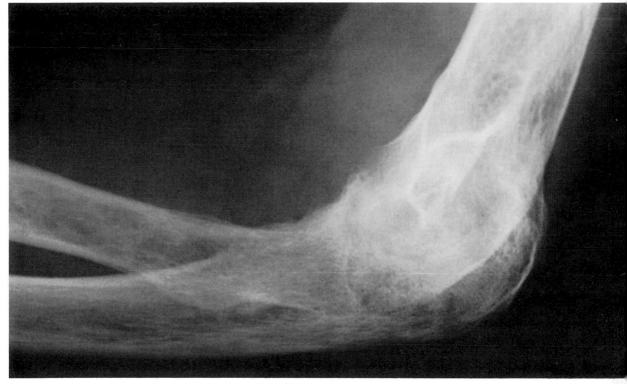

E8–6C.

E8–6. Juxta-articular demineralization, loss of the sharp cortical margins and an out-of-focus appearance of the ends of the bones reflect hyperemia and rapid bone demineralization. The narrowed joint space provides the clue that cartilage is being rapidly destroyed as well, and thus from a sterile picture the diagnosis of a bacterially contaminated joint must be suspected. Joint aspiration revealed the presence of acid fast bacilli. Despite therapy, total destruction of the joint necessitated surgical intervention and a synovectomy seven months later (Fig. 8–6B and C). Although it is unusual for such rapid destruction to be seen in *tuberculous arthritis*, a more virulent picture occasionally occurs. Examination of the synovium demonstrated classic tuberculous granulomas, verifying the initial diagnosis and reinforcing the necessity for joint aspiration in monarticular arthritis.

Chapter 9

THE SHOULDER, ACROMIOCLAVICULAR AND STERNOCLAVICULAR JOINTS

Accurate diagnosis of diseases affecting the shoulder is a challenging task. A patient with a painful shoulder is difficult to examine and position accurately for a routine AP and internal or external rotation examination. Often the study is compromised because of a sling, a "frozen shoulder" or inability to cooperate because of pain with motion. To compound the difficulties, the routine films that are generally done in radiology departments never view the cartilage space tangentially and generally yield a series of overlapping shadows of the articulating bones. Although the shoulder is subject to the same diseases and the same changes as other, previously illustrated regions, the early diagnostic clues provided by changes in the cartilage and cortical margins of bone are obscure on film. Hence disease processes invoke changes in the shoulder that are *radiographically* detectable at a much later stage.

Fortunately, the shoulder joint is rarely the primary site of polyarticular arthritis, and films of other affected joints may be relied on for diagnosis. Monarticular disease of the shoulder, such as calcific tendinitis or infectious arthritis, can be diagnosed by using a combination of information from the patient and films.

The mechanical difficulties may be obviated by a simple method of filming the patient which completely eliminates the need for movement of the shoulder and, in addition, displays the anatomic components of the shoulder far better than the routine generally employed. To evaluate the joint space, a film perpendicular to the glenoid articulation is obtained by angling the patient 20 degrees with his back against the film. Figure 9–1A illustrates the cartilage space and the articulating surfaces of bone. It is apparent that loss of cartilage and early erosions in the shoulder may be detected as easily as in the hand, the knee or the hip if this projection is obtained.

To separate the overlapping shadows of the posterior and anterior elements of the scapula, the acromion and coracoid processes, an additional view is obtained by radiographing the body of the scapula end on and the glenoid fossa en face (Fig. 9–1B). This is easily accomplished by turning the patient so that he faces the film at a 60 degree angle and the shoulder that is to be filmed touches the cassette. A normally aligned humeral head will be directly superimposed upon the glenoid fossa, as in this example, and the acromioclavicular joint will be located posteriorly and superiorly to the glenoid fossa. The coracoid processes will project anteriorly and superiorly.

It is important to remember that pain in the shoulder may be referred from the brachial plexus or the cervical area. Thus

354

Figure 9–1. Normal shoulder.
A. A 20 degree angulation with the back against the cassette allows a tangential view of the shoulder joint and better evaluation of the cartilage width and the articular margins of bone.

B. When the patient faces the film and is steeply angled (approximately 60 degrees), the X-ray beam sites down the scapula and superimposes the head of the humerus on the glenoid fossa.

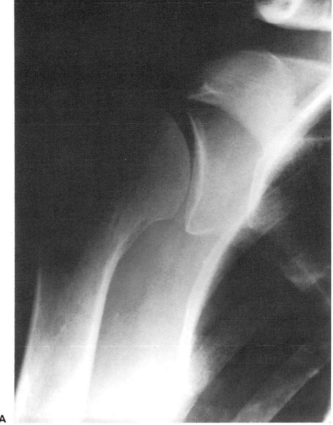

A

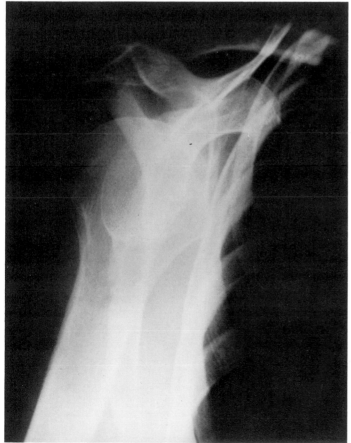

B

355

a normal-appearing radiographic study of a painful shoulder must be followed by adequate assessment of these regions.

ANATOMY OF THE SHOULDER

Although the shoulder joint has essentially the same type of ball and socket articulation as the hip, a much greater range of motion is provided by the shallow glenoid fossa and its fibrocartilaginous extension, the glenoid labrum. The joint capsule is attached superiorly to the circumference of the glenoid and inferiorly along the anatomic neck of the humerus. This is demonstrated by an arthrogram of a normal joint (Fig. 9–2). Additional support of the humeral head is given by the flat tendons of the muscles that make up the rotator cuff: by the supraspinatus superiorly, and the infraspinatus and teres minor posteriorly, all three of which attach to the greater tuberosity; and anteriorly, by the subscapularis, which attaches to the lesser tuberosity. Despite the encircling tendinous cuff, the laxity of the joint capsule allows a large range of motion and separation of the articulating bones that compose the shoulder joint.

The synovial membrane lines the inner surface of the capsule and extends downward as a pouch around the tendon of the long head of the biceps within the intertubercular groove (arrow). Additional synovium-lined bursae lie beneath the acromion (the subacromial bursa and its lateral extension, the subdeltoid bursa), just above the acromion (the subcutaneous acromial bursa) and beneath the coracoid process (the subcoracoid bursa).

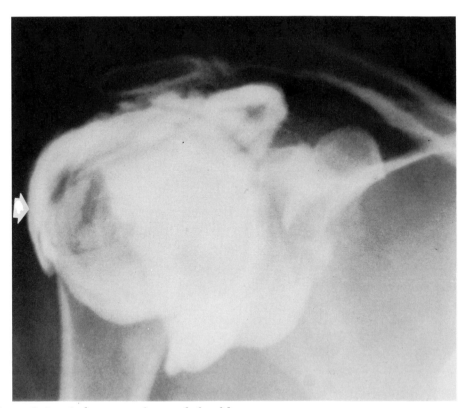

Figure 9–2. Arthrogram of normal shoulder.
The extent of the joint capsule is delineated by contrast material. A prominent subscapular extension of the capsule is seen projecting toward the axilla. Filling of the subacromial bursa may occasionally occur normally. Extension of the capsule as a pouch around the long head of the biceps (arrow) demarcates the intertubercular groove.

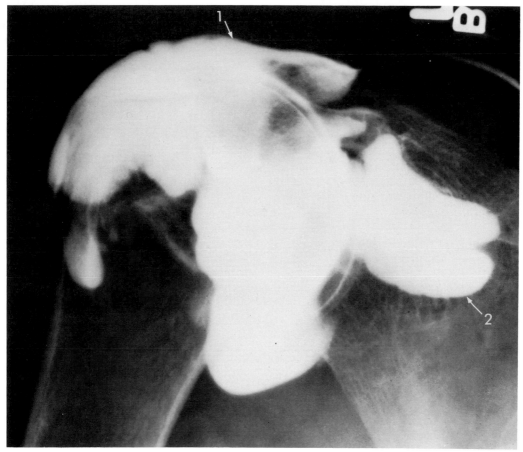

Figure 9–3.   Rotator cuff tear.
Filling of (*1*) the subacromial bursa superiorly and (*2*) the subcoracoid bursa inferiorly indicates tear of the rotator cuff. The normal hyaline articular cartilage is seen as a radiolucent crescent over the head of the humerus.

The subacromial bursa may rarely communicate with the joint capsule in a normal shoulder without a rotator cuff tear. Since the tendon of the supraspinatus muscle separates the subacromial bursa from the joint capsule superiorly, any tear in the rotator cuff at this point results in communication between the two spaces, easily diagnosed by an arthrogram and by the patient's inability to abduct his arm.

Rotator Cuff Tear. By injecting water-soluble contrast material into the joint the extent of the capsule is delineated. The radiolucent crescents that parallel the head of the humerus and the glenoid fossa represent the hyaline articulating cartilage and are separated by a thin white line of contrast material (Fig.

9–3). Normally two outpouchings fill with contrast—the bicipital portion that extends along the intertubercular or bicipital groove, and a subscapular extension. A rotator cuff tear has resulted in communication of the joint capsule with the subacromial bursa superiorly and the subcoracoid bursa inferiorly (arrows). The important anatomic relationships of capsule, bursae and bones are exceptionally well delineated on this single film.

SOFT TISSUE CALCIFICATION OF THE SHOULDER

Abnormal calcifications of the shoulder are similar in character to those of the hip, and the same diagnostic criteria can be used to suggest an etiology.

Calcific Tendinitis. Most commonly, collection of calcium in the shoulder is due to calcific deposits within the tendons of the rotator cuff. Figure 9–4 radiographically illustrates an amorphous collection adjacent to the greater tuberosity. Although this is the site of three tendinous insertions, that of the supraspinatus is the most frequently involved. Calcifications in the other two tendons are slightly more inferior; however, this is often difficult to assess precisely in the highly mobile shoulder joint.

Two additional calcific deposits are present in the subcutaneous tissue. Their radiolucent centers and round appearance typify injection granulomas, and deposits of this type are frequently present in the hip and shoulder, the common areas of injection.

Dermatomyositis. A single view of the shoulder of an eight year old girl illustrates the extensive and diffuse collections of calcium throughout the muscles of the shoulder (Fig. 9–5). A film taken one year earlier had shown only a trace of calcium, and the rapidity of its deposition was echoed in other regions of her body.

Synovial Osteochondromatosis. True synovial osteochondromatosis is a disease of unknown etiology, generally affecting the shoulder, hip or knee. Calcification and ossification of synovium may also follow multiple episodes of trauma to a joint, and the radiographic appearance is similar. The loose bodies may be larger and less numerous in the post-traumatic joint, but the distinction is academic.

Numerous fragments of ectopic bone and cartilage are scattered through the fibrotic synovium taken from a joint sub-

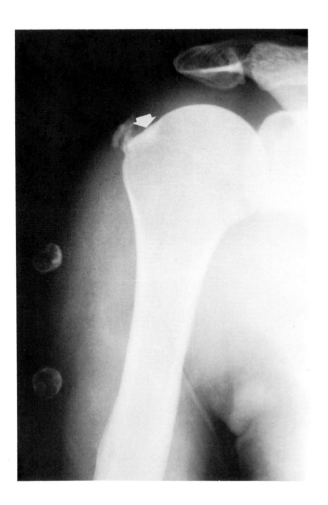

Figure 9–4. Calcific tendinitis. Amorphous calcification in the soft tissues adjacent to the greater tuberosity occurs most commonly in the supraspinatus tendon. The flattened, sclerotic superior margin of the humeral head (arrow) mimics the changes of a Hill-Sachs deformity. This often precedes calcification of the tendon and is helpful in diagnosing tendinitis from a radiograph. The two additional calcifications are injection granulomas.

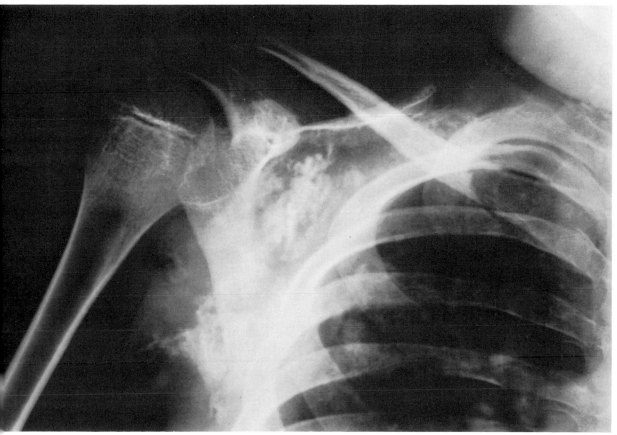

Figure 9–5. Dermatomyositis.
Extensive soft tissue calcification developed over a one year period in an eight year old girl.
It is best seen in the axillary region and is also superimposed on the shadows of the scapula and lung.

jected to past trauma (Fig. 9–6). The appearance is not unlike what would be seen in the following example of synovial osteochondromatosis.

Typical degenerative joint disease of the shoulder is manifested by the prominent osteophytes and lipping of the inferior glenoid labrum (Fig. 9–7). Large calcified loose bodies are seen within the joint capsule in the shoulder of a wrestler. Both the location and the character of the calcification distinguish this picture from the previous example of the amorphous muscle calcification of dermatomyositis.

The curvilinear calcification paralleling the superior margin of the humeral head suggests calcification within the articular cartilage (arrow). Since the most common cause of chondrocalcinosis is degenerative cartilage, it is not surprising that this severely damaged and traumatized joint demonstrates this finding.

ALIGNMENT ABNORMALITIES OF THE SHOULDER

It is extremely difficult to judge abnormalities of alignment in the shoulder because of the huge range of motion that it normally undergoes. Often an interpretation of a dislocated shoulder is made by the uninitiated when viewing the shoulder on a routine chest film. The

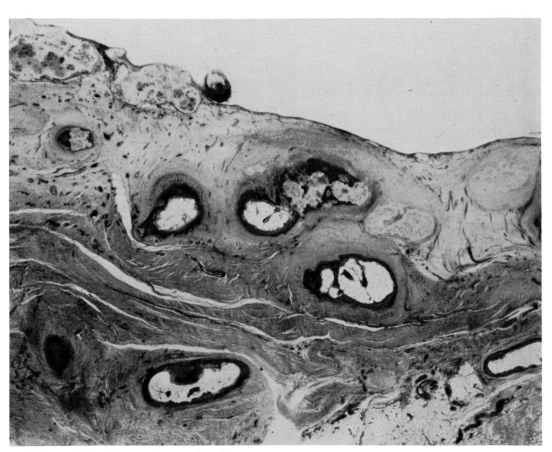

Figure 9–6. Synovial osteochondromatosis.
Numerous fragments of ectopic bone and cartilage are scattered throughout the fibrotic synovium, as seen on a photomicrograph of a specimen of synovium removed from a joint subjected to past trauma. (Courtesy of The Arthritis Foundation.)

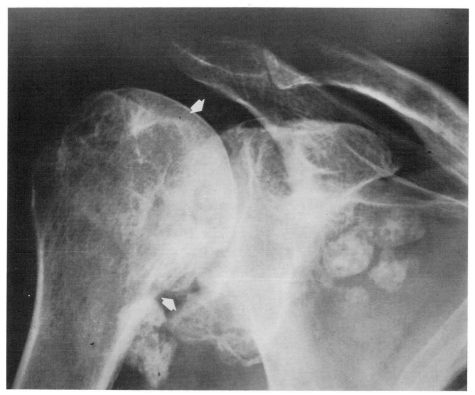

Figure 9–7. Synovial osteochondromatosis.
Large intraarticular ossifications are more characteristic of osteochondromatosis secondary to trauma than to the findings of idiopathic synovial osteochondromatosis. Multiple episodes of trauma to this wrestler's shoulder resulted in cystic changes of the humeral head, proliferative new bone extensively deforming the inferior lip of the glenoid and calcification of the articular cartilage (arrows). This is an unusually advanced example of osteoarthritis, which rarely occurs in the shoulder.

inferior position and overlap of the humeral head on the scapula looks like a dislocation as the patient rotates his scapulae off the lung fields in his enthusiasm to cooperate with the x-ray technician.

Alignment abnormalities are easy to detect by the two oblique views of the shoulder that were previously described. The steep, 60 degree PA view reveals the true relationship of the glenoid fossa to the humeral head and establishes its posterior or anterior location.

Anterior Dislocation. On a routine AP view of the shoulder in which anterior dislocation has occurred, the humeral head is displaced inferiorly and medially and is superimposed over the scapula. Figure 9–8 illustrates the abnormal alignment as well as an additional

important radiographic finding. The superior border of the humerus is scalloped, owing to compression of bone at the level of the greater tuberosity as it impacts against the inferior margin of the glenoid. Since this defect will persist following reduction of the dislocation, it will alert the radiologist to the history of a dislocation.

Seen more frequently than a scalloped contour is an area of condensed bone. This is the result of a fracture that has caused compression of bone at the level of the greater tuberosity. The irregularity or impacted bone is known as the Hill-Sachs or Bankhart deformity. It is most easily observed following reduction, when the arm can be abducted and internally rotated 60 degrees. It must be dis-

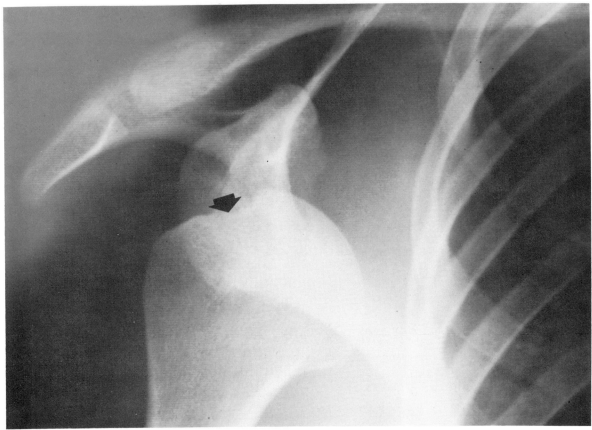

Figure 9–8. Anterior dislocation.
Inferior and medial dislocation of the humeral head is easily detected on a routine AP view of the shoulder. The saucerlike depression of the superior margin of the humeral head (arrow) has resulted from a compression fracture in which the humerus impacted against the scapular margin. Its appearance mimics that of an inflammatory erosion.

tinguished from the small erosions and sclerosis of the greater tuberosity from an adjacent tendinitis.

Posterior Dislocation. Posterior dislocation of the shoulder is difficult to recognize on a routine view of this joint. Lack of parallelism between the humeral head and the glenoid suggests the diagnosis, but superimposition of the two bones occurs normally from positional changes alone. An abnormally shaped humeral head is often the only hint of defect; this occurs because of the rotation that accompanies the dislocation. To compound the diagnostic dilemma, soft tissue swelling frequently obscures the clinical signs of the posteriorly situated humeral head, making it impossible to palpate. Figure 9–9A illustrates the difficulty in recognizing an abnormality on a routine view. The axillary projection (Fig. 9–9B) clarifies the relationship of the articulating bones, but is a far more confusing film and a more painful procedure for the patient than a 60 degree PA view. The humeral head does not articulate with the glenoid fossa but instead is superimposed on the scapula. A large compression defect of the humeral epiphysis is present. Both the relationship of the two bones and the large bony defect were unrecognizable on a single projection of the shoulder. A normal axillary view is included for comparison (Fig. 9–10).

Figure 9–9. Posterior dislocation.

A. A routine AP view is remarkably normal in a posteriorly dislocated shoulder. Because of the concomitant *internal* rotation, however, the humeral head is more club-shaped than normal. Overlap of the shadows of the glenoid and the humeral head may be seen normally and offer no clue to the extensive pathology present.

B. An axillary view demonstrates the posterior position of the humeral head in relation to the glenoid fossa and also reveals a large compression fracture (arrows) which was completely obscured on the routine view. *1*, glenoid fossa; *2*, acromion; *3*, clavicle; *4*, coracoid process.

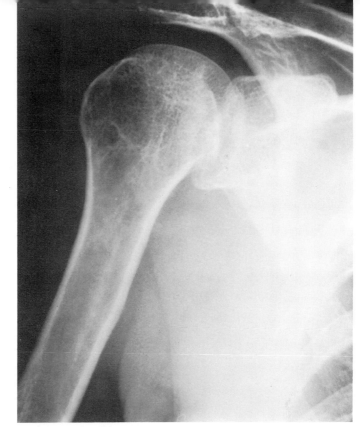

A

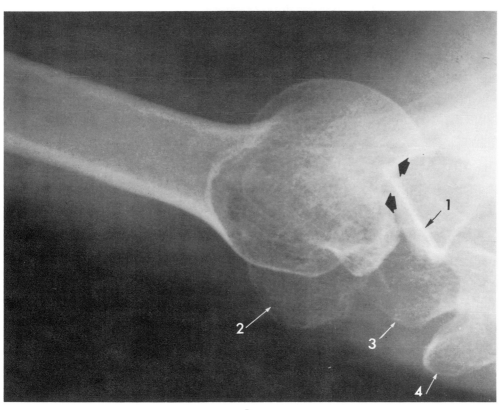

B

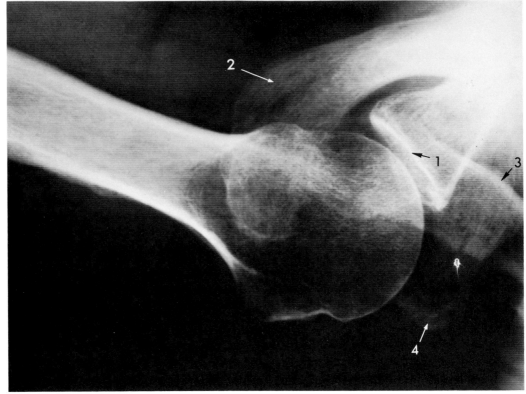

Figure 9–10. Normal axillary view of shoulder.
The glenoid fossa articulates with the smooth round cortical margin of the humerus. The acromioclavicular joint is hidden behind the humeral head, and the coracoid process is faintly seen anteriorly. *1*, glenoid fossa; *2*, acromion; *3*, clavicle; *4*, coracoid process.

ABNORMAL MINERALIZATION OF THE SHOULDER

The trabeculae of the bones of a normal shoulder are sharp, fine, white structures so numerous that they appear as a closely woven mesh. The solid white cortex of the shaft of the humerus casts a wide, distinct shadow as it encroaches on the spongiosa. As the bone loses calcium, the trabeculae become thin and sparse, and the cortex narrows. Tiny holes may appear in the shaft of bone if the process is rapid, whereas a homogeneous ground glass appearance indicates chronic loss of bone.

Sudeck's Atrophy. The etiology of Sudeck's atrophy is uncertain. Clinically there may be either soft tissue swelling or wasting, accompanied by pain. The prominent radiographic finding is that of severe, rapid demineralization. Pain in the humerus prompted a film of a patient with bronchogenic carcinoma (Fig. 9–11). Although the moth-eaten appearance of the diaphysis suggests marrow invasion by carcinoma, it is actually a reflection of rapid bony demineralization secondary to brachial plexus involvement by tumor. The bone changes of Sudeck's atrophy appear radiographically as patchy holes mimicking metastatic carcinoma or multiple myeloma.

Hyperparathyroidism. Demineralization is so extensive in a patient with hyperparathyroidism that the moth-eaten appearance of the shaft of the humerus is similar to that in Sudeck's atrophy (Fig. 9–12). The curvilinear calcification of chondrocalcinosis parallels the humeral

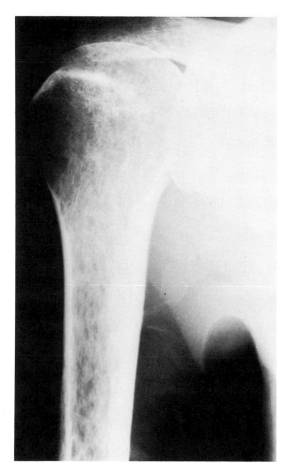

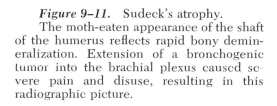

Figure 9–11. Sudeck's atrophy.
The moth-eaten appearance of the shaft of the humerus reflects rapid bony demineralization. Extension of a bronchogenic tumor into the brachial plexus caused severe pain and disuse, resulting in this radiographic picture.

head. Although it is far more common to find chondrocalcinosis as the *only* radiographic abnormality in the joints of patients with primary hyperparathyroidism, the combination of chondrocalcinosis, abnormal bony mineralization and absence of subchondral erosions eliminates as diagnostic possibilities the other causes of calcified cartilage and leads the clinician to search for the parathyroid adenoma.

An amorphous calcific deposit is barely visible adjacent to the greater tuberosity and represents calcific tendinitis. This is not uncommonly seen in the shoulder of patients with this metabolic disorder, but it is such a common occurrence in the general population that it may be only a chance association rather than an accompaniment of the propensity to metastatic calcification.

ABNORMALITIES OF THE GLENOHUMERAL JOINT SPACE

Cystic Erosions and Cartilage Destruction

In contrast to the other regions of the body in which the joint space is a well-defined and fixed distance between articulating bones, the great mobility of the shoulder allows separation and overlap of the bones on an AP view of the joint. Any abduction, adduction or internal or external rotation will alter the relationship of their shadows on a film. It is impossible to diagnose destruction of the water-density cartilage until the disease process has extended into the articulating bone. Furthermore, this is extremely difficult to appreciate when the articulating bones

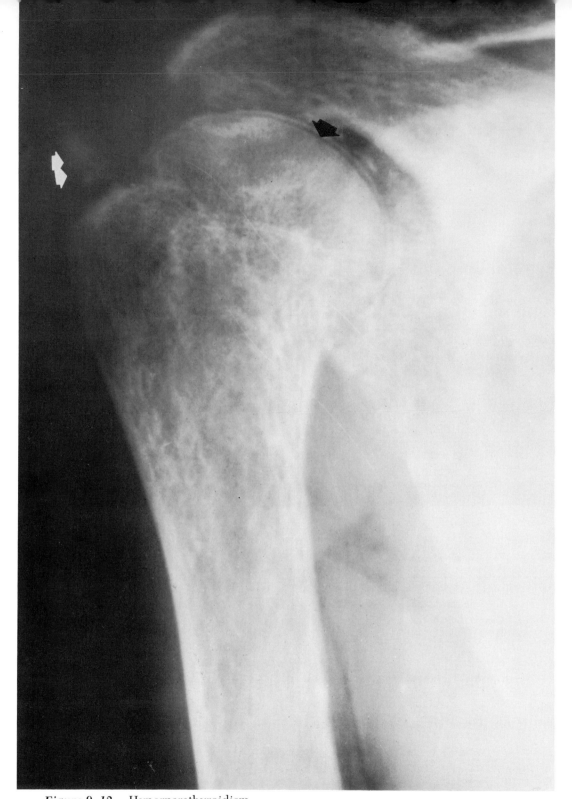

Figure 9–12. Hyperparathyroidism.

    The mottled texture of the bones and the cortical thinning reflect the underlying metabolic abnormalities of calcium and phosphate metabolism. Chondrocalcinosis is a frequent accompaniment of hyperparathyroidism and can be seen paralleling the head of the humerus (arrow). An amorphous collection of calcium in the soft tissue adjacent to the greater tuberosity represents calcific tendinitis (double arrow).

overlap and obscure fine detail. When a 20 degree AP view is obtained the joint is viewed tangentially, and early erosions are more easily detected.

Any disease that causes synovial proliferation will destroy the cartilage and erode the adjacent bones. Therefore the radiographic findings of irregular cortical margins are nonspecific, as will be seen in the following examples.

Hemophilia. The saucerlike defect deforming the head of the humerus in Figure 9–13 is similar in appearance to the compression deformity from repeated episodes of shoulder dislocation. The most important radiographic clue as to the etiology of the deformity lies in whether the abnormality is confined to a single bone or involves both articulating bones. In this example, similar erosions have caused large radiolucent defects in the glenoid fossa, and a smaller erosion deforms the inferior margin of the hu-

meral head. When both articulating surfaces are affected, an inflammatory process with synovial hypertrophy is a far more likely cause than a localized process such as trauma.

Rheumatoid Arthritis. Figure 9–14 shows, above the greater tuberosity, a rat bite shallow erosion from rheumatoid arthritis. There is nothing to distinguish this erosion from those seen in other diseases, either in its location or in its appearance. One additional important finding is included on the film, however, which establishes the problem as a systemic disorder: similar erosive changes are present along the inferior articulating edge of the clavicle. Thus multiple joint involvement is helpful in ruling out a disease that tends to be monarticular, such as an infectious arthritis. In general, determination of whether there have been pathologic changes of both sides of a joint or in a number of joints is critical

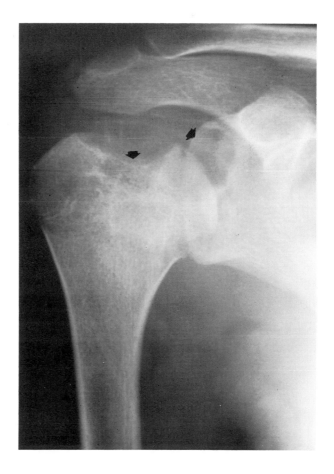

Figure 9–13. Hemophilia.
Large erosions deform both the humeral head and the glenoid fossa (arrows) following multiple episodes of intra-articular hemorrhage. The destruction is nonspecific and could be duplicated by any condition that results in a hypertrophied synovium.

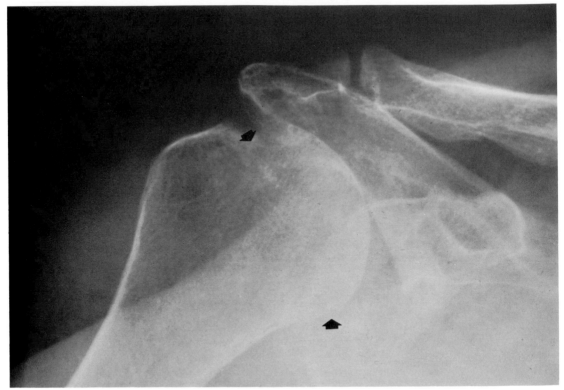

Figure 9–14. Rheumatoid arthritis.

Marginal erosions, often the earliest signs of an inflammatory arthritis, occur at the vulnerable point where the protective cap of articular cartilage ends. They are present both superiorly and inferiorly (arrows) in this patient. Although changes of the glenoid labrum are not apparent at this stage, an inferior erosion of the distal clavicle attests to the systemic nature of the inflammatory condition and excludes diseases that are generally monarticular.

in narrowing the list of diagnostic alternatives so that one may consider appropriate disease possibilities.

Films of a young woman with rheumatoid arthritis (Fig. 9–15) show arthritic changes in both shoulders as well as in the acromioclavicular joints. Resorption of the distal clavicle (Fig. 9–15B) has resulted in a tapered or whittled contour. This is a frequent finding in rheumatoid arthritis but is by no means pathognomonic of that disease. It may be present in progressive systemic sclerosis and in hyperparathyroidism and was seen in the past in patients with poliomyelitis.

As a rule, rheumatoid arthritis does not stimulate osteoblastic activity at the site of erosions. However, cystic changes in the subchondral bone may have well-defined sclerotic borders when the general bony mineralization is normal. This was illustrated by the film of the wrist of a laborer with rheumatoid arthritis, in Chapter 4 (Fig. 4–12), and is seen here in a shoulder (Fig. 9–16). In the absence of detectable erosions of the glenoid fossa and clavicle, the changes in the humeral head are so nonspecific that a precise diagnosis cannot be made. Similar changes from degenerative joint disease, hemophilia and gout may be identical.

Gout. The similarity of cystic lesions and the nonspecificity of the sclerotic borders are apparent when the shoulder changes of a patient with gout (Fig. 9–17) are compared with those seen in the preceding example of rheumatoid arthritis. Again, the changes are confined to a single bone, and without the information

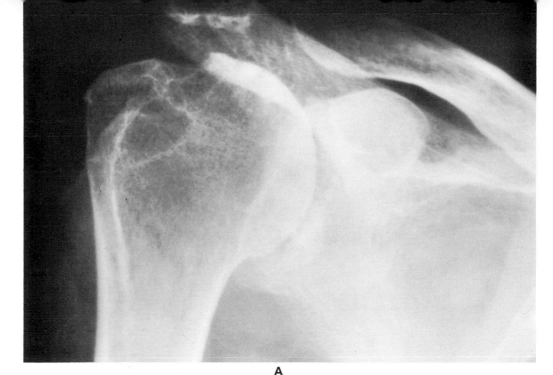

A

Figure 9–15. Rheumatoid arthritis.

A. A large cortical erosion of the right humeral head, widening of the acromioclavicular joint and tapering of the distal clavicle reflect inflammatory changes.

B. Small cystic changes in the glenoid margin of the left shoulder can be seen in addition to the erosions of the humerus and tapering of the distal clavicle.

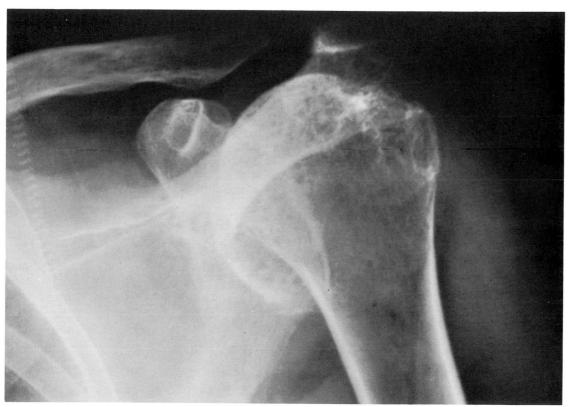

B

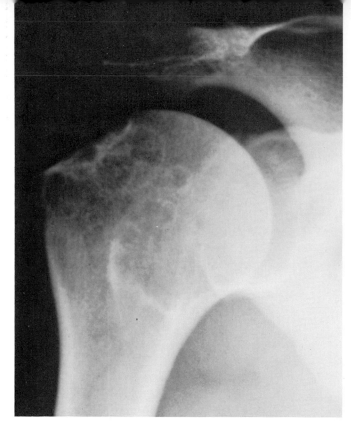

Figure 9–16. Rheumatoid arthritis.

Occasionally the cystic erosions of rheumatoid arthritis have a well-defined sclerotic margin, and the findings are indistinguishable from any chronic arthritis.

Figure 9–17. Gout.

Well-circumscribed cysts are characteristic of gout, and their sclerotic border indicates production of trabeculae adjacent to the tophaceous deposit. Since gout rarely affects the shoulders except in patients with chronic tophaceous gout, the disease is usually well-documented before the radiograph and differential diagnosis is not a problem.

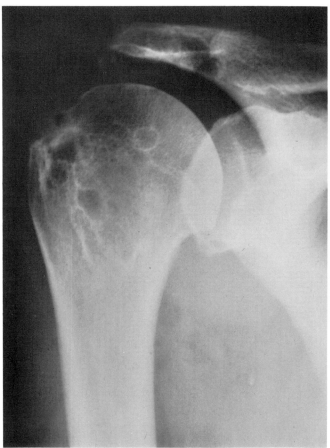

from appropriate laboratory studies and knowledge of the distribution of the disease in the patient, the diagnosis of gout cannot be made.

Additional radiographic clues, as in Figure 9–18A, must be present to allow the diagnosis of a specific arthritis. A patient with chronic tophaceous gout has both soft tissue changes as well as bony erosions. The cystic erosions have the typical sclerotic border that is more commonly seen in gout than in rheumatoid arthritis. A large erosion has deformed the superior margin of the humerus, and adjacent to it is a cloudlike collection of calcium. Only when the soft tissue mass demonstrates the typical characteristics of a chronic tophus with deposition of calcium can gout be suggested.

A mutilating arthritis may result from long-standing tophi and contiguous erosion of the adjacent bone. Figure 9–18B, the same shoulder nine years later, illustrates massive deformity of the soft tissues by a huge tophus. Calcium is scattered throughout the mass. The humeral head is absent, an unusual occurrence from pressure erosion alone. It may be that avascular necrosis, a rare but reported complication of gouty arthritis, has contributed to the total dissolution of the humeral head.

In addition to the changes in the glenohumeral joint, there are widening of the acromioclavicular joint and erosion of the end of the clavicle. The splayed appearance of the erosion, again, is typical of gout and indicates the production of new bone at the margin of the tophus. It is not exuberant enough to be characterized as an overhanging edge, but the pathologic implication is the same.

Avascular Necrosis

Whenever pathologic changes are confined to the epiphysis, and there is no evidence of cartilage destruction or changes of the opposite articulating bone, a primary epiphyseal abnormality must be considered rather than an arthritis.

Congenital abnormalities, such as epiphyseal dysplasia, and growth disturbances, as in cretinism (congenital hypothyroidism), deform the epiphyses and are limited to one side of the joint until a superimposed degenerative arthritis complicates the radiographic picture.

Avascular necrosis will cause areas of rarefaction and sclerosis limited to the humeral head that mimic the erosions that accompany synovial proliferation. The combination of a flattened, deformed epiphysis and absence of abnormalities in the glenoid distinguishes primary epiphyseal problems from the erosions and cystic changes that accompany an arthritis. This pair of findings may be the result of many different diseases. In clinical practice, the most frequent underlying disease conditions associated with this finding are sickle cell or S-C disease, adrenocorticosteroid therapy, pancreatitis, alcoholism and systemic lupus erythematosus. It is seen more frequently in the latter disease in association with adrenocorticosteroid therapy, but this is by no means necessary to cause the complication of avascular necrosis.

In all of the conditions leading to avascular necrosis, the primary pathophysiologic mechanism appears to be that of obstruction of the vascular supply to the bone, with subsequent ischemia and necrosis. Although the precise mechanisms are incompletely known, it is convenient to consider that obstruction of the blood supply by abnormal red blood cells as in sickle cell and S-C disease and sickle thalassemia, or by fat particles in pancreatitis and alcoholism, results in an avascular state. The avascular necrosis of Gaucher's disease stems from occlusion by the abnormal marrow cells. The bubbles of nitrogen in the blood of tunnel workers suffering from "the bends" or caisson disease occlude vessels either intraluminally or from extravascular compression; such episodes thus cause avascular necrosis of bone. In systemic lupus erythematosus the underlying vasculitis may result in obliteration of the blood supply with similar pathologic and radiographic results.

The pathophysiologic mechanism in

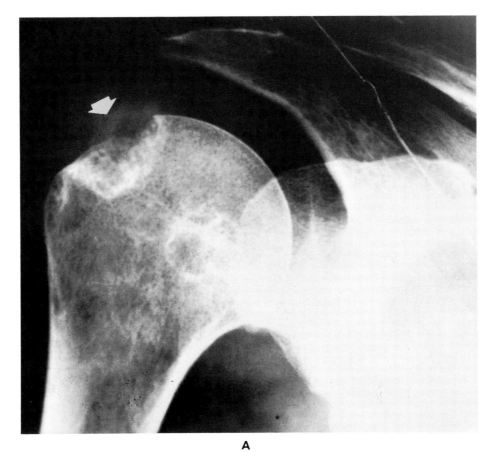

A

Figure 9–18. Chronic tophaceous gout.
   A. A large intraosseous cyst with sclerotic margins and a well-defined erosion with an adjacent tophus (arrow) are pathognomonic of gout when the soft tissue mass contains calcium, as in this example.

steroid production of avascular necrosis is more theoretical. The radiographic appearance of the bone is identical to that in other conditions resulting in avascular necrosis; thus it is logical to assume that epiphyseal changes seen in steroid administration are related to avascular necrosis. This may result from a mechanism similar to that in alcoholism and pancreatitis, with mobilization of fat and consequent occlusion of the vessel. On the other hand, fractures of bone are a well-known complication of the osteoporotic changes due to steroids as seen, for example, in the vertebral bodies. The cortical breaks and radiolucent subchondral lines may thus represent epiphyseal fractures and explain the more frequent

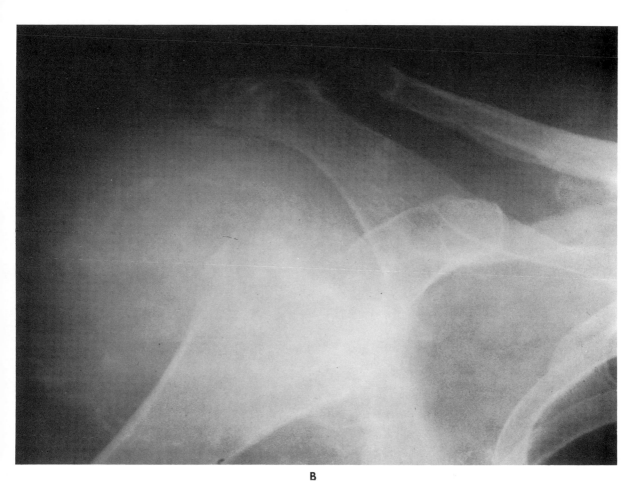

B

Figure 9–18.   Continued.
   B. Nine years later, massive soft tissue tophi, faintly calcified, distort the shoulder. Extensive loss of bone of the humeral head is out of proportion to the typical erosions and may reflect a concomitant avascular necrosis, a rare but reported occurrence in gouty arthropathies. Widening of the acromioclavicular joint and erosion of the margin of the clavicle documents an additional site of involvement in this patient.

occurrence of avascular necrosis in the weight-bearing hip joints.

Sickle Cell Disease.   In addition to the nonhomogeneous appearance of the head of the humerus, there is deformity of its contour, with loss of the round, smooth appearance (Fig. 9–19). These changes are identical to the changes of avascular necrosis in the hip. Absence of changes in the glenoid fossa supports the supposition that the changes are from a primary abnormality of the humeral epiphysis. Unlike the weight-bearing hip joint, superimposed degenerative changes in the shoulder are less likely to follow avascular necrosis.

Sickle Thalassemia.   Although avascular necrosis is more common in sickle cell disease and S-C disease, it occasionally is found in patients with sickle thalassemia. Figure 9–20 is an example of the early changes of avascular necrosis

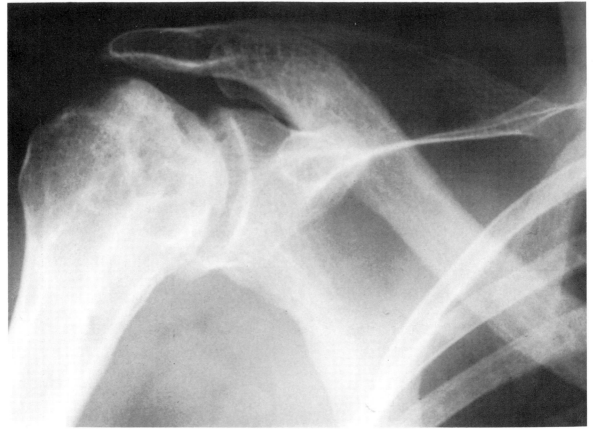

Figure 9–19. Sickle cell disease.
Localization of pathologic changes to the head of the humerus, with alternating areas of mottled sclerosis and rarefaction and a flattened contour of the humeral head, is diagnostic of avascular necrosis. This may complicate many of the hemoglobinopathies, as in this patient with sickle cell disease.

in a patient with this blood dyscrasia. Only the break in the cortex and the radiolucent line in the epiphysis indicate the crumbling necrotic bone. The configuration mimics a traumatic fracture but is too close to the articulating margin of the bone for this etiology to be very likely. Since sclerotic new bone is a sign of healing, its absence indicates the early stage at which this film was taken.

Epiphyseal Overgrowth

Deformity of the epiphysis may result from abnormal rates of growth as well as destructive processes. Both hemophilia and juvenile rheumatoid arthritis are characterized by stimulation of epiphyseal growth. Because of the thick cartilage in the joints of children, the articulating ends of the bones are protected from erosions to a greater extent than in adults. Hence the only evidence of a previous inflammatory disease or episodes of intra-articular bleeding may be a deformed epiphysis and minimal joint space narrowing.

Juvenile Rheumatoid Arthritis. Alterations in the contour of the humeral head are common sequelae of juvenile rheumatoid arthritis. Because of the overgrowth of the epiphysis and the tendency for early epiphyseal fusion, bizarre con-

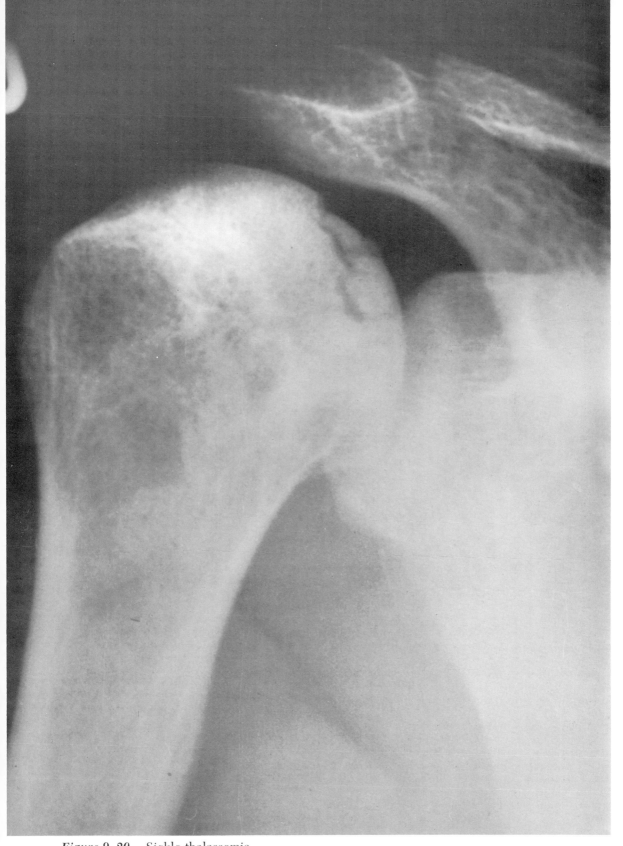

Figure 9–20. Sickle thalassemia.

When films are taken early in the course of avascular necrosis, the cortical break in the humeral head may be the only indication of its presence. Lack of mottling or sclerosis of the humeral head suggests that healing has not begun.

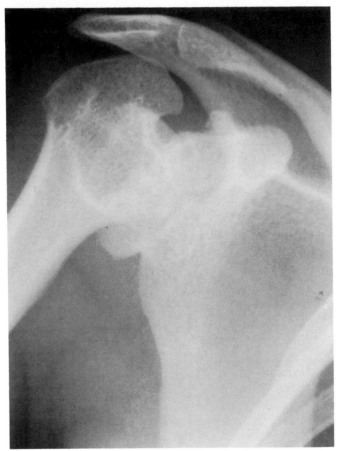

Figure 9–21. Juvenile rheumatoid arthritis.
    A bizarre configuration of the articular end of the bone may be the only stigma of the juvenile onset of an arthritis. Epiphyseal overgrowth in the area of the greater tuberosity has resulted in this peculiar hatchet-shaped appearance.

figurations of the ends of the bones may be seen. Figures 9–21 and 9–22 are radiographs of two different patients with juvenile rheumatoid arthritis. Both examples demonstrate the loss of a normal round contour of the humeral head and minimal joint space narrowing. The notched configuration between the superior and inferior borders of the humeral head in Figure 9–21 is not dissimilar to that seen in the compression fracture that occurred from trauma (see Figure 9–9*B*). Recognition of the peculiar changes that are seen in arthritides with a childhood onset is essential to correctly evaluate the radiographic findings.

Resorptive Arthropathy

Although resorptive arthropathies are rare, when they occur they are most frequently seen in patients with rheumatoid and psoriatic arthritis or are associated with a Charcot joint.

Rheumatoid Arthritis. There are no radiographic clues to distinguish rheumatoid from psoriatic arthritis in the large joints, as there are in the hands and feet. A patient with rheumatoid arthritis illustrates the changes that may occur in the shoulders when severe resorption of bone plays a primary role (Fig. 9–23). Because of the shallow glenoid fossa and

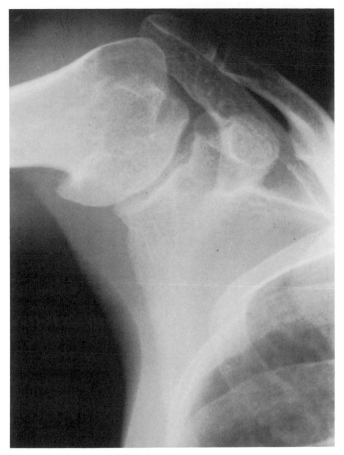

Figure 9–22.   Juvenile rheumatoid arthritis.
Epiphyseal overgrowth and residual irregularities of both the humeral head and the glenoid labrum reflect a burned-out inflammatory arthritis.

the large range of motion of the shoulder, unusual pressure from adjacent bones is an unlikely cause of the uniform circumferential resorption.

Figure 9–23A shows not only resorption of the entire humeral head but tapering of the distal clavicle and the superior margins of the third and fourth ribs. Pressure from the scapula on the osteoporotic bones has been postulated as the mechanism for the *rib erosion,* and exaggerated resorption of bone at the point of muscle attachment may accentuate this phenomenon. The unusual and severe destruction of the proximal humerus may have a similar inciting cause. Both clavicular and rib resorption are seen in hyper-

parathyroidism as well as in rheumatoid arthritis, and the findings are indistinguishable although the pathogenesis may be quite different.

Figure 9–23B, of the patient's opposite shoulder, offers an opportunity to view the resorptive changes at an intermediate stage. Tapering of the clavicle and superior rib erosion are also present and reflect the generalized tendency in this patient toward bone resorption.

Charcot Joint.   A neuropathic shoulder is practically always associated with syringomyelia. The radiographic manifestations are the same in this joint as in the knee, elbow or hip. Complete disorganization of the joint, with resorp-

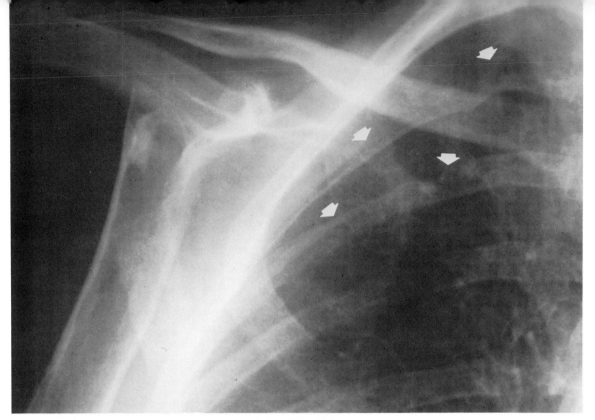

A

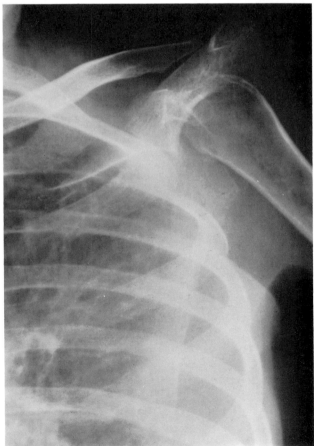

B

Figure 9–23. Rheumatoid arthritis.

A. Occasionally a resorptive arthropathy occurs in the shoulder; when it does, it is most commonly associated with either rheumatoid arthritis or a Charcot joint. Total dissolution of the humeral head is apparent, and tapering of the distal clavicle and superior rib erosions (arrows) attest to the generalized tendency toward loss of bone.

B. The left shoulder demonstrates similar changes, although at an earlier stage. Minimal tapering of the clavicle, with resultant widening of the acromioclavicular joint, is present. Although there is circumferential loss of volume of the humeral head, it is only beginning to show a tapered configuration.

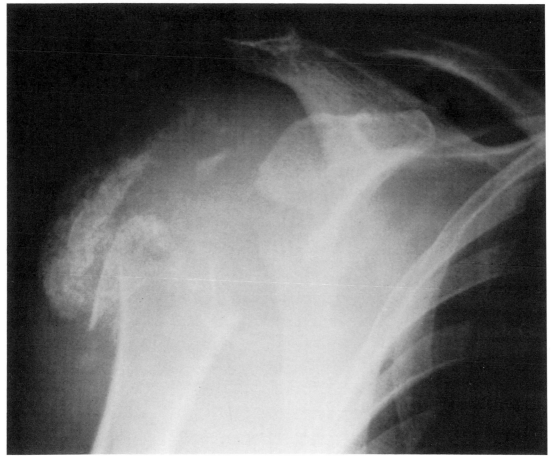

Figure 9–24. Syringomyelia.
Resorption of the end of the humerus, fragmentation and soft tissue calcification characterize a neuropathic joint.

tion of the articulating bones and formation of ectopic new bone, characterizes a Charcot joint (Fig. 9–24).

THE ACROMIOCLAVICULAR JOINT

Although the acromioclavicular joint is separate from the glenohumeral joint, it is included on films of the shoulder; it is thus appropriate to discuss pathologic changes occurring here in conjunction with diseases of the shoulder joint itself. The presence of simultaneous abnormalities of the two regions is helpful in suggesting a systemic problem as the culprit and in excluding such localized processes as avascular necrosis and infection.

Abnormalities of the soft tissue and bones of the acromioclavicular joint have the same implications as in other joints of the body. Several representative examples are demonstrated.

Soft Tissue Calcification

Myositis Ossificans. Both soft tissue and alignment abnormalities are seen in Figure 9–25. There is separation of the acromioclavicular joint due to previous

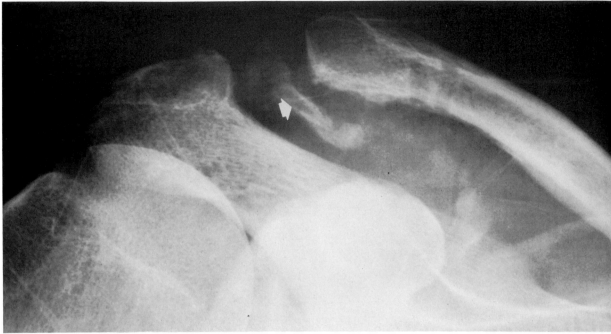

Figure 9–25. Traumatic acromioclavicular joint separation.

Widening of the joint space and an avulsion fracture can be seen (arrow). The soft tissue calcification, representing myositis ossificans, is in the area of the conoid ligament and within the acromioclavicular joint.

trauma. An avulsion fracture of the inferior border of the clavicle is seen (arrow), in addition to extensive ossification adjacent to it. The widened space between the articular ends of the bones is obvious in this example. Occasionally the separation is subtle and must be exaggerated by placing weights in the patient's hands, but usually the weight of the unsupported arm itself is enough to demonstrate the abnormal articulation. Loss of alignment of the *inferior* surfaces of the acromion and clavicle support the suspicion of a joint separation when the interpretation is equivocal.

Progressive Systemic Sclerosis. Two signs of scleroderma may be seen in the acromioclavicular joint: tapering or whittling of the distal clavicle, and deposition of calcium around the joint. Progression of the pathologic changes is illustrated by two films taken three years apart. Massive calcium deposits are seen and reflect similar changes in the rest of this patient's body (Fig. 9–26). In the absence of resorptive changes of the clavicle, the presence of calcium is nonspecific and might reflect anything that causes deposition of calcium in the para-articular tissues—for example, trauma, gout or hyperparathyroidism.

Gout. Splaying of the end of the clavicle (Fig. 9–27) suggests the presence of an intra-articular mass and contiguous pressure erosion. Only when the hazy increase in density associated with calcium within a tophus is present, as in Figure 9–28, can gout be suggested as the underlying arthritis. Since tophi stimulate new bone production, splaying and sclerosis of the base of an erosion are helpful radiographic signs in the absence of the telltale calcium deposition.

A microscopic section through a tophaceous deposit illustrates the sharp continuous line of new bone that outlines and sharply demarcates the tophus (Fig. 9–29).

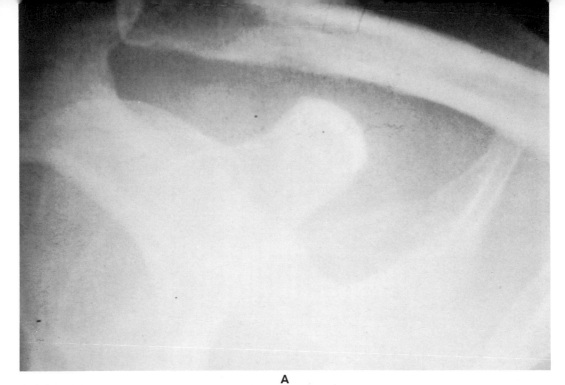

A

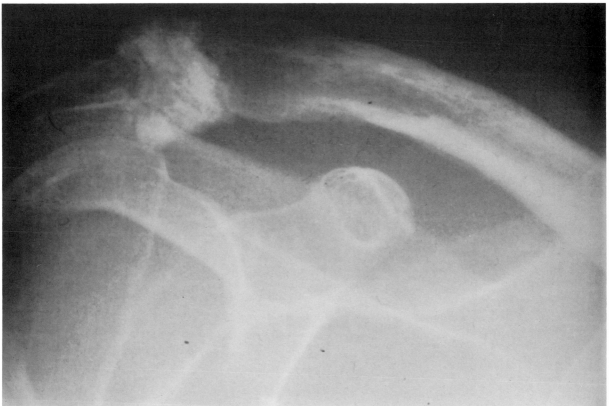

B

Figure 9–26. Progressive systemic sclerosis.

A. The acromioclavicular joint is normal.

B. Extensive para-articular calcification developed over a three year period. Its amorphous character is similar to that seen in the hands, elbow and knee. Pressure erosion of the distal clavicle is apparent when compared to the normal film.

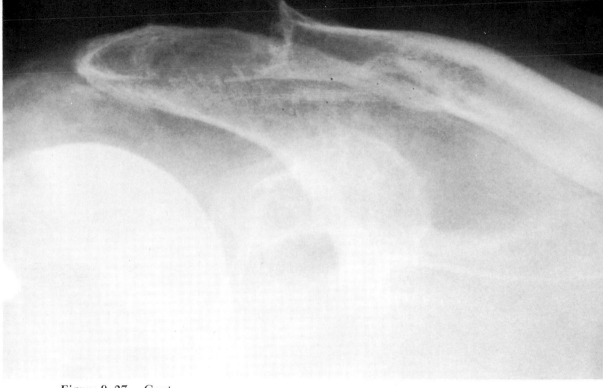

Figure 9–27. Gout.
Splaying of the end of the clavicle and a sclerotic margin suggest an intra-articular mass and differ from the tapered configuration of rheumatoid arthritis.

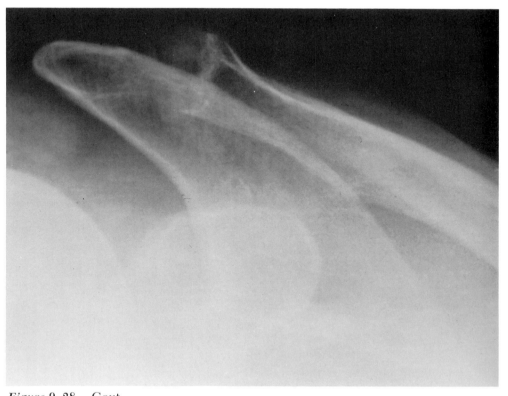

Figure 9–28. Gout.
A faintly calcified intra-articular tophus is present adjacent to the scooped-out, sclerotic end of the clavicle.

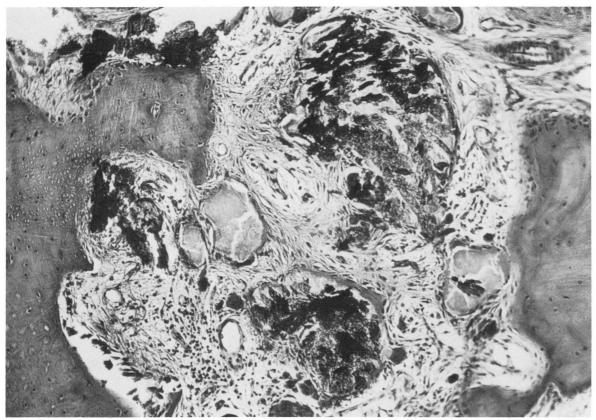

Figure 9–29. Gouty tophus.
A continuous margin of new bone (gray in the photomicrograph) surrounds a subchondral tophus and illustrates the sharply defined character so prominent on a radiograph. (Courtesy of The Arthritis Foundation.)

Osteomyelitis

Coccidioidomycosis. If the radiographic abnormality is confined to a bone and the articular margins of the acromion and clavicle are normal, a primary bone disease rather than an arthritis must be considered. Granulomatous diseases and cystic degeneration may both appear as well-circumscribed cystic lesions. The large size of the lytic bone lesion in Figure 9–30 cannot be attributed to degenerative change. The sclerotic margin typifies the response of bone to a low-grade or indolent infection, as in this example of coccidioidomycosis osteomyelitis.

THE STERNOCLAVICULAR JOINT

Occasionally the sternoclavicular joint may be involved in an inflammatory process, and destruction of the cartilage and the articular ends of the bones progresses in the same manner as in other joints. Such involvement is most frequently seen in rheumatoid arthritis and in infectious processes. Juvenile rheumatoid arthritis and ankylosing spondylitis rarely involve this region.

Although the patient may be very precise as to the location of his pain, the area of the sternoclavicular joint is extremely difficult to examine well by routine radiographs. Superimposition of the mediastinal structures, the vertebral bodies and the ribs obscure the joint no matter how many attempts are made to rotate the patient for optimal visualization. For this reason, when disease of the sternoclavicular joint is suspected, tomograms must be obtained to blur out the superimposed structures. If this is not done, the outcome is *always* a delay in

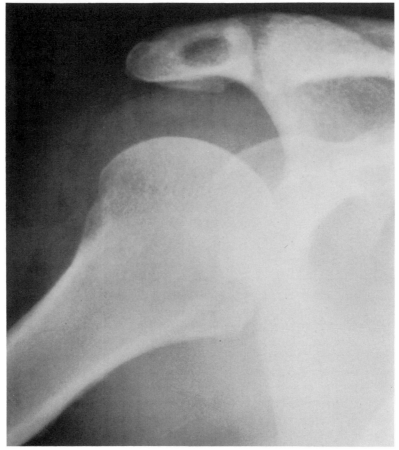

Figure 9–30. Coccidioidomycosis osteomyelitis.
A large, well-circumscribed radiolucent defect in the acromion represents a granulomatous infection. The adjacent acromioclavicular joint is uninvolved.

diagnosis and treatment of the underlying pathology.

Inflammatory Arthritis

Pseudomonas Arthritis. Pain and swelling developed in a heroin addict and multiple oblique views of both sternoclavicular joints were taken. Although the detail is difficult to determine, absence of the sharp margin on the right (Fig. 9–31A) indicates inflammation with loss of the articular cortex. The left side (Fig. 9–31B) is normal, as demonstrated by the intact thin white cortical margin. Widening of the joint space and cartilage destruction are far easier to detect if to-

mograms are taken and direct comparison of the left and right sternoclavicular joints made. The inflammatory process involving the right side was found to be caused by Pseudomonas organisms.

A second example of infectious arthritis of the sternoclavicular joint shows how tomography enhances one's ability to evaluate the extent of destruction. The chest film (Fig. 9–32A) demonstrated an increased density overlying the right upper lung, but the tomogram (Fig. 9–32B) documented its origin in the anterior first rib. Extensive erosion of the manubrium as well as the first rib is best appreciated by comparing the silhouette to the normal left side. Demineralization of the proximal right clavicle is also ap-

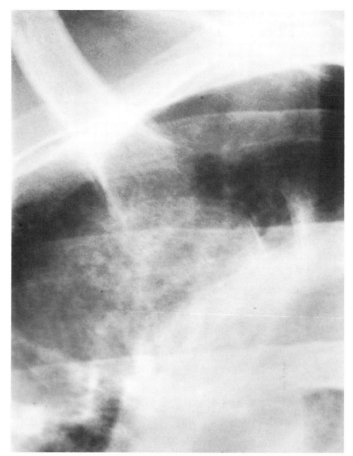

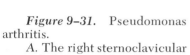

Figure 9–31. Pseudomonas arthritis.

A. The right sternoclavicular joint of a heroin addict illustrates loss of the sharp cortical margin on an oblique view.

B. By comparison, the left joint is normal.

A

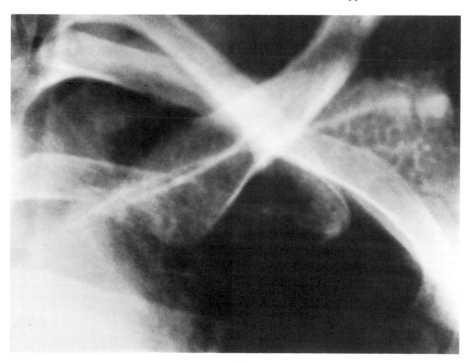

B

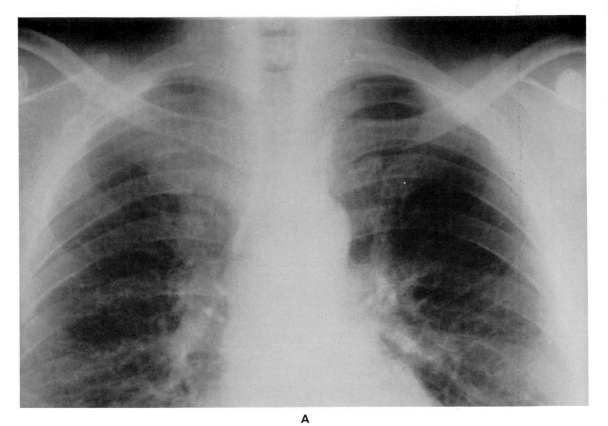

A

Figure 9–32. Sternoclavicular joint infection.
A. A film demonstrates an increased density of the right upper chest but fails to reveal the bony skeleton as the source.

parent, reflecting the infectious process. The shadow on the chest film was cast by an associated abscess.

Tuberculous Arthritis. Localized swelling anterior to the xyphosternal junction is apparent on a lateral view of the sternum (Fig. 9–33). Increased retrosternal soft tissue is also evident. Well-circumscribed areas of destruction of the inferior third of the sternum and the upper portion of the body of the xyphoid are typical of the chronic slow changes of tuberculosis.

Coccidioidomycosis Osteomyelitis. The distinction between infectious arthritis and osteomyelitis is evident when one compares the preceding example with Figure 9–34, a film showing granu-

loma of the body of the sternum. Like the lesion in the acromion (Fig. 9–30), the sharply demarcated sclerotic margin here indicates the slow rate of growth and the bone's ability to contain the pathologic process.

Resorptive Arthropathy

Rheumatoid Arthritis. Although resorptive changes of the distal clavicle are more common, the medial clavicle may be whittled in a similar fashion, causing widening of the sternoclavicular joint (Fig. 9–35). The changes at the acromioclavicular joint are frequently noticed on a routine chest film. The difficulty in

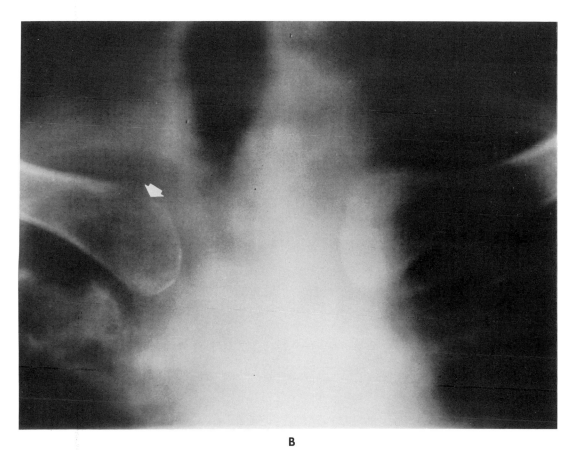

B

Figure 9–32. Continued.
B. A tomogram shows destruction of the anterior first rib on the right, demineralization of the proximal end of the clavicle with a break in its cortex (arrow) and widening of the distance between the clavicle and the manubrium. At surgery, extensive infection necessitated resection of both bones together with the extraosseous soft tissue mass.

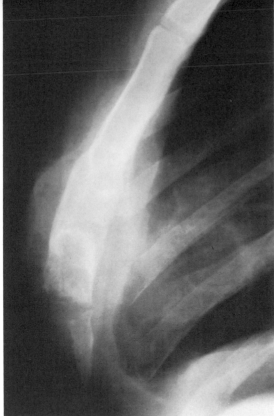

Figure 9–33. Tuberculous infection of the sternum.

Irregular destruction of the articular bones at the xyphosternal junction and presternal as well as retrosternal soft tissue swelling are the radiographic signs of a destructive process. Biopsy is necessary for diagnosis, as metastatic disease and lymphoma may give a similar picture.

Figure 9–34. Coccidioidomycosis osteomyelitis.

Well-circumscribed holes in the body of the sternum are typical of an indolent infection.

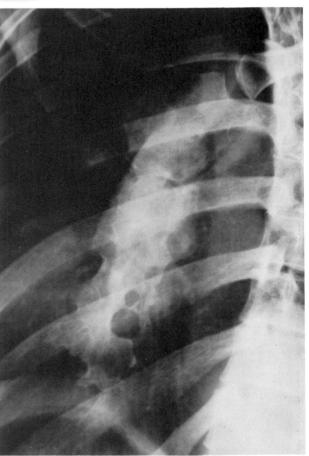

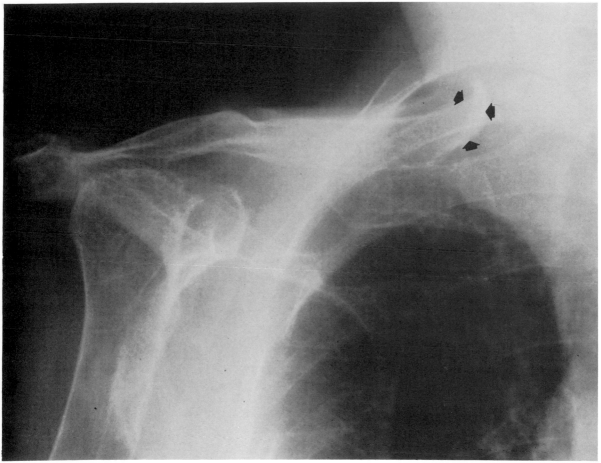

Figure 9-35. Rheumatoid arthritis.
Resorptive changes of the medial clavicle may occur, giving the bone a whittled appearance (arrows). The distal clavicle and humeral head also reflect extensive bone loss in this patient.

evaluating the medial end of the clavicle from a routine projection may contribute to the seeming rarity of involvement of this region. The resorptive changes of the clavicle do not occur in juvenile rheumatoid arthritis or ankylosing spondylitis; hence, their appearance may be helpful in distinguishing rheumatoid arthritis from these two entities, since all three may cause identical changes in the cervical spine.

SUGGESTED READING

Kotzen, L. M. Roentgen diagnosis of rotator cuff tear. Report of 48 surgically proven cases. Amer. J. Roentgen. *112*:507 (1971).

Moseley, H. F. *Shoulder Lesions.* Baltimore, Williams and Wilkins Co., 1969.

Weston, W. J. The enlarged subdeltoid bursa in rheumatoid arthritis. Brit. J. Radiol. *42*:481 (1969).

Zanca, P. Shoulder pain: involvement of the acromioclavicular joint (analysis of 1000 cases). Amer. J. Roentgen. *112*:493 (1971).

EXERCISES

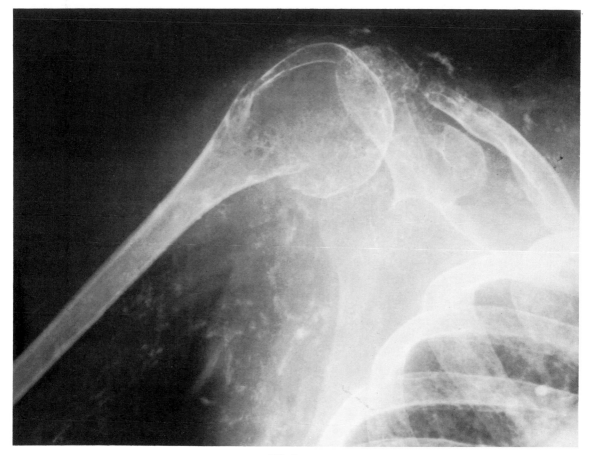

E9–1.

E9–1. "To behold is not necessarily to observe."*

Be careful! The dramatic soft tissue calcifications and severe osteoporosis overshadow more subtle findings, but the category of alignment is where one will find the answer to this young woman's cause of pain. A fracture of the humeral head through the severely osteoporotic bone can be seen as an interrruption in the cortical margin of bone and a varus angulation of the shaft. Years of adrenocorticosteroid therapy for *dermatomyositis* have established a bony background ripe for a pathologic fracture.

*W. Humboldt

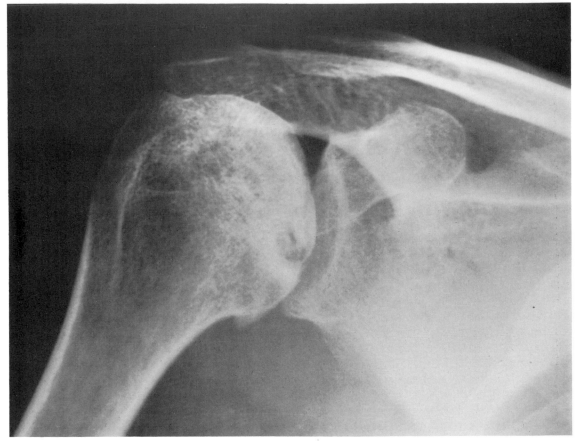

E9–2.

E9–2. The shoulder and the hip are the joints most commonly affected by avascular necrosis. Any patient on steroids, with acute onset of pain in either of these two areas, should be suspected of having this complication. Flattening of the epiphysis, a break in the cortical margin and a mottled increase in density in the presence of a normal joint space are the radiographic criteria of *avascular necrosis* and are present in the shoulder of this young woman with *systemic lupus erythematosus.*

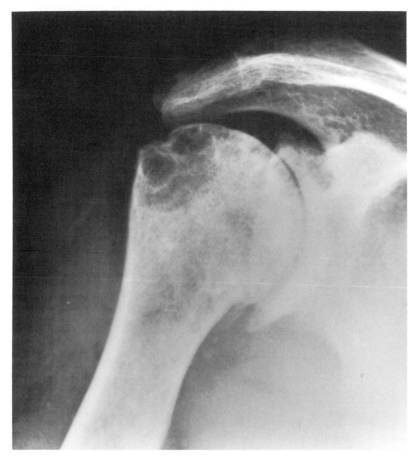

E9–3.

E9–3. Identical cystic changes occur in such a spectrum of conditions affecting the shoulder that other clues must be found to distinguish one arthritis from another. Narrowing of the joint space, as in this example, implies only far-advanced cartilage destruction. The presence of osteophytes which extend the lower lip of the glenoid margin speaks of osteoarthritis. It is so rare to see degen-erative joint disease in the shoulder that, unless a specific history of trauma can be elicited, a primary epiphyseal abnormality or a metabolic condition causing early degenerative changes in cartilage (such as acromegaly or ochronosis) must be suspected. In this case, the patient had *Morquio's disease;* his hips and spine have been shown in the Exercises following Chapter 7.

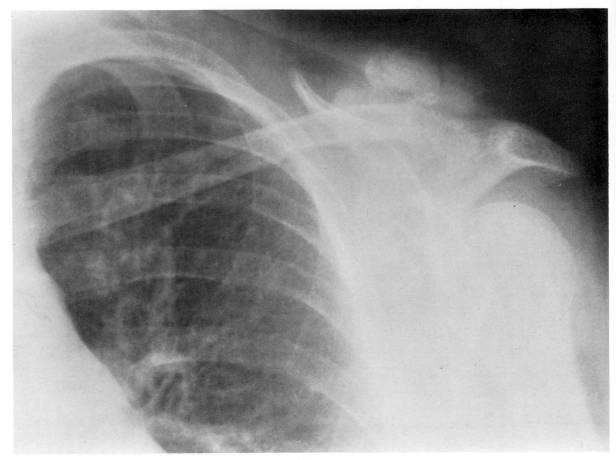

E9–4.

E9–4. Without a history, the differential diagnosis of para-articular calcification is only an intellectual exercise. With the information that the patient has chronic renal disease and is on dialysis, the film takes its rightful role as an indicator of malfunction of calcium metabolism and of the parathyroid glands, signaling an elevated calcium phosphate product in the blood stream. Para-articular depos- its mirror similar collections in critical organs undetectable radiographically and provide an indicator for prompt intervention designed to lower the blood phosphate levels. In this case, conservative medical measures to counteract the effects of *hyperparathyroidism* failed, and surgical extirpation of the massively hypertrophied parathyroid glands was necessary.

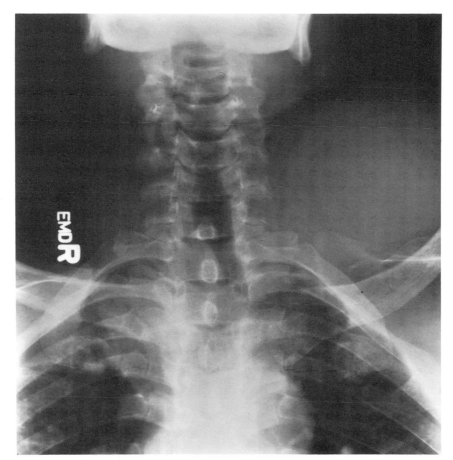

E9–5A.

Exercise continued on following page.

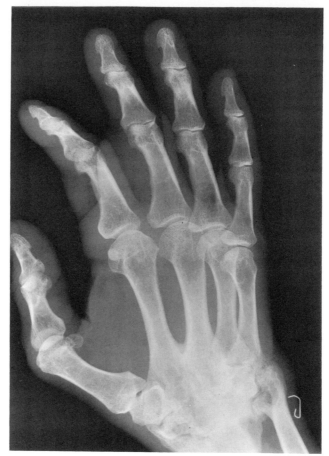

E9–5B.

E9–5. Three seemingly disparate findings provide the clues to this man's diagnostic problem. Widening of the superior mediastinum with displacement of the trachea to the left, marked swelling of the supraclavicular soft tissues on the left and an infiltrate in the apex of the right lung all may be due to *tuberculosis*, as they were in this case. Although an archaic term, "scrofula" denotes a contemporary problem, and tuberculous adenitis may occasionally be a prominent clinical feature of the disease.

In addition to swelling of his neck, this man had a localized mass involving his middle finger (E9–5B) that had been there for three years and for which he had refused treatment. Its chronicity is re-flected in the saucerlike erosion of the adjacent proximal phalanx. The curiosity of the physician overcame the reluctance of the patient, and a needle biopsy established the diagnosis of "a cold abscess characteristic of tuberculosis."

A well-documented episode of tuberculous arthritis of the wrist years ago left as its aftermath irregular destruction of the carpal bones and erosion and dislocation of the distal ulna. Although mimicking the destructive changes of rheumatoid arthritis, the monarticular distribution and the irregular loss of cartilage between the carpal bones makes this case most typical of a chronic infectious arthritis.

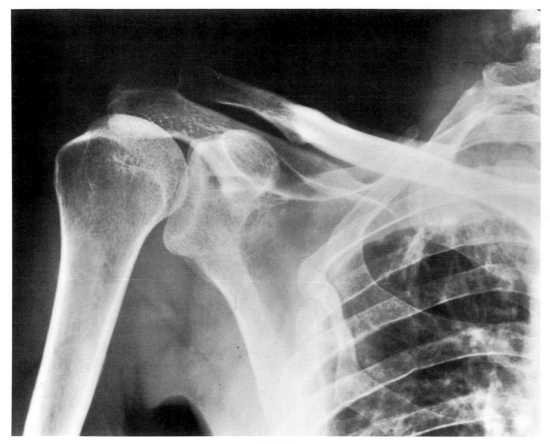

E9–6.

E9–6. The frustration of finding a normal shoulder radiograph when the patient insists he has pain is outweighed by the satisfaction of a successful search for the answer. At times one must look as high as the upper cervical spine to find the bony spur catching the nerve root at the intervertebral foramen. Sometimes it is much easier, as in this example, because the answer may lurk in the corner of the film. The white shadow of a *Pancoast tumor* has filled in the apex of the lung, has involved the brachial plexus and has caused shoulder pain and the mistaken impression of joint disease.

Chapter 10

THE SPINE, THE SACRO-ILIAC JOINTS AND THE SYMPHYSIS PUBIS

Back pain is a frequent problem, and the diagnostic possibilities range from malingerer to malignancy. The ability to recognize early signs of disease in the spine is predicated on a thorough knowledge of normal radiographic anatomy. With use of the same scheme of analysis that has been followed throughout this monograph, many of the previously discussed manifestations of the arthritides will be noted in the spine, and these same signs will be helpful in diagnosing the cause of the abnormality.

As in the other regions of the body, arthritis involving the spine may result from trauma, from infection, from connective tissue disorders and from degenerative changes. A knowledge of the characteristic types of changes, as well as the frequency with which different conditions affect the spine, is helpful in making a specific diagnosis.

Rather than dividing the discussion into abnormalities of soft tissue, alignment, bony mineralization, and cartilage destruction, as in the earlier chapters, it will be more helpful to contrast the changes in each region of the spine that occur with different diseases.

CERVICAL SPINE

Anatomy

A radiograph of a normal lateral spine illustrates the alignment of each vertebra and the appearance of the articulating processes (Fig. 10–1). The superior and inferior articulating facets are parallel to each other, and there is a well-defined, uniform joint space between them. The odontoid process lies in close approximation to the anterior ring of the first cervical vertebra. It is held in place firmly by a strong transverse ligament that attaches to each side of the ring and thus prevents its separation during flexion and hyperextension of the neck. Since these areas, as well as the joints of Luschka (the pointed projections at the posterior superior margins of the vertebral bodies) are synovium-lined joints, they must be closely scrutinized when diseases accompanied by synovitis are suspected.

SUBLUXATION

Any of the connective tissue disorders may cause synovitis and erosive changes in the cervical spine. In addition, the transverse ligament is affected by the inflammatory process. Ligamentous laxity results, and motion of the odontoid process occurs when the neck is flexed. Rheumatoid arthritis is the most frequent offender, but it is also seen in psoriatic arthritis and juvenile rheumatoid arthritis. Rarely, it occurs in ankylosing spondylitis.

Rheumatoid Arthritis. Figure 10–2 is a film of the lateral cervical spine of a patient with rheumatoid arthritis. Although the film was taken with the neck in flexion to exaggerate the malalignment, the similarity to the normal neck is obvious. There is one important dif-

398

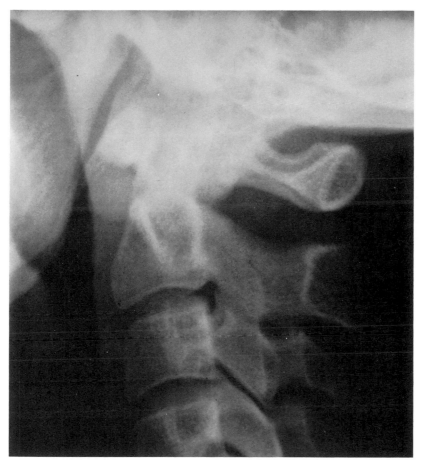

Figure 10–1. Normal cervical spine.

The prevertebral soft tissue measures only a few mm and contains no abnormal calcifications. Lines drawn through the anterior and posterior margins of the vertebral bodies as well as the anterior margin of the dorsal spines form smooth, continuous arcs. The odontoid process is separated from the anterior ring of the first cervical vertebra by no more than 2.5 mm. The apophyseal joints are sharply defined and uniform in width.

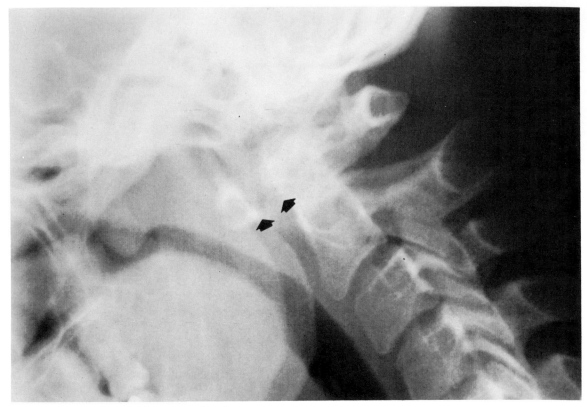

Figure 10–2. Rheumatoid arthritis.
　　Although no demineralization or erosions are present to suggest the diagnosis of rheumatoid arthritis, subluxation of C2 on C1 indicates inflammatory changes of the transverse ligament. One cm separates the odontoid process from the ring in the flexed position (arrows).

ference, however. The space between the odontoid process and the anterior ring of the first cervical vertebra is much greater than the normal separation of 2.5 mm seen in adults. This increased distance indicates anterior subluxation of the first cervical vertebra. When atlanto-axial subluxation occurs, the dorsal spine of the first cervical vertebra is displaced anteriorly, causing the spinal cord to take an erratic course from the foramen magnum through the upper cervical canal. It is not surprising that patients with this defective alignment develop symptoms of numbness and tingling of the fingers or even sudden quadriplegia.

A similar subluxation of the first cervical vertebra is illustrated in Figure 10–3. The separation of the odontoid process from the anterior ring is exaggerated in this patient by an accompanying synovitis which has eroded the bone and left only an amputated stump. In addition to the changes in the first cervical vertebra, there is an anterior subluxation of the fifth cervical vertebra, altering the alignment of the articulating facet as well. Changes throughout the cervical spine are commonly seen in rheumatoid arthritis and often are accompanied by disc space narrowing. The absence of prominent degenerative spurs distinguishes these changes from spondylosis.

Occasionally degenerative changes may be superimposed on the underlying inflammatory arthritis, and osteophytes associated with disc space narrowing may be the predominant radiographic finding. A film of an elderly man with rheumatoid arthritis demonstrates these changes between the third and fourth as well as the fourth and fifth cervical vertebrae (Fig. 10–4). In addition, there is marked erosive destruction of the odon-

Figure 10–3. Rheumatoid arthritis.

Subluxation due to rheumatoid arthritis may be seen in the cervical spine, in addition to the frequent atlantoaxial dislocation. Although the remaining vertebral bodies appear well-aligned, an offset of the dorsal spines of C3 and C4 and the posterior margins of the vertebral bodies of C5 and C6 indicate additional levels of subluxation (arrows). Erosions have deformed the fifth dorsal spine and amputated the odontoid. The widened space behind the anterior ring of C1 is due to erosion as well as subluxation.

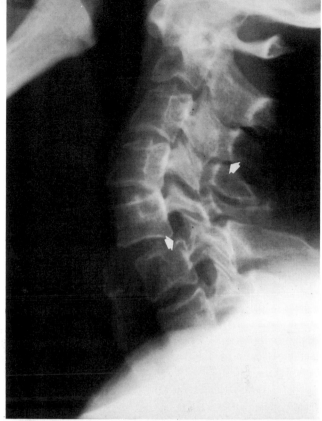

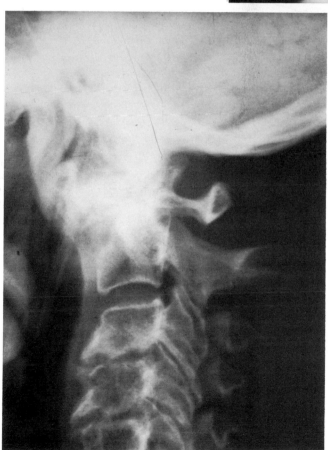

Figure 10–4. Rheumatoid arthritis.

The erosion of the odontoid process and subluxation of C2 on C1 is similar to that seen in the preceding example (Fig. 10–3). However, extensive destructive changes of the vertebral end plates and loss of the disc spaces at multiple levels indicate additional sites of inflammatory disease. A superimposed osteoarthritis is present, and osteophytes have developed at the levels of C3, C4 and C5.

toid process, similar to that seen in the preceding film, and never seen in an uncomplicated spondylosis. The changes of the intervertebral spaces are indistinguishable from those that accompany a degenerative process, but the disc spaces involved and the atlantoaxial subluxation differentiate an inflammatory arthritis from spondylosis. Degenerative changes of the cervical spine tend to begin at the intervertebral space between the fifth and sixth cervical vertebrae, the level of the greatest amount of pivotal motion. Whenever similar changes are present diffusely throughout the cervical spine or, as in this case, where they *spare* the intervertebral disc space between the fifth and sixth cervical vertebrae, other

arthritides, or previous trauma, must be suspected.

Congenital Absence of the Dens. Destruction of the dens from a localized synovitis must not be confused with its congenital absence. Figure 10–5 illustrates the smooth rounded surface and sharp cortical margin of the underdeveloped odontoid. Often, tomography must be employed in order to elucidate the margins of the dens and exclude the presence of erosion.

Psoriatic Arthritis. Psoriatic arthritis may affect the entire spine and duplicate the appearance of ankylosing spondylitis, or it may be limited to the cervical spine in a pattern identical to that of rheumatoid arthritis. In the latter case, inflamma-

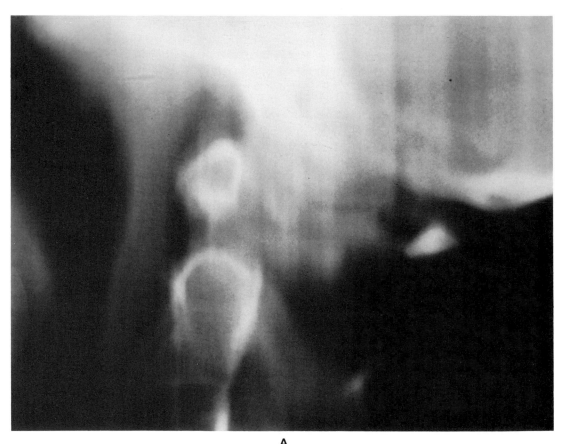

A

Figure 10–5. Congenital absence of the dens.
A. Lateral tomography of the cervical spine illustrates the smooth, rounded contour of the underdeveloped odontoid process.

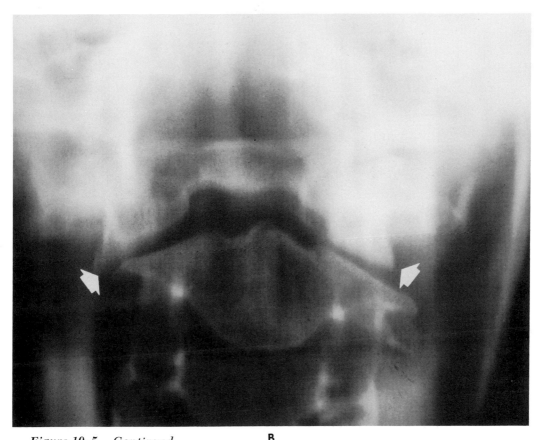

Figure 10–5. Continued.   **B**
B. An AP tomograph demonstrates the appearance on a frontal projection and also shows the offset between the first and second vertebral bodies (arrows).

tory involvement of the transverse ligament results in laxity and subluxation, as illustrated in the preceding patients with rheumatoid arthritis. Involvement of the synovial joints of Luschka and the apophyseal joints posteriorly will cause erosions of the articular bones, narrowing of the inflamed joint spaces and subluxations. This malalignment is often exaggerated in flexion and extension, and when it is clinically suspected, radiographic films in these positions should be obtained.

A patient with psoriatic arthritis was filmed in a neutral position (Fig. 10–6A). Although narrowing of the intervertebral space between the third and fourth cervical vertebrae is apparent, the excessive mobility is only appreciated when the spine is viewed in a flexed or hyperextended position (Fig. 10–6B and C). It is apparent that the spinal cord must go wherever the malaligned cervical vertebrae go; therefore, nodding "yes" may be a hazardous motion for these patients.

BONY ANKYLOSIS

Complete bony ankylosis may occur in ankylosing spondylitis, juvenile rheumatoid arthritis and, less commonly, in rheumatoid and psoriatic arthritis. When the ankylosis is confined to the apophyseal joints, three connective tissue disorders must be considered: juvenile rheumatoid arthritis, rheumatoid arthritis and psoriatic arthritis. Paravertebral calcification is more prominent in ankylosing spondylitis and is only occasionally seen in patients with psoriatic arthritis. Both patterns of ankylosis convert the spine to a rigid structure and make it extremely vulnerable to severe injury even with mild forms of trauma.

Ankylosing Spondylitis. Although fusion of the apophyseal joints is commonly seen in ankylosing spondylitis, it is not

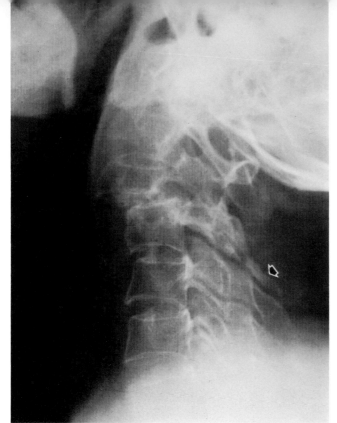

A

Figure 10–6. Psoriatic arthritis.

A. Changes may exactly mimic rheumatoid arthritis, as in this example. An erosion of the dorsal spine of C4 is seen (arrow), as well as subluxation of the vertebral body.

B. The subluxation of C3 on C4, and C4 on C5, is exaggerated by flexing the head.

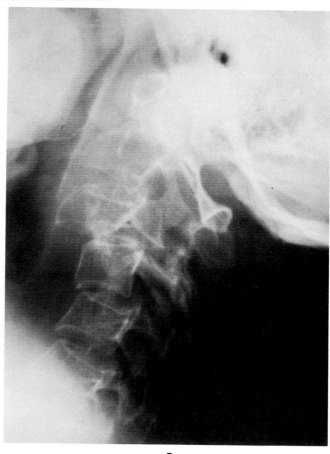

B

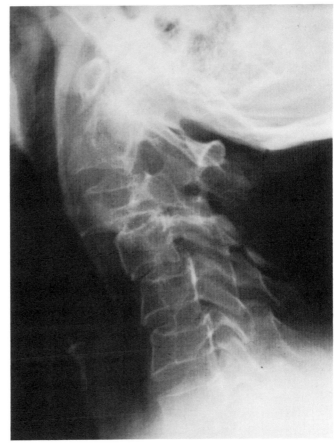

Figure 10-6. Continued.
C. It is only partially restored when the neck is hyperextended.

C

always present; the extensive paravertebral calcification anteriorly is often the more dramatic radiographic finding, as seen in Figure 10-7. This pattern of fusion is easily distinguished from that of rheumatoid arthritis. The vulnerability of a rigid spine to injury from minor trauma is illustrated by this example. The minimal jarring forces that occurred in mowing grass resulted in a horizontal fracture through the bridging bone anterior to the vertebral bodies and extending through the intervertebral space between the fourth and fifth cervical vertebrae (arrow). The hazards in minor stressful activities that occur daily must constantly be kept in mind by such patients, and radiographs of their cervical spine must be thoroughly examined for evidence of fractures. At times it is difficult to detect a break in the bone through the maze of extra shadows in patients with ankylosis

of the spine. If clinically suspected, a fracture that cannot be seen on routine films may necessitate tomography to clarify it.

Juvenile Rheumatoid Arthritis. Juvenile rheumatoid arthritis affecting the spine follows the pattern of adult rheumatoid arthritis, involving the *cervical spine,* sparing the thoracic and lumbar spines and occasionally resulting in inflammatory changes of the sacroiliac joints. Inflammatory changes of the apophyseal joints may result in bony ankylosis with subsequent intervertebral space narrowing. Growth disturbances may foreshorten the vertebral bodies, adding to the deformity.

A film of a 30 year old woman illustrates the classic findings of juvenile rheumatoid arthritis (Fig. 10-8). Inflammatory changes begin at the upper cervical vertebrae and may progress to involve the

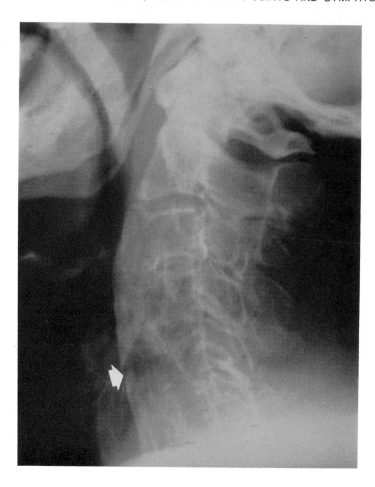

Figure 10–7. Ankylosing spondylitis.

Paravertebral calcification has transformed this into a bamboo spine. Minor trauma has resulted in a fracture through the fifth cervical vertebra and the adjacent syndesmophyte (arrow).

entire cervical spine. Apophyseal fusion of the upper cervical vertebrae has occurred, leading to severe narrowing of the intervertebral spaces. The decreased anterior-posterior dimensions of the cervical vertebrae occur when the arthritis has its onset during the growth period and thus are helpful in implicating the juvenile onset of rheumatoid arthritis.

Congenital Block Vertebrae. Failure of the spine to become normally segmented in the fetal period results in a configuration which may mimic severe disc space narrowing or an acquired fusion of the vertebral bodies (Fig. 10–9). There are two important features which distinguish congenital block vertebrae from these conditions. Where fusion of the vertebral bodies is acquired, as in inflammatory arthritides, destruction of the disc space must have occurred. The height of the fused vertebrae will therefore be decreased by the amount of disc and bone loss. The height of block vertebrae, on the other hand, will equal the height of the two vertebral bodies plus

Figure 10–8. (Facing page) Juvenile rheumatoid arthritis.

Typically the inflammatory changes of juvenile rheumatoid arthritis begin with the most cephalad apophyseal joints and gradually involve the lower cervical vertebrae. Fusion often results, and secondary narrowing of the intervertebral spaces mimics the changes of disc disease. The decreased AP diameter of the vertebral bodies reflects the childhood onset of the arthritis and the subsequent growth disturbance. In the absence of a history, this finding indicates a juvenile onset of an inflammatory arthritis.

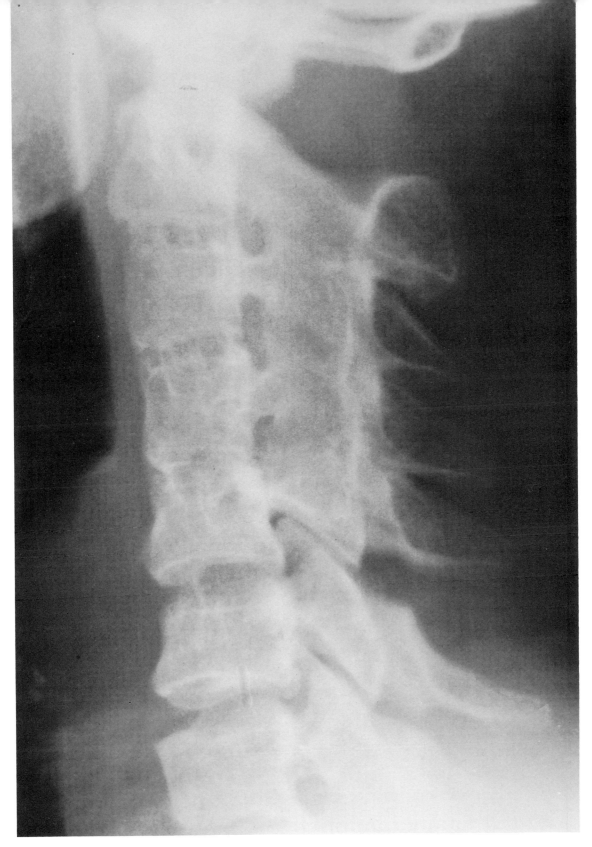

Figure 10–8. *See legend on opposite page.*

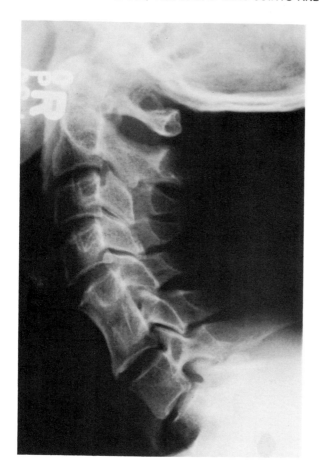

Figure 10–9. Congenital block vertebrae.

The smooth, concave appearance of the anterior border of the fused vertebrae, and the fact that their height equals that of both vertebral bodies *plus* a disc space, distinguish failure of segmentation from inflammatory changes with intervertebral space destruction.

the undeveloped intervertebral space. In addition, a block vertebra has a smooth, continuous, concave anterior margin that is markedly different from the irregular line of an acquired fusion.

OSTEOPHYTES

Degenerative disease of the spine has manifestations very different from the rheumatoid diseases and is diagnosed by three radiographic signs: (1) narrowing of the intervertebral space; (2) osteophytes along the border of the vertebral bodies; and (3) narrowing and sclerosis of the apophyseal joints. The term osteoarthritis should be used to designate only the changes in the apophyseal joints. A "true" arthritis (one with a component of inflammation) does not occur along the vertebral bodies in degenerative disease: the development of osteophytes signals an underlying discogenic process. This may be a result of trauma, of senescent

changes in the cartilage or the healing stages of infection. Since osteophytes form in response to degenerative cartilage, even in the absence of intervertebral space narrowing, the presence of these bony spurs points to an underlying abnormality. For this reason, *spondylosis* is a more precise term than *degenerative arthritis* for describing this condition.

Spondylosis. The maximum motion in flexion and extension of the cervical spine occurs at the level of the fifth and sixth cervical vertebrae. Routine films of this region in the middle-aged population group generally demonstrate mild changes of intervertebral space narrowing and osteophyte formation. The spurs are most easily seen anteriorly, as in Figure 10–10, on a lateral view of the spine. They may occur posteriorly, however, encroaching on the intervertebral foramina and causing nerve root signs. The

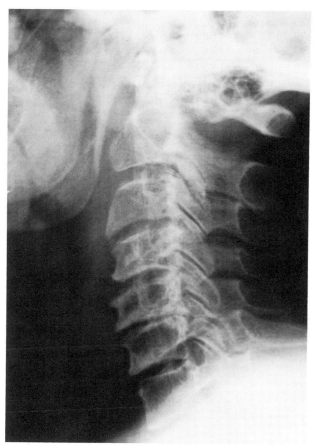

Figure 10–10. Spondylosis.
Narrowing of the intervertebral space between the fifth and sixth cervical vertebrae is the common site of degenerative changes of the cervical spine. Early signs of narrowing along the posterior margin of the intervertebral space of C4-C5 are also present. Small osteophytes accompanying the disc space narrowing complete the typical picture of spondylosis.

intervertebral foramina are visualized en face in oblique projections of the cervical spine, and small but significant bony projections may be diagnosed with ease using these views.

Any condition which hastens the degenerative changes in the disc spaces may result in spondylosis. Underlying inflammatory conditions such as rheumatoid arthritis may have a superimposed spondylosis (see Figure 10–4). Localized trauma with transient subluxation may damage the disc and initiate early degenerative changes. Patients with Parkinson's disease may have extensive spondylosis throughout the cervical spine because of the constant motion of the neck.

Ankylosing Hyperostosis (Forestier's disease). Exuberant osteophyte formation and degenerative changes in the disc characterize the condition known as Forestier's disease. New bone formation around the degenerative cartilage is excessive and bridging of the intervertebral spaces common, resulting in a condition which superficially resembles ankylosing spondylitis. However, the osteophytes are thicker and more anterior, and although the new bone may incorporate the anterior longitudinal ligament and the outer fibers of the annulus, its appearance is very different from that in ankylosing spondylitis. When this condition occurs in the cervical spine, the patient's primary complaint is frequently the feeling that food sticks in his throat. It is evident in examining the spine of such a patient (Fig. 10–11) that the bony projections encroach on the soft tissue space occupied by the esophagus. A barium swallow study would demonstrate anterior displacement of the esophagus by the extrinsic mass of new bone.

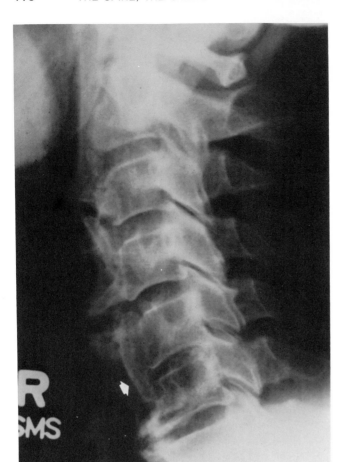

Figure 10–11. Forestier's disease.

Exuberant osteophytes anteriorly encroach on the soft tissue space occupied by the esophagus. Absence of degenerative changes of the intervertebral spaces and apophyseal joints are typical of this form of spondylosis, as is the "additive" nature of the osteophytes. Sparing of the sacroiliac joints distinguishes this entity from ankylosing spondylitis, even though the osteophytes may be vertically oriented, similar to a syndesmophyte, as at C5-C6 (arrow).

THORACOLUMBAR SPINE

Infectious Arthritides: Localized

Several features distinguish suppurative from granulomatous infections in the spine. One of these is the rate at which bone and cartilage is destroyed: granulomatous infections develop much more slowly. Another distinguishing feature is the presence of a localized cold abscess associated with bone destruction. This is a typical accompaniment of tuberculosis; however, a small paravertebral abscess may also be seen in association with a gram negative infection. Finally, early formation of osteophytes adjacent to a destroyed disc indicates healing and is typically seen in suppurative infections. Although osteophytes may be associated with tuberculous spondylitis, they are a very late occurrence in this disease.

Tuberculous Spondylitis. Because of the paucity of symptoms in tuberculous spondylitis, not infrequently the initial manifestation of infection is observed on a routine chest film as a localized paraspinal mass. The abscess of a young child with this disease extends from the seventh thoracic vertebra to the first lumbar vertebra (Fig. 10–12A, arrows). Involvement of the bone is present, as seen by loss of height of the tenth thoracic vertebra. Its dramatic reduction to a thin wedge is better appreciated on the lateral view (Fig. 10–12B, arrows). Not only does the indolent nature of the infection result in merely minor symptomatology, but the pathologic changes are slow, and the intervertebral spaces characteristically are involved late in the course of the disease.

Figure 10–12.   Tuberculous spondylitis.

A. A large paravertebral mass extends from the seventh thoracic vertebra to the first lumbar vertebra (arrows).

B. Bone and disc changes are difficult to evaluate on an AP view but are clear on the lateral projection. The tenth thoracic vertebra has collapsed, widening the adjacent disc spaces (arrows). The gouged-out defects of the anterior margins of the ninth and eleventh thoracic vertebrae are typical of the changes of tuberculous osteomyelitis.

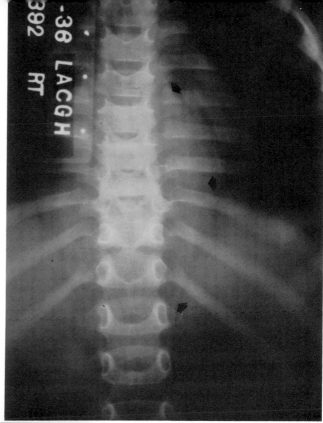

A

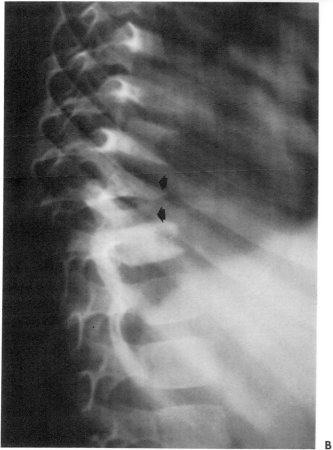

B

411

In this example, destruction of the vertebral body has resulted in widening of the adjacent intervertebral spaces. Preservation of the disc space is more common in granulomatous than in pyogenic diseases, since proteolytic enzymes are not produced and the fragmented cartilage remains. In addition, deposition of granulation tissue adds to the soft tissue shadow between the vertebral bodies.

In this example, additional bone destruction involves the vertebral bodies above and below the tenth thoracic vertebra. The gouged appearance is typical of the manner in which tuberculosis affects the spine, as it often involves the anterior portion of the vertebral body before the end plates.

The prominent paravertebral mass associated with tuberculous spondylitis and the complete vertebral destruction that may occur is dramatically illustrated in a pathologic specimen (Fig. 10–13). Posterior displacement of the spinal cord indicates the extent of the abscess.

The end stage of a healed tuberculous spondylitis is illustrated in Figure 10–14. Because of the destroyed intervertebral space and the destructive changes of the anterior vertebral bodies, kyphosis de-

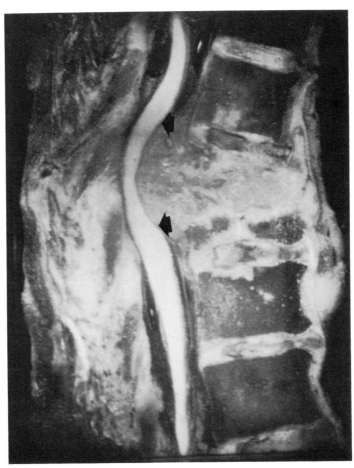

Figure 10–13. Tuberculous spondylitis.
A pathologic specimen of the lower thoracic spine shows a large paravertebral cold abscess displacing the spinal cord posteriorly (arrows). Complete destruction of the adjacent vertebral body and the beginning of a kyphotic deformity are apparent. The persistent space between the destroyed vertebral body and its adjacent vertebra reflects the absence of proteolytic enzymes and illustrates the accumulation of granulomatous tissue and bony and cartilaginous fragments. (Courtesy of The Arthritis Foundation.)

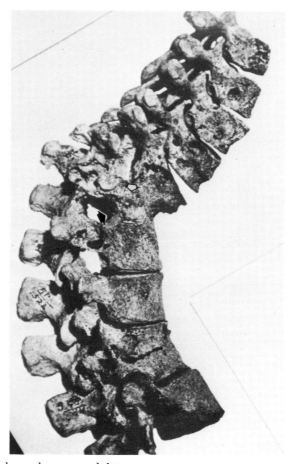

Figure 10–14. Tuberculous spondylitis.
  Collapse of the twelfth thoracic vertebra to a thin wedge (arrows) and fusion with adjacent vertebral bodies has resulted in a severe kyphotic deformity. (Courtesy of The Arthritis Foundation.)

velops and bony ankylosis may fuse two adjacent vertebrae.

In a quarter of patients with tuberculosis, new bone forms during the healing phase, and prominent osteophytes associated with a wedge-shaped vertebral body remain as hallmarks of an earlier tuberculous infection. For this reason, the presence of osteophytes, as in Figure 10–15A, does not necessarily indicate a suppurative infection or exclude the diagnosis of tuberculosis. The formation of osteophytes is a late occurrence in this disease, distinguishing it from the serial changes that rapidly take place in a suppurative infection. The pattern can be differentiated from spondylosis by the marked destructive changes in the vertebral body that accompany the osteophytes, best seen on a lateral projection (Fig. 10–15B). An identical picture, however, may occur from a traumatic fracture with wedge collapse and subsequent healing.

Suppurative Spondylitis Following Drug Abuse. It is *essential* to detect any infection of the spine at the earliest possible moment and thus diagnose and initiate treatment at the onset of disease. Otherwise, irreparable damage will ensue. In the past, the most frequent infections of the spine were tuberculous or staphylococcal. Today, with the rise in intravenous drug abuse, it is much more common to culture Pseudomonas or Klebsiella than any other bacterial agent.

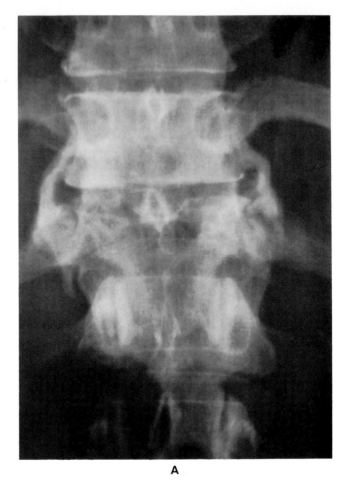

A

Figure 10–15. Tuberculous spondylitis.
A. The end stage of a tuberculous osteomyelitis may be identical to that of a pyogenic infection, with bony destruction and osteophytes. However, these changes appear after months or years.

The radiographic changes in such infections are similar to those in tuberculosis except that the rate of change is measured in weeks and months rather than in years.

An initial film of the lumbar spine following the onset of back pain in a young man was normal (Fig. 10–16A). Two weeks later, destruction of the vertebral end plates of the third and fourth lumbar vertebrae and concomitant loss of the intervertebral cartilage became apparent (Fig. 10–16B). Two *months* later, despite treatment, progressive rapid loss of bone and destruction of the disc were evident. Anterior osteophytes had formed, bridg-

ing the intervertebral space (Fig. 10–16C and D). This pattern of change and the brief period over which they occurred are characteristic of both staphylococcal and gram negative infections.

In the majority of patients with a history of drug abuse who develop osteomyelitis, as in the preceding case, a transient septicemia establishes the infection in the vertebral body, and spread to the adjacent vertebra quickly follows via the interconnecting arterial supply. Occasionally, the sternoclavicular joint, the sacroiliac joint or a peripheral joint may be involved. This pattern, similar to that of deposition of metastatic tumor,

Text continued on page 418.

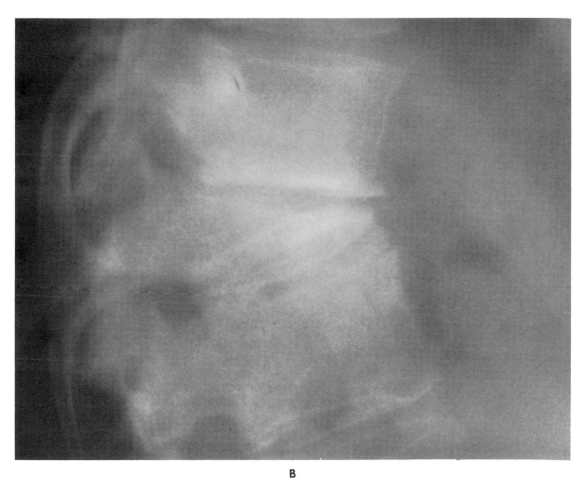

B

Figure 10–15. Continued.
B. The lateral view documents the extensive loss of height of the twelfth thoracic vertebra. Slight narrowing of the adjacent intervertebral spaces accompanies the change.

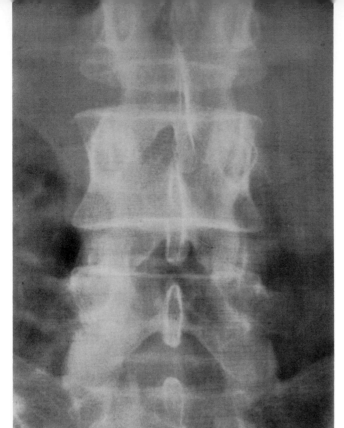

Figure 10–16. Pseudomonas osteomyelitis.

A. Often a film of the spine will be normal at the onset of back pain.

B. Within two or three weeks, however, a pyogenic infection will cause radiographic blurring and irregularity of the sharp cortical margin of the vertebral end plate and narrowing of the disc space (arrow).

A

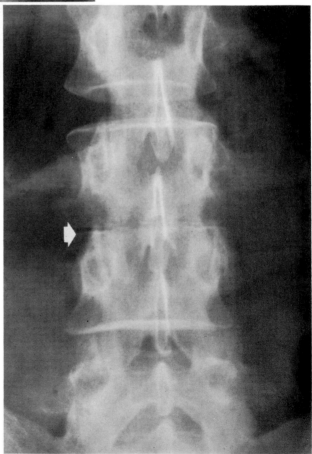

B

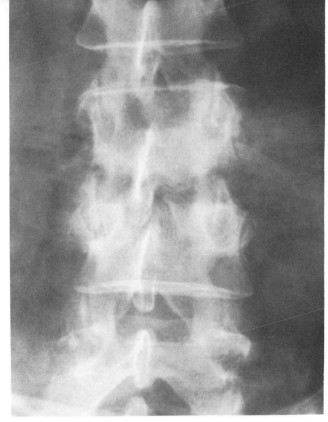

Figure 10–16. Continued.
C and *D*. Rapid destruction of bone and cartilage is characteristic of pyogenic infections; in this patient, the damage has occurred over a two month interval.

C

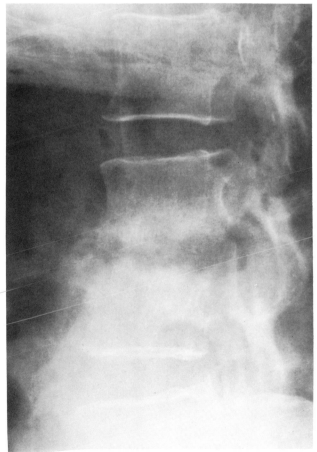

D

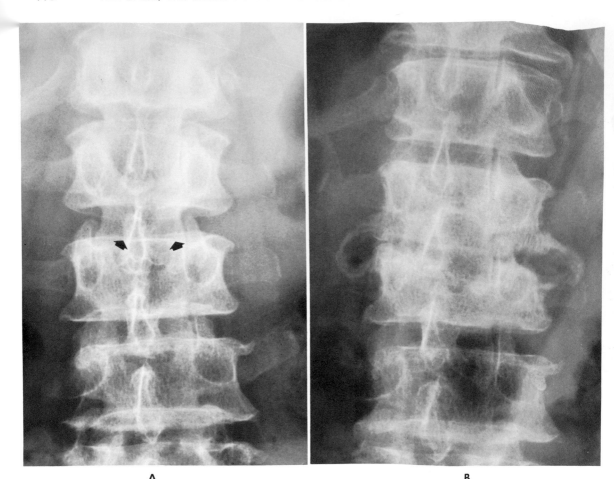

A   B

Figure 10–17.   Suppurative spondylitis following fracture.
   A. A break in the white line of the vertebral end plate (arrows) reflects an anterior superior fracture of the vertebral body.
   B. Four months later, extensive destruction of the vertebral end plates, loss of the intervertebral space and evidence of prominent lateral osteophytes signal a superimposed infection.

presumably relates to blood flow and the presence of hemopoietically active marrow. Any bone that has an increased metabolic activity or localized hyperemia is also vulnerable to the deposition of metastasizing tumor or bacteria, as illustrated by the following case.

Suppurative Spondylitis Following Fracture.   Trauma to the lumbar spine in an osteoporotic 55 year old woman resulted in a fracture of the anterior superior margin of the second lumbar vertebra. Although the findings were extremely subtle on a frontal projection of the spine, the break in the cortical line indicated the compression fracture (Fig.

10–17A, arrows). Persistence of her back pain led to a second examination four months later (Fig. 10–17B). Extensive destruction of adjacent vertebral bodies, loss of the intervertebral disc space and rapid development of bridging osteophytes attested to the presence of a superimposed bacterial infection.

Fracture with collapse of the involved vertebral bodies may widen the disc space but never obliterates it. To attribute loss of disc space and growth of osteophytes to trauma alone is a great error; radiographic changes such as those evident in the preceding patient should always suggest a superimposed infection.

To illustrate the possible different findings associated with loss of vertebral height, a film of a patient with severe osteoporosis from long-term adrenocorticosteroid use is presented (Fig. 10–18A). In this example, both central and anterior collapse are present throughout the spine, frequent complications of this severe degree of osteoporosis. However, in spite of the destruction of the vertebrae, it is apparent that the intervertebral space is maintained or even widened.

Radiographing a pathologic specimen clarifies the anatomic detail of the collapse by eliminating the overlying shadows of bowel gas and soft tissues (Fig. 10–18B). Infractions through the thin, fragile cortex of multiple vertebral bodies are present.

Infectious Arthritides: Disseminated

Suppurative Spondylitis Involving Multiple Vertebral Bodies. Multiple levels of the spine may be involved by infection. For example, a heroin user developed acute onset of back pain. Radio-

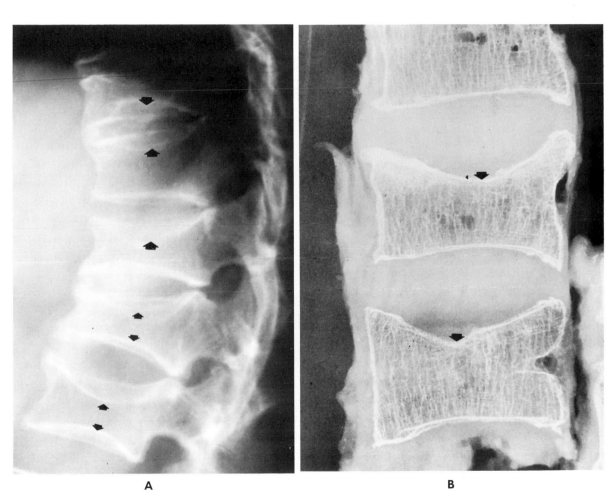

A **B**

Figure 10–18. Osteoporosis with compression fractures.

A. A thin cortex and "ground-glass" matrix are characteristic of osteoporosis; in this patient with systemic lupus erythematosus they have resulted from prolonged adrenocorticosteroid therapy. Central collapse (arrows) of the brittle bones has caused widening of the intervertebral spaces.

B. The pencil-thin, white cortex and sparse, lacy trabeculae give little support against the stress of weight bearing. Compression fractures with loss of vertebral height (arrows) are evident in this pathologic specimen. Widening of the intervertebral disc spaces accompanies the fractures. (Courtesy of Roger Terry, M.D.)

graphic examination of his spine demonstrated loss of the disc space at three levels, with adjacent bone destruction (Fig. 10–19). Despite the prominent finding of disc narrowing, it is rare for infection to be established in the relatively avascular cartilage, and a primary osteomyelitis with herniation of the disc into the destroyed vertebral end plates is the most likely explanation for the findings. The distinction between osteomyelitis and cartilage infection is critical when diagnostic procedures are planned. Biopsy of the disc space is frequently nonproductive, and a bone biopsy may be necessary to provide a bacterial diagnosis.

Disseminated Tuberculous Spondylitis. The gouged appearance of the anterior vertebral bodies is evident at multiple levels in a film of a 63 year old woman with disseminated tuberculosis (Fig. 10–20).* Despite extensive involvement of her spine for a year prior to treatment, the destructive changes are limited to the anterior vertebral bodies, and the disc spaces have not yet become involved. The slow progression of the disease characterizes granulomatous infections of the spine and distinguishes them from the previous examples of suppurative spondylitis. Despite the passing of a year, only minimal increase in the size of the lytic areas was apparent. The destruction of bone and sparing of the disc spaces indicate the pathophysiologic mechanism of the infection: an osteomyelitis occurs primarily and disc destruction follows.

---

*This patient's hand was illustrated in Chapter 3, Fig. 3–13.

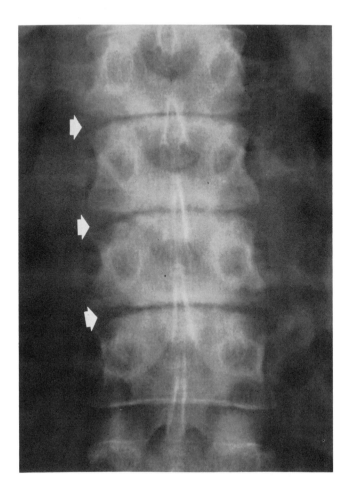

Figure 10–19. Spondylitis. Loss of the sharp cortical margins of L1, L2, L3 and L4 (arrows) and intervertebral narrowing are particularly dramatic when contrasted with the normal intervertebral space at L4-L5. The increased density of bone along the involved vertebral end plates indicates a reactive osteitis.

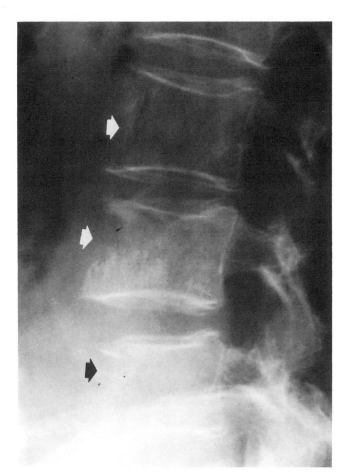

Figure 10-20. Tuberculous spondylitis.

Because of the anterior vertebral arterial plexus, infection may spread to contiguous bones, simulating spread from a primary focus within the disc space. Lytic areas of destruction are present in the anterior portions of three contiguous vertebral bodies (arrows). Preservation of the disc space early in the course of infection is characteristic of tuberculosis because of the absence of proteolytic enzymes.

Ankylosing Spondylitis

Undoubtedly the most underdiagnosed arthritis of the spine is ankylosing spondylitis. It occurs in young men as early as adolescence and is characterized by intermittent back pain. The full-blown radiographic picture is pathognomonic of this disease when bony bridging converts the separate vertebral bodies into a bamboo spine. The diagnostic dilemma, however, occurs early in the disease when back pain first begins. Later, the patient may even walk into the office with a typical thoracic kyphosis, flexed hips and poker spine, and yet the radiographs of his back appear normal.

In order to illustrate the pathologic changes associated with ankylosing spondylitis, a series of patients with progressively more subtle findings in the lumbar spine are presented.

BAMBOO SPINE

The typical bamboo spine is created from extensive soft tissue calcification within the outer fibers of the annulus of the vertebral disc and the fibers of the anterior and lateral vertebral ligaments. The new bone bridges the intervertebral space and fuses the spine into a rigid unit, as in Figure 10–21. This anterior and lateral new bone is characteristic of ankylosing spondylitis and is called a syndesmophyte. Its vertical axis distinguishes it from the more horizontal orientation of an osteophyte.

A dried preparation of the spine of a patient with ankylosing spondylitis illustrates the anatomic location of the interconnecting bony bridges (Fig. 10–22).

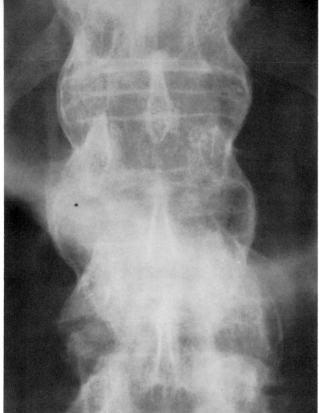

Figure 10–21. Ankylosing spondylitis.

Syndesmophytes developing in the outer layers of the disc and on the inner surface of the longitudinal ligaments bridge the intervertebral spaces and fuse the spine into a rigid structure.

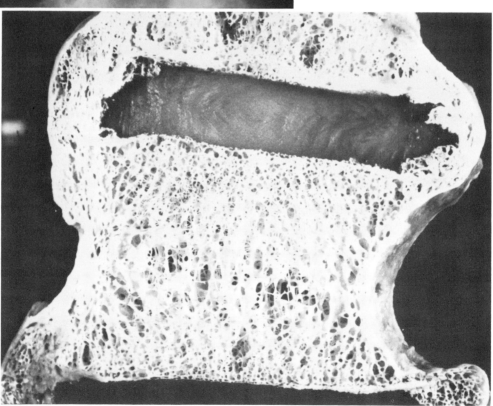

Figure 10–22. Ankylosing spondylitis.

A macerated preparation illustrates the characteristic vertical orientation of the syndesmophytes and their location in the outer aspects of the annulus. (Courtesy of The Arthritis Foundation.)

The anterior extent of the annulus is apparent from a specimen of the vertebral bodies and intervertebral disc of a child (Fig. 10–23). That the new bone is within the annulus is more apparent when the anterior and lateral extent of the fibrocartilage is appreciated.

In addition to new bone surrounding the vertebral body, posterior ossification forms within the interspinous ligaments, fusing the spinous processes. When it is viewed on a frontal projection, as in Figure 10–24A, a solid vertical white shadow is seen running down the midline of the vertebral bodies. Ankylosing spondylitis typically begins symmetrically in the sacroiliac joints and methodically progresses up the spine. In this example, the intervertebral spaces are all bridged by new bone laterally, resulting in a bamboo spine. The lateral view (Fig. 10–24B) illustrates the peripheral calcification of the outer fibers of the disc and graphically demonstrates the difference in location of the pathologic changes in this disease and in Forestier's disease, in which the osteophytes tend to develop anterior to the ligaments.

APOPHYSEAL FUSION

In addition to soft tissue calcification around the vertebral bodies, synovitis accompanies ankylosing spondylitis and frequently results in bony fusion of the apophyseal joints. The tendency, again, is to begin in the lower lumbar spine and to gradually involve higher vertebrae until finally the cervical spine may become affected. Wherever arthritis affects

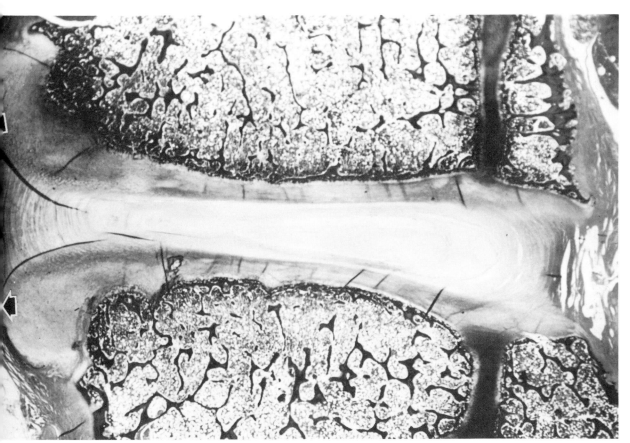

Figure 10–23. Normal disc.
A lateral projection of an intervertebral disc from a child documents the anterior extent of the fibrocartilage (arrows) and makes it easier to understand the location of syndesmophytes in this peripheral portion of the annulus. (Courtesy of Roger Terry, M.D.)

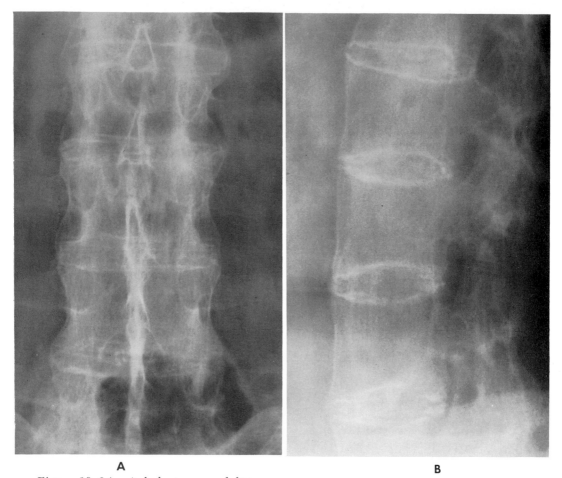

A **B**

Figure 10–24.   Ankylosing spondylitis.

A. The AP view illustrates syndesmophytes bridging the intervertebral spaces laterally and also demonstrates a continuous line of bone fusing the spinous processes. Ankylosing spondylitis typically begins at the sacroiliac joints and progressively involves more proximal vertebral bodies.

B. The lateral view demonstrates the typical squared appearance of the anterior vertebral silhouette from erosion of the corners due to an osteitis. Early syndesmophyte formation is present. Complete obliteration of the apophyseal joints is apparent, with bony ankylosis of the spine posteriorly.

these posterior joints, a secondary narrowing of the intervertebral space follows. If the evidence of arthritic changes were overlooked, it would be easy to assume that a primary disc problem was responsible for the abnormal intervertebral space. Although the changes in the apophyseal joints are identical to those occurring in rheumatoid arthritis, their presence in the lumbar spine differentiates ankylosing spondylitis from this disease.

Characteristically, ankylosing spondylitis begins symmetrically at the sacroiliac joints and progresses in a cephalad direction. Most frequently the disease burns itself out, and changes are limited to the sacroiliac joints and the lower lumbar vertebrae. However, occasionally the entire spine will be involved. Figure 10–25A illustrates bony bridging anteriorly and fusion of the apophyseal joints posteriorly. The lateral view of the cervical spine (Fig. 10–25B) demonstrates early involvement of the posterior elements with fusion of the lower apophyseal joints between the fifth and sixth cervical vertebrae, and narrowing and irregularity of the joint space immediately above (arrow). A syndesmophyte has formed, bridging the space between the fourth and fifth cervical vertebrae.

OSTEITIS

The most subtle manifestation of ankylosing spondylitis is the radiographic appearance of osteitis. This affects the anterior corners of the vertebral bodies and causes destruction of bone. Normally, the lumbar vertebrae have a concave anterior margin and the superior and inferior corners project anteriorly. The result of osteitis is a squared-off appearance of the silhouette on the lateral view of the spine, as in Figure 10–26. This is an early manifestation of ankylosing spondylitis and must be searched for if the disease is to be detected at its onset. (This same finding was also present in Figures 10–24 and 10–25.)

As healing of the osteitis occurs, new bone forms along the anterior border of the vertebral body, and the concave silhouette reappears. At first, the syndesmophyte casts a separate shadow, but eventually it fuses imperceptibly with the underlying bony cortex, as in Figure 10–27 (arrow).

Spondylosis

Osteophyte formation is stimulated by the presence of degenerative cartilage,

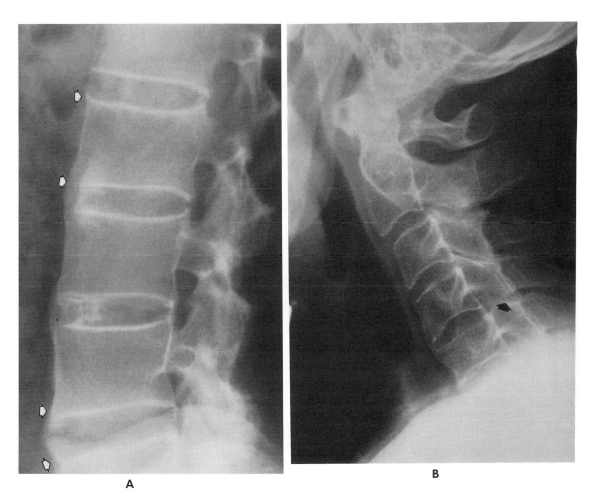

A

B

Figure 10–25. Ankylosing spondylitis.

A. As healing follows the initial osteitis, syndesmophytes develop and restore the concave configuration of the anterior vertebral borders (arrows).

B. Ankylosing spondylitis typically progresses proximally, and the entire spine in this patient is involved by spondylitis to the level of C4, where syndesmophytes and apophyseal joint abnormalities end (arrow).

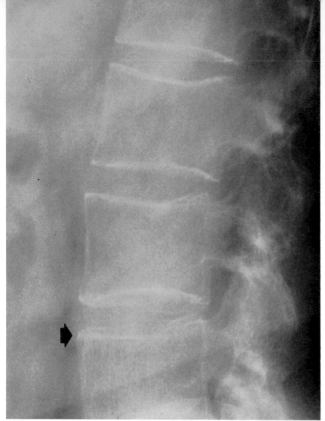

Figure 10-26. Ankylosing spondylitis.

The importance of recognizing the earliest manifestation is essential in correctly interpreting the cause of back pain. Squaring of the lower vertebral body (arrow) indicates the presence of an active inflammatory process and must not be overlooked. Substantiating the presence of ankylosing spondylitis is the change in the apophyseal joints, resulting in obliteration of the synovial joints of the lower lumbar spine.

Figure 10-27. Ankylosing spondylitis.

Syndesmophytes bridge the anterior disc spaces. In addition, an osteophyte has formed (arrow), illustrating the difference in appearance between a degenerative and an inflammatory response of bone. Its horizontal orientation is distinctive from the vertical projection of the syndesmophytes.

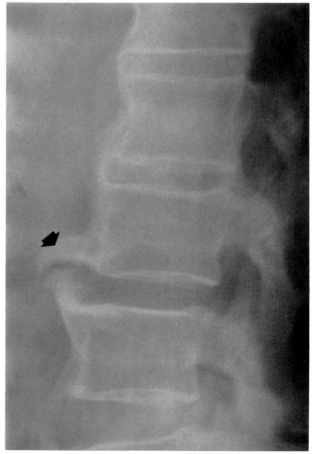

and it signifies discogenic disease. The difference between a syndesmophyte, the sine qua non of ankylosing spondylitis, and an osteophyte is illustrated by a single film (Fig. 10–27) and an accompanying gross pathologic specimen (Fig. 10–28). A patient with ankylosing spondylitis and a bamboo spine demonstrates the vertical orientation of syndesmophytes, but in addition, discogenic disease has resulted in a prominent osteophyte formed around the degenerative cartilage (arrow). The horizontal projection of the bony spur is in striking contrast to the appearance of the syndesmophytes and emphasizes the difference between their development.

Intervertebral disc space narrowing indicates loss of substance of the disc and is additional evidence of discogenic disease. Figure 10–29A demonstrates both intervertebral space narrowing and osteophytes throughout the lumbar spine. There is an additional radiographic finding which is pathognomonic of disc disease because it represents pathologic changes of the cartilage: the black line in the intervertebral spaces, seen on both the frontal and lateral views (Fig. 10–29B) and called a vacuum disc. Although its exact pathologic nature is not known, the name of this phenomenon implies gas within the disc itself. Since it is a persistent finding, unlike the transient crescent

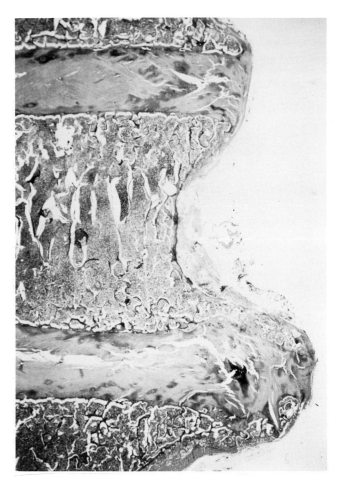

Figure 10–28. Osteophytes.
Large horizontal projections of new bone are separated by cartilage and are identical to the radiographic changes of spondylosis. Degenerative changes in the cartilage accompany the developing osteophytes. (Courtesy of The Arthritis Foundation.)

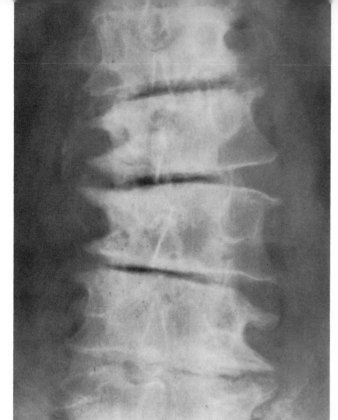

Figure 10–29. Spondylosis.
A. Degenerative changes of the spine are characterized by narrowing of the disc space and osteophyte formation. They differ in pattern from spondylitis by preservation of the vertebral end plates and by more horizontally directed productive new bone that appears to buttress or compensate for the areas of interspace narrowing and vertebral collapse. Frequently a "vacuum disc" is seen as a radiolucent line between the vertebral bodies. This probably represents accumulation of lipid material in the degenerative nucleus pulposus.
B. The vacuum discs are equally well seen on a lateral view.

A

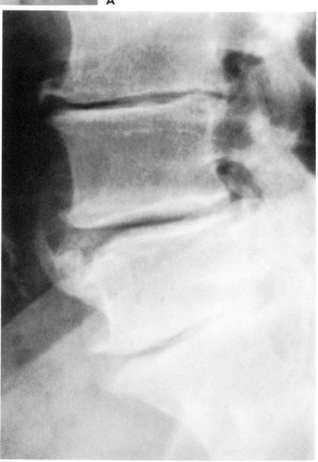

B

of gas that occurs in the large joints during moments of reduced intra-articular pressure, the term is probably a misnomer. The black line more likely represents collections of lipid material within the degenerative disc which cast a radiolucent shadow similar to gas. Whatever the pathophysiologic mechanism, its presence is always indicative of disc disease.

Figure 10–30 demonstrates a vacuum disc between the fifth lumbar vertebra and the sacrum. Accompanying this sign of disc disease is slight narrowing of the intervertebral space. The interspace between the fifth lumbar vertebra and the sacrum is notoriously difficult to evaluate and frequently appears minimally narrowed in normal patients on the lateral view of the spine. In the absence of osteophytes, the presence of the horizontal lucent line allows an unequivocal diagnosis of disc disease at a level that is otherwise easy to misdiagnose.

A third example of spondylosis illustrates another radiographic sign of discogenic disease (Fig. 10–31). In addition to prominent *osteophytes* and nonuniform *narrowing* of multiple intervertebral spaces, a *vacuum disc* is present at the intervertebral space between the second and third lumbar vertebrae. The fourth sign of cartilage destruction is seen between the third and fourth lumbar vertebrae as a *calcified disc.* It should not be surprising to find calcification within the degenerative cartilaginous disc, since calcification of dystrophic cartilage may occur anywhere in the body.

Ochronosis. Wherever extensive disc disease is present and is associated with universal calcification of the cartilage, an

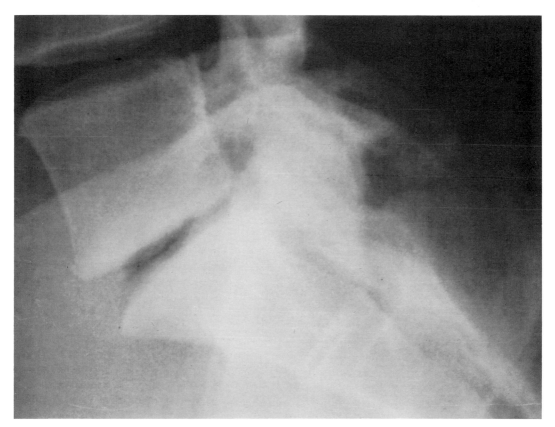

Figure 10–30. Vacuum disc.
An unequivocal diagnosis of degenerative disc disease can be made if a vacuum disc is present, despite only minimal evidence of disc space narrowing.

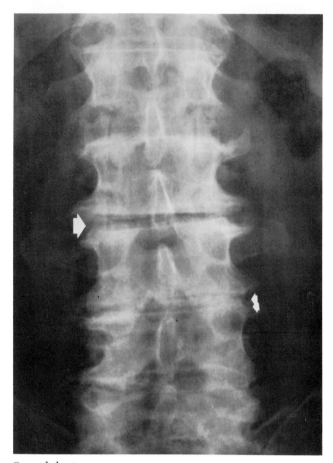

Figure 10–31. Spondylosis.
Irregular narrowing of the intervertebral spaces and osteophytes are present at all levels of the lumbar spine. A vacuum disc is present at L2-L3 (arrow). Calcification of cartilage occurs from any cause of degeneration and is not pathognomonic of ochronosis. Extensive calcification within the disc is seen at L3-L4 (double arrows).

etiology of ochronosis is likely. Figure 10–32 illustrates these findings. There is severe superimposed degenerative disease with marked narrowing of the disc spaces, osteophytes and eburnation of the vertebral end plates. The calcified cartilage is present but must be searched for to distinguish it from adjacent sclerotic new bone.

Figure 10–33 shows the pathologic specimen from another patient with ochronosis. The dense pigmentation of the cartilage and the irregular narrowing of the intervertebral spaces diffusely through the spine are changes identical to those revealed by the radiographs. In addition, calcification within the disc space is apparent (arrow).

Acromegaly. Overgrowth of bone and cartilage are the hallmarks of acromegaly, and they occur in the spine as in the other regions of the body. A lateral view of the spine illustrates apposition of new bone at the periphery of the vertebral bodies. This alters their shape, giving the bones an increased anterior-posterior dimension (Fig. 10–34). Because of the circumferential formation of new bone, the vertebrae may occasionally appear as a bone within a bone, although it is not apparent in this example. Untimely degenerative changes accompany the cartilaginous overgrowth, signified in this case by osteophytes, intervertebral space narrowing and calcification within the disc cartilage.

Figure 10–32. Ochronosis.

A. Deposition of pigment within the disc cartilage causes destruction and subsequent narrowing of the intervertebral spaces. Calcification is common and can be seen paralleling the vertebral end plates, almost hidden by the eburnation that has occurred.

B. The typical horizontally directed osteophytes can be seen anteriorly at the margins of the narrowed disc spaces.

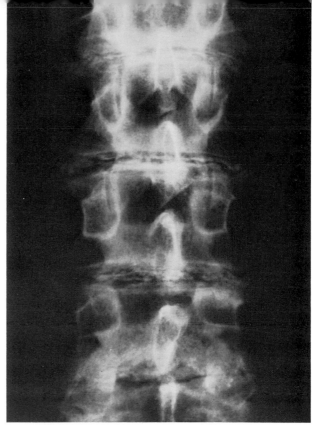

A

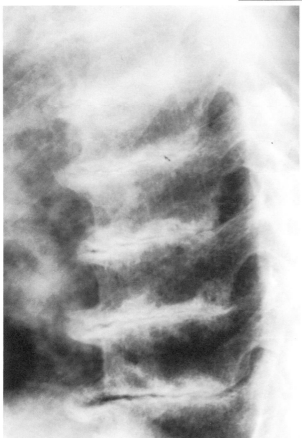

B

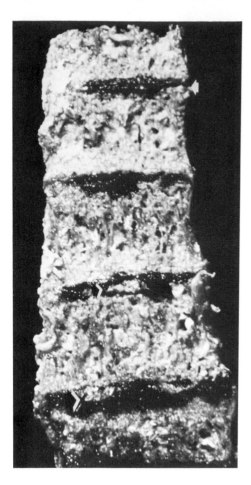

Figure 10–33. Ochronosis.

The pathologic specimen is similar to the radiograph of the spine. Black pigment has darkened the discs, and irregular narrowing of all the intervertebral spaces is present. Chondrocalcinosis is present (arrows). (Courtesy of The Arthritis Foundation.)

Figure 10–34. Acromegaly.

A lateral view of the spine illustrates multiple levels of degenerative disc disease and osteophytes, reflecting the early senescence that accompanies this endocrine disorder. The increased AP diameter of the vertebral bodies from bony overgrowth distorts their normal shape.

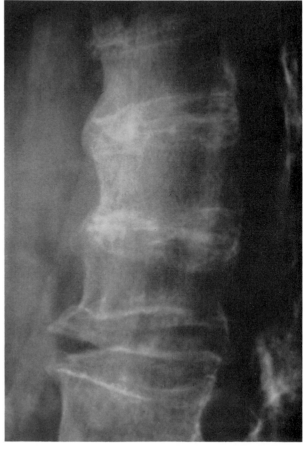

THE SACROILIAC JOINTS

The ease with which small or subtle abnormalities may be detected on an examination of the lumbar spine is in striking variance with the difficulty of evaluating the sacroiliac joints. Their oblique course results in superimposition of the two articulating bones on each other on a frontal projection, and hence, the joint space is never viewed tangentially. Any suspicious abnormality must be further evaluated by additional projections in order to avoid the hazard of diagnosing disease where there is none or to delineate the abnormal finding to its best advantage. This may be done either by obtaining oblique views of each joint, in order to "sight down" the cartilage space, or by angulation of the x-ray tube 30 degrees toward the patient's head to obtain a supine AP angled view of both sacroiliac joints simultaneously.

Even though the supine view of the sacroiliac area is difficult to evaluate, there are definite criteria of normality that can be judged on this projection. The importance of recognizing them becomes evident when it is realized that the opportunity of evaluating early signs of an abnormality generally must be done from supine views of the sacroiliac joints on spine series, abdominal series and films from colon and kidney examinations.

Normal Sacroiliac Joint. An appreciation of the criteria that establish a normal sacroiliac joint on a less than ideal projection is important because it enables one to recognize minimal deviations and thus detect the subtle signs of early pathologic changes. In a normal joint, the articulating margins of bone are sharply defined by a continuous subchondral white line, and the width of the sacroiliac joint is uniform throughout (Fig. 10–35).

Traumatic Dislocation. The fre-

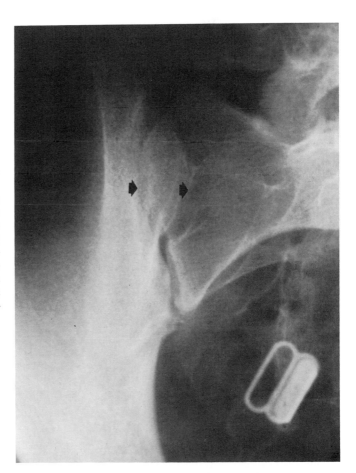

Figure 10–35. Normal sacroiliac joints.

Sharp, smooth outlines of the articulating bones and a cartilage space uniform in width are the two criteria for a normal joint. Because of the obliquity, the superior margins of the bones are viewed twice (arrows). The upper third of bone is bound by interosseous ligaments and is not part of the synovium-lined joint.

quency of pelvic fracture in accidents in today's high-speed auto and motorcycle traffic is accompanied by a high incidence of traumatic changes in the sacroiliac joints. Because the pelvis is a ring, a break in one side is almost always accompanied by a second break or diastasis of one of the joints.

Widening of the sacroiliac joint and a fracture fragment of the inferior margin are seen in Figure 10–36, a film taken following a motorcycle accident. There is a vertical fracture of the ilium superimposed over the sacroiliac joint (arrow). The severity of the displacement is appreciated by noting the wide separation of the superior borders of the ilium and sacrum. Although healing may take place with no residual evidence of the previous trauma, permanent alignment abnormalities and degenerative changes may ensue.

Osteitis Condensans Ilii. Although the term osteitis implies inflammation, the clinical history of postpartum back pain in young women and the radiographic appearance of sclerosis of the ilium in association with a normal cartilage space suggest a reaction to stress as the pathogenesis of osteitis condensans ilii. This condition is practically always bilateral and symmetrical in its appearance and is rarely seen in men. The changes seem to regress spontaneously later in life and hence are not normally present on films of postmenopausal women.

Figure 10–37 illustrates the classical

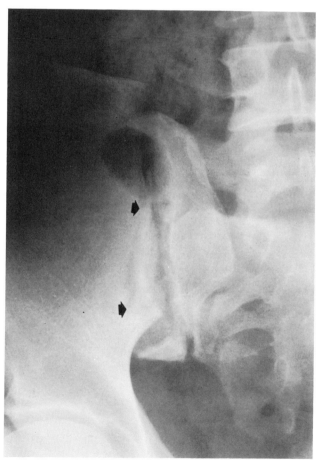

Figure 10–36.   Sacroiliac trauma.

Separation of the joint, a triangular fracture fragment inferiorly and an adjacent vertical fracture through the ilium (arrows) have resulted from a motorcycle accident. Additional fractures or joint diastasis usually accompanies a break in the pelvic ring and, in this patient, was seen as a wide separation of the symphysis pubis (see also Figure 10–46).

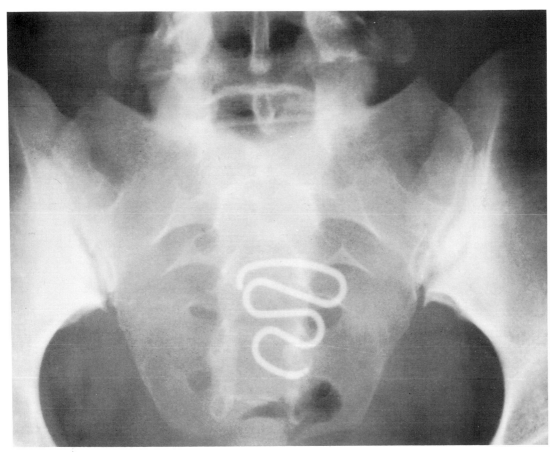

Figure 10–37. Osteitis condensans ilii.

Bilateral sclerosis limited to the iliac sides of the sacroiliac joints is not uncommonly present in young women and may be associated with trauma from childbearing. It is easily distinguishable from the healed stage of an inflammatory arthritis by the normal cartilage space.

appearance of osteitis condensans ilii in a woman of childbearing age (as well as her intrauterine device). Bilateral involvement, sclerosis limited to the iliac bones, and normal sacroiliac joints are pathognomonic of this condition.

This illustration is also useful in delineating the extent of the sacroilac joint, as the sclerosis defines the limits of the articulating bone. It should be recalled that the upper third of the sacrum and ilium do not articulate but are joined by a strong sacroiliac ligament. Hence, the changes of osteitis condensans ilii stop short of this level. The extent of involvement is markedly different from that in the rheumatoid diseases. In these, ligamentous involvement is a prominent component of the pathophysiologic changes, and therefore the upper third of the sacrum and ilium exhibit inflammatory changes in addition to the true joint space.

Unilateral Osteitis Condensans Ilii. Very rarely, osteitis condensans ilii may occur unilaterally, as seen in Figure 10–38. The sclerosis may be identical to the end stage of a unilateral infection; optimal views of the cartilage space are necessary to assure that the joint itself is normal. Unilateral osteitis condensans ilii is sometimes associated with contralateral hip disease, suggesting once more that the pathologic changes may be a result of undue stress on the sacroiliac joint with a subsequent reactive osteitis.

Unilateral Sacroiliitis

INFLAMMATORY ARTHRITIS

Involvement of the sacroiliac joint by infection or by one of the inflammatory arthritides, such as ankylosing spondylitis, is an easy diagnosis to make when enough time has elapsed to allow signs of healing to appear on the radiograph. However, it is critical that one be able to appreciate the earliest signs of inflammatory involvement and instigate treatment at a stage in which it can alter the course of the disease.

The earliest sign of sacroiliitis is *widening* of the joint space. Because of the inflammation, this is generally accompanied by demineralization of the articulating bones, which is reflected in a loss of the sharp cortical margin. Thus, the space is irregularly widened and fuzzy in its appearance. Sclerosis, narrowing of the joint space and bony ankylosis are manifestations of healing; they occur late in the course of an inflammatory arthritis.

Tuberculous Sacroiliitis. The signs of early joint inflammation are present in the left sacroiliac joint of a 15 year old boy with tuberculous arthritis (Fig. 10–39A). Although the findings appear to be subtle, they are dramatic when compared to the normal right side. There is irregular widening and loss of the sharp white cortical margin. Following tuberculostatic therapy, early signs of healing appear as sclerosis along the iliac side of the joint (Fig. 10–39B). Four months later, the sclerotic new bone has become the predominant radiographic finding (Fig. 10–39C) and appears similar to that seen in osteitis condensans ilii. Irregular widening of the joint, however, implicates an inflammatory origin of the disease.

Although the age and sex of this patient are consistent with the pattern associated with ankylosing spondylitis, the unilaterality of involvement excludes this diagnosis.

Another example of tuberculous arthritis shows the second pattern of an end-stage inflammatory arthritis. Figure 10–40 illustrates the appearance of complete obliteration of the sacroiliac joint and bony ankylosis. The upper third of the sacrum is spared since the infectious process was limited to the joint and did not involve the ligament.

Tomography is often helpful in delineating the degree of joint destruction in this difficult area. Figure 10–41 illustrates the tomographic appearance of bony ankylosis as well as the normal sacroiliac joint.

Text continued on page 441.

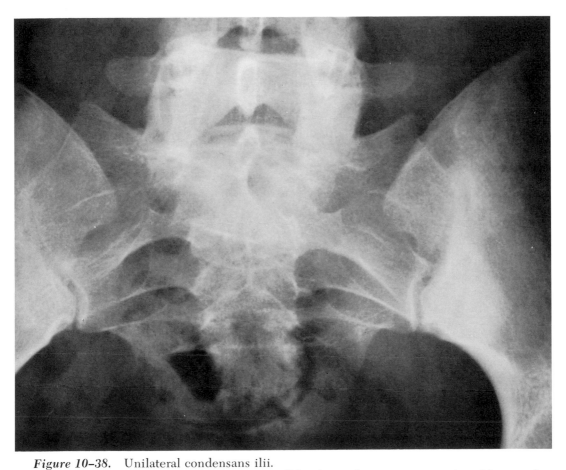

Figure 10-38. Unilateral condensans ilii.

Sclerosis of the inferior articulating margin of the ilium of a young woman is evident on the left. The joint itself shows no evidence of previous inflammation. The unilaterality is unusual, but occasionally is seen and may be associated with contralateral hip disease. In this case there was no detectable symptomatology referable either to the sacroiliac or hip joint, and the finding was a chance observation on a film from a kidney study.

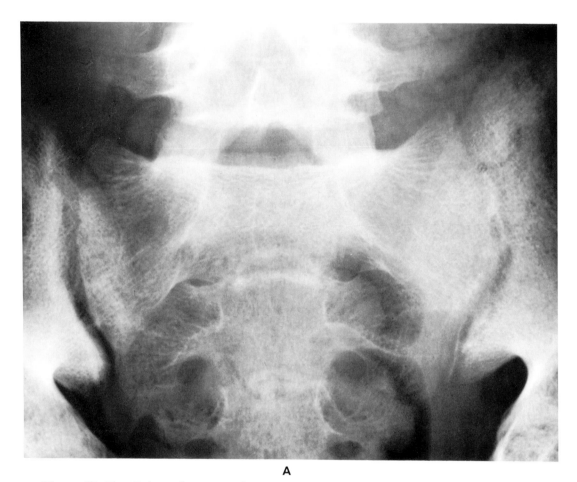

A

Figure 10–39. Tuberculous sacroiliitis.
A. Unilateral sacroiliitis is manifested by widening of the cartilage space on the left and erosions of the articulating edges of bones.

Figure 10–39. *Continued*

B. A year later, marked sclerosis is apparent, indicating healing. Although the sclerosis appears to be limited to the iliac side of the joint, the widened and irregular sacroiliac joint cannot be confused with the appearance of osteitis condensans ilii.

C. The final healed picture illustrates permanent sclerosis and a widened, irregular sacroiliac joint.

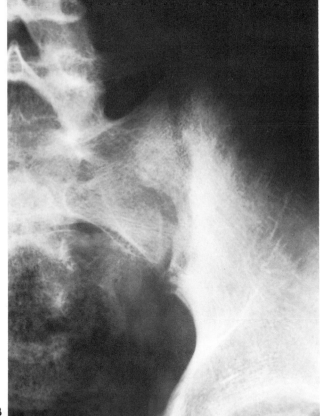

B

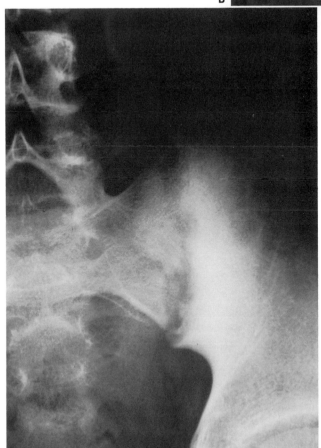

C

439

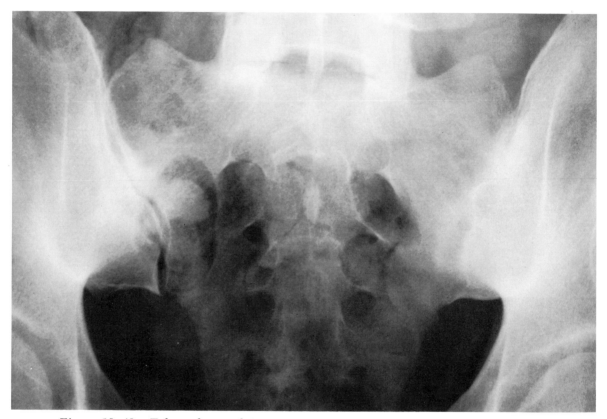

Figure 10–40. Tuberculous arthritis.

The healed stage of a tuberculous arthritis may result in bony ankylosis with complete obliteration of the joint space. Sclerotic changes of the ilium are present, as in the preceding figure.

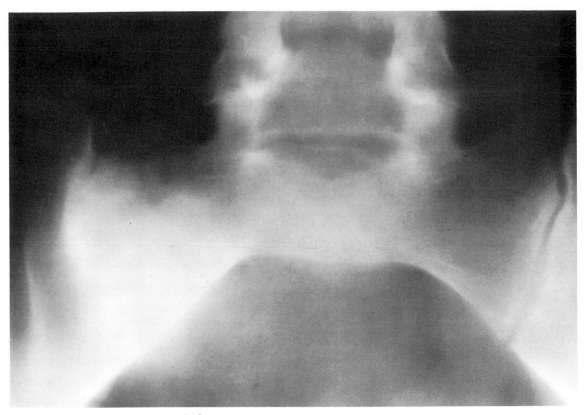

Figure 10–41. Bony ankylosis.
Tomography is often helpful in establishing the presence of bony ankylosis, as seen here in the right sacroiliac joint. The normal tomographic appearance of a sacroiliac joint is seen on the left side. The sharp margins and uniform width of the articular cartilage are evident.

Bilateral Sacroiliitis

Ankylosing Spondylitis. Ankylosing spondylitis may occasionally begin in one sacroiliac joint, but it is rare for films to be taken at a sufficiently early stage to record the unilaterality. By the time patients seek medical help the disease has involved both joints, and any difference in degree of destruction is virtually impossible to detect. Even young military recruits, who are universally known to seek aid for their back pain far earlier than the general population, manifest *bilateral* sacroiliac involvement on the earliest film if ankylosing spondylitis is the culprit.

Bilateral bony ankylosis of the sacroiliac joints and bony bridging of the intervertebral spaces between the lower lumbar vertebrae characterize the classic radiographic changes of ankylosing spondylitis (Fig. 10–42). The residual Pantopaque in the neural canal and the radiolucent bone defect superimposed on the fourth and fifth vertebrae attest to the difficulties in diagnosing early signs of ankylosing spondylitis. Twenty years earlier, this 40 year old man underwent laminectomy to "correct" his back pain. Unfortunately, this is not an uncommon story, and not infrequently the telltale sign of an old laminectomy is superimposed on the full-blown picture of ankylosing spondylitis, mute testimony of an earlier diagnostic dilemma. Since disc space narrowing accompanies fusion of the apophyseal joints, the confusion with disc disease in the course of ankylosing spondylitis can be appreciated.

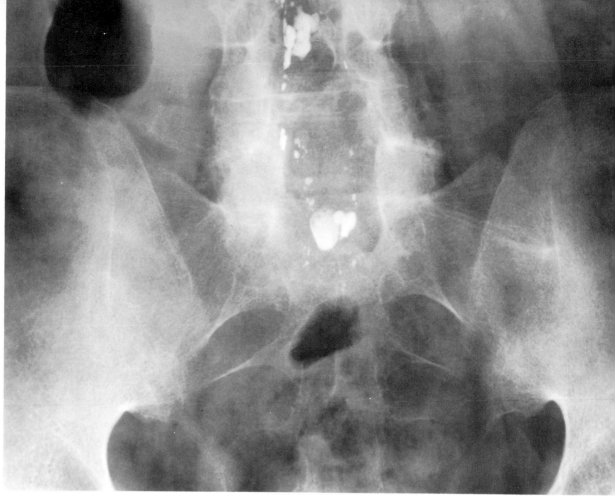

Figure 10–42. Ankylosing spondylitis.

Bilateral bony fusion of the sacroiliac joints is most commonly associated with ankylosing spondylitis. Misdiagnosis of the cause of back pain early in the course of the disease led to a laminectomy. The large surgical defect can be seen. Residual Pantopaque from a myelogram is superimposed on the laminectomy defect.

Occasionally, the radiographic signs of ankylosing spondylitis are seen in patients with gastrointestinal disorders. These findings may be identical to ankylosing spondylitis. They are characterized by bilateral involvement of the sacroiliac joints and progressive changes of the spine which may ascend to the thoracic and cervical levels.

Ulcerative Colitis. Ankylosing spondylitis accompanies ulcerative colitis more frequently than it does Crohn's disease. In both conditions it affects the sacroiliac joints symmetrically and tends to be self-limiting, with little or no involvement of the lumbar spine. Occasionally, however, there may be extensive involvement indistinguishable from the radiographic changes of ankylosing spondylitis.

A film of a middle-aged man with ulcerative colitis illustrates bilateral sacroiliitis with sclerosis as the predominant finding (Fig. 10–43). Although the bilaterality and sclerosis are similar to the findings in osteitis condensans ilii, the sex of the patient and the changes in the joint space, as well as sclerosis of both the sacrum and the ilium, easily distinguish the two conditions.

ASYMMETRIC INVOLVEMENT OF THE SACROILIAC JOINTS

Rheumatoid arthritis, juvenile rheumatoid arthritis, psoriatic arthritis and Reiter's syndrome may affect only one sacroiliac joint, but they frequently in-

442

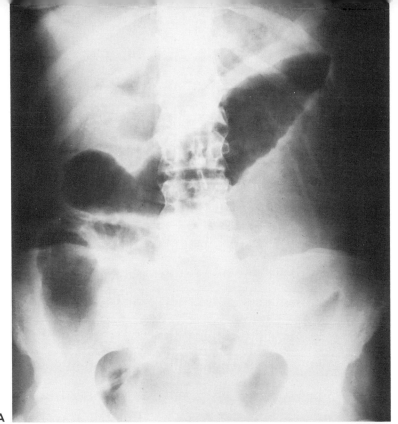

A

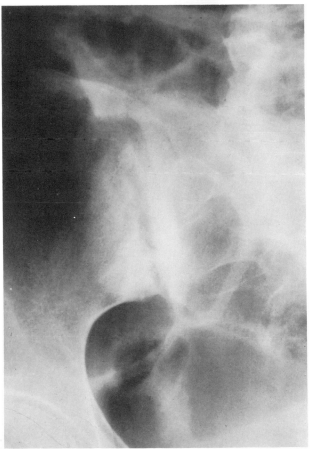

B

Figure 10–43. Ulcerative colitis.

A. Bilateral sacroiliitis is present, as well as a dilated transverse colon showing the soft tissue shadows of pseudopolyposis. Toxic megacolon and ankylosing spondylitis may both complicate the picture of ulcerative colitis.

B. A close-up of the right sacroiliac joint shows the irregularity of the joint space as well as sclerosis of both sacrum and ilium, differentiating the picture from osteitis condensans ilii.

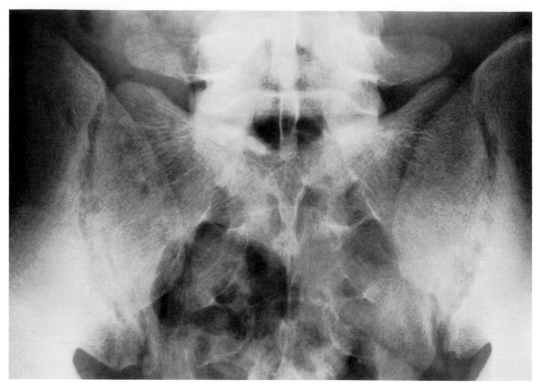

Figure 10–44. Reiter's syndrome.

Although the changes in the sacroiliac joints may be indistinguishable from those of anky-losing spondylitis, when Reiter's syndrome affects these joints they are frequently involved asymmetrically, as in this example. Irregular widening of the joint space and sclerosis are present bilaterally but are more extensive on the left. Bony ankylosis is very rare in Reiter's syndrome. Most frequently the end result of the inflammatory process is irregular widening and sclerosis of the adjacent bone.

volve both. Unlike ankylosing spondy-litis, these conditions all have a tendency for asymmetric involvement. Hence, bi-lateral sacroiliitis with different degrees of destruction should suggest one of these four entities rather than ankylosing spondylitis.

Reiter's Syndrome. The asymmetric sacroiliac joint involvement of Reiter's syndrome is illustrated in Figure 10–44. There is irregular widening of the left sacroiliac joint and sclerosis of both ar-ticular bones. The right sacroiliac joint is only minimally involved, and the fuzzy outline of the bony margins is the only indication of inflammation.

Gout. The rarest cause of sacroili-itis is gout; this should be the last diag-nostic consideration in a patient with back pain. Unfortunately, the use of

aspirin to decrease the discomfort of sa-croiliac pain may elevate the serum uric acid level, and laboratory studies may falsely suggest gouty arthropathy as the diagnosis.

When gout affects the lumbosacral spine, the same radiographic changes that occur in peripheral joints are found here: soft tissue tophi; contiguous bony erosions with sclerotic margins; and splayed or overhanging edges. Two films taken several years apart illustrate the mutilating effects that can occur from chronic tophaceous gout. Inflammatory changes of both sacroiliac joints are seen in Figure 10–45A. There are erosions with sclerotic margins. Similar findings are also present in the posterior elements of the fifth lumbar vertebra. Involvement of the fourth lumbar vertebra and the supe-

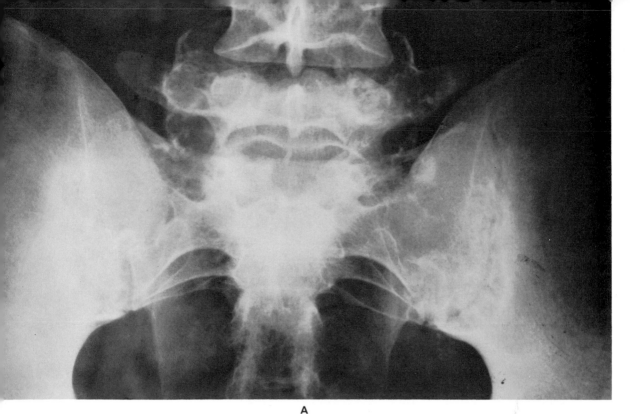

A

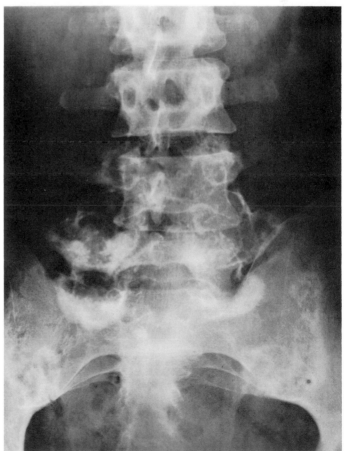

B

Figure 10–45. Gout.

A. Asymmetric involvement of the sacroiliac joints with erosions and productive new bone has caused a mottled appearance of the articulating bones. Distortion of the posterior portions of L5 is also the result of tophaceous deposits.

B. Nine years later, progressive expansion of the pedicle and transverse process of L5, involvement of the pedicles of L4 and more extensive sclerotic new bone along the superior margin of the sacrum and both sacroiliac joints give a bizarre appearance to the spine.

rior margin of the sacrum, and extensive sclerosis including the sacroiliac joints, is seen on the later film (Fig. 10–45B).

THE SYMPHYSIS PUBIS

The articular bones of the pubis are covered by hyaline cartilage and are separated by a fibrocartilaginous disc. Occasionally, this joint is involved by arthritis, and the changes are identical to those seen in other joints.

Traumatic Separation. Fracture of the pelvis may be accompanied by diastasis of the pubis, as is seen in Figure 10–46. Healing may take place with no residua. Often, however, there will be a permanent offset of the margins of the bones or minimal sclerotic changes along the articular margins, indicating the previous episode of trauma.

Osteitis Pubis. Low-grade infection

of the symphysis pubis may follow instrumentation of the urethra or vaginal delivery. It is characterized by irregular erosion of the pubic bones and sclerosis. Rarely, as in Figure 10–47, "gas" may be present in the fibrocartilage; it is similar in radiographic appearance to that seen in degenerative disc disease.

Chondrocalcinosis. As in other joints, the fibrocartilage in the symphysis pubis may calcify. The thin vertical calcific density should not be confused with the frequently observed shadow of superimposed buttock folds. Calcified cartilage within the symphysis in a patient with hyperparathyroidism is illustrated in Figure 10–48. The extent of calcification is demarcated by the margins of the bones superiorly and inferiorly. The confusing buttock shadow that is sometimes seen on pelvic films will extend beyond these limits and is therefore easily distinguished.

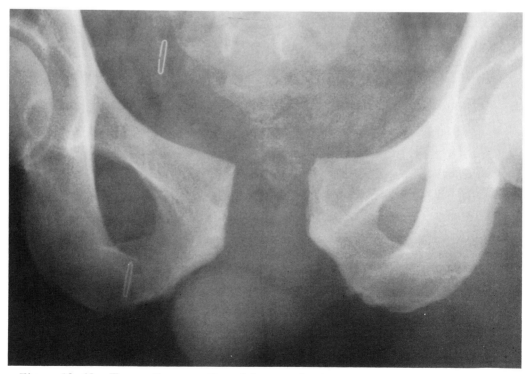

Figure 10–46. Traumatic separation of the symphysis.
Fracture of the pelvis is not infrequently accompanied by diastasis of the sacroiliac joints or, as in this example, by separation of the symphysis pubis.

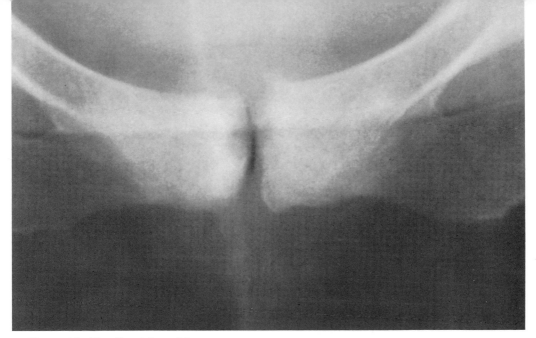

Figure 10–47. Osteitis pubis.
Erosions and reactive sclerosis indicate an underlying inflammatory process. Degenerative changes of the cartilage are apparent both in the irregular narrowing and in the radiolucent line similar to the vacuum disc of the spine.

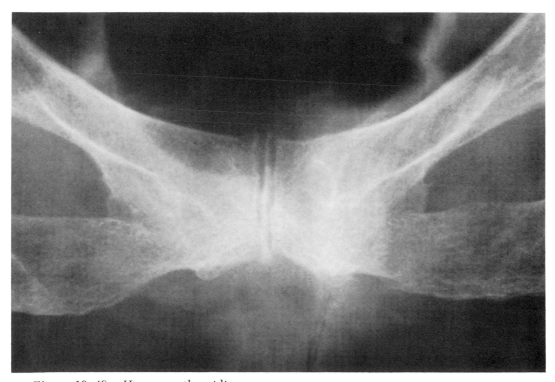

Figure 10–48. Hyperparathyroidism.
The fibrocartilage of the symphysis pubis is a frequent site of chondrocalcinosis. It is occasionally mimicked by a dense vertical skinfold, but restriction of the shadow to the length of the joint distinguishes true calcification.

447

SUGGESTED READINGS

Cliff, J. M. Spinal bony bridging and carditis in Reiter's disease. Ann. Rheum. Dis. 30:171 (1971).

Cohen, A. S., J. M. McNeill, E. Calkins, J. T. Sharp, and A. Schubart. The "normal" sacroiliac joint: Analysis of 88 sacroiliac roentgenograms. Amer. J. Roentgen. 100:559 (1967).

Doyle, F. H., D. H. Gutteridge, G. F. Joplin, and R. Fraser. An assessment of radiological criteria used in the study of spinal osteoporosis. Brit. J. Radiol. 40:241 (1967).

Dunn, A. W., and H. D. Morris. Fractures and dislocations of the pelvis. J. Bone Joint Surg. (Amer.) 50A:1639 (1968).

Good, A. E. Involvement of the back in Reiter's syndrome: Followup study of 34 cases, Ann. Int. Med. 57:44 (1962).

Good, A. E. Reiter's disease and ankylosing spondylitis. Acta Rheum. Scand. 11:305 (1965).

Jajic, I. Radiologic changes in the sacroiliac joints and spine of patients with psoriatic arthritis and psoriasis. Ann. Rheum. Dis. 27:1 (1968).

Jayson, M. I. V., and I. A. D. Bouchier. Ulcerative colitis with ankylosing spondylitis, Ann. Rheum. Dis. 27:219 (1968).

Martel, W. Cervical spondylitis in rheumatoid disease: A comment on neurologic significance and pathogenesis. Amer. J. Med. 44:441 (1968).

Martel, W., and G. G. Bole. Pathologic fracture of the odontoid process in rheumatoid arthritis. Radiology 90:948 (1968).

McEwen, C. Arthritis accompanying ulcerative colitis. Clin. Orthop. 57:9 (1968).

McEwen, C. Arthritis accompanying ulcerative colitis. Clin. Orthop. 57:9 (1968).

McEwen, C., D. Di Tata, C. Ling, A. Porini, A. Good, and T. Rankin. Ankylosing spondylitis accompanying ulcerative colitis, regional enteritis, psoriasis and Reiter's disease: A comparative Study. Arthritis Rheum. 14:291 (1971).

Meijers, K. A. E., S. F. Van Voss, and R. J. Francois. Radiological changes in the cervical spine in ankylosing spondylitis. Ann. Rheum. Dis. 27:333 (1968).

Numaguchi, Y. Osteitis condensans ilii, including its resolution. Radiology 98:1 (1971).

Soren, A. Joint affections in regional ileitis. Arch. Int. Med. 117:78 (1966).

Vix, V. A., and Chi Yol Ryu. The adult symphysis pubis, normal and abnormal, Amer. J. Roentgen, 112:517 (1971).

Wright, V., and G. Watkinson. Sacroileitis and ulcerative colitis. Brit. Med. J. 2:675 (1965).

Zvaifler, N. J., and W. Martel. Spondylitis in chronic ulcerative colitis. Arthritis Rheum. 3:76 (1960).

EXERCISES

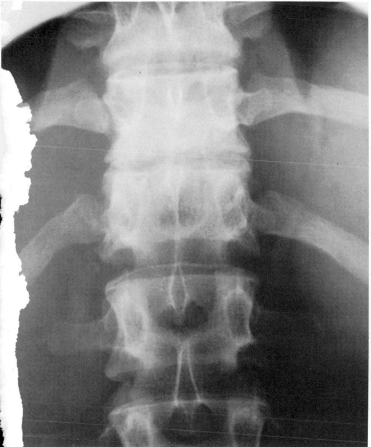

E10–1A.

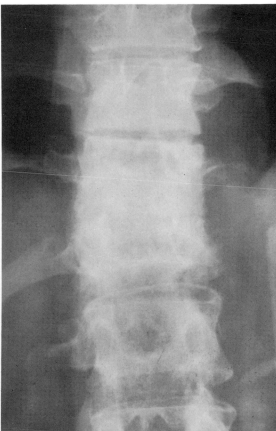

E10–1B. One year later.

E10–1. A paraspinous mass and adjacent intervertebral space narrowing advertise the presence of an infectious spondylitis. The mycobacterium is the most frequent offender when a localized abscess is associated with a spondylitis. An identical combination of findings, however, may occasionally accompany a gram negative infection.

Slow but relentless destruction of the disc space and adjacent bones occurred over a year, as seen by a later film of this patient with tuberculous spondylitis (E10–1B). Surgical drainage (note the resected eleventh and twelfth ribs on the left) has eliminated a large percentage of the abscess, but a persistent displacement of the mediastinal stripe can still be seen.

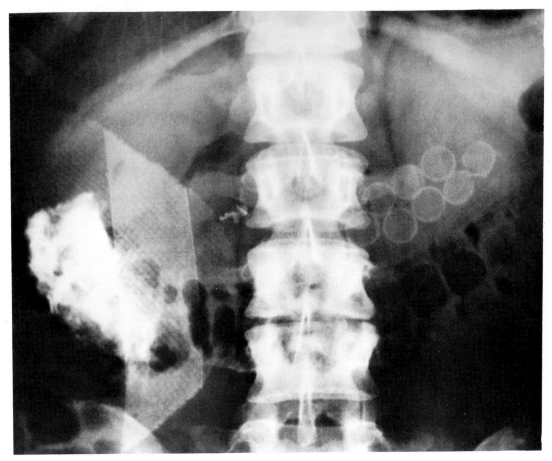

E10–2.

E10–2. With only a single glance, one might overlook the narrowed intervertebral disc space between the third and fourth lumbar vertebrae because the margins of the bones are still sharp. The confusing collection of white mesh and moulage to the right of the spine represents a contrast-filled sinus tract and abscess pocket from the psoas muscle to the gauze covered flank. The Sherlock Holmes reader will tie these clues together and make the bacterial diagnosis using the additional evidence of eight para-aminosalicylic acid pills in the antrum of the stomach: the case is clearly one of *tuberculous spondylitis.*

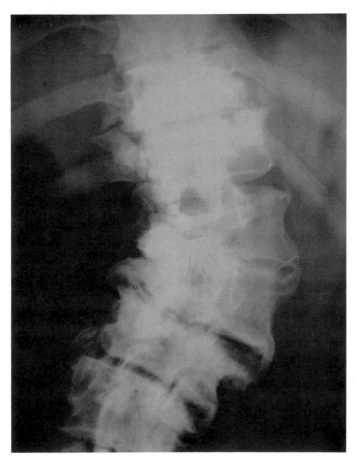

E10–3.

E10–3. Exaggerated degenerative changes deforming extensive areas of the spine should always suggest *tabes dorsalis*. Combined with fragmentation, paravertebral ossification and increased density of the vertebral bodies, it is almost unnecessary to order the confirmatory laboratory studies.

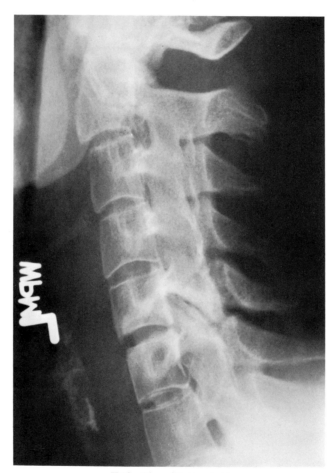

E10–4A.   (Patient A)

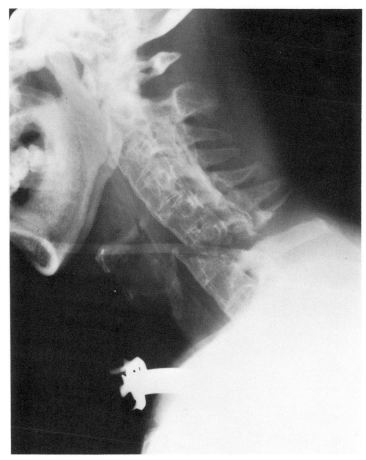

E10–4B. (Patient *B*)

E10–4. "The obvious is that which is never seen until someone expresses it simply."*

Bony ankylosis of the apophyseal joints of the cervical spine should always suggest *rheumatoid arthritis*. Whenever there is trauma to such a poker spine, no matter how minimal, it spells danger. No obvious fracture was apparent after a minor whiplash injury, yet there is evidence on this lateral view of significant trauma. The wide prevertebral soft tissue shadow extending the length of the cervical vertebrae reflects edema or hemor-

*Kahlil Gibran

rhage when it occurs immediately after a neck injury, as in this man. Knowing the vulnerability of a rigid spine and with a high index of suspicion of the possibility of a fracture, tomography is indicated to assure detection of an occult fracture.

Complete ankylosis of the apophyseal joints in a patient with ankylosing spondylitis (E10–4B) is identical to the example of rheumatoid arthritis (E10–4A). What distinguishes the two conditions is the paravertebral ossification encasing the vertebral bodies. The bipartite nature of this poker spine was caused by falling out of bed. The spinal cord faithfully followed the acute angulation of the neural canal at the sixth cervical vertebra, resulting in sudden quadriplegia.

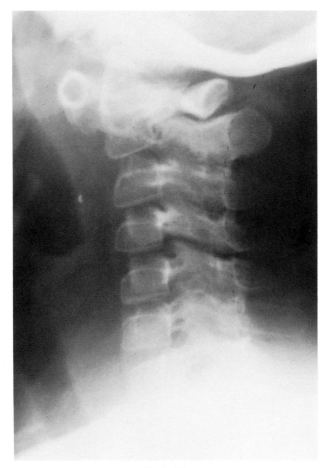

E10–5A.

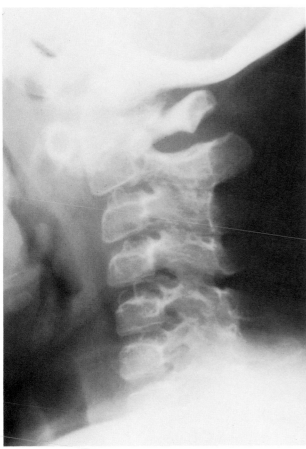

E10–5B. One year later.

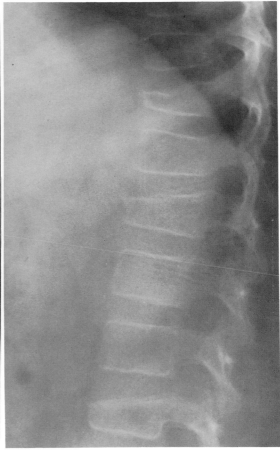

E10–5C.

E10–5. Two films separated by a year's time reveal progressive narrowing and erosions of the apophyseal joints and increasing involvement of the lower cervical spine, summarizing the pathophysiologic changes of *juvenile rheumatoid arthritis* as it affects this region. The earlier film demonstrates atlantoaxial subluxation, implicating an additional site of inflammatory involvement in the transverse ligament. Although the separation of the odontoid from the anterior ring of the first cervical vertebra is normally greater in children than in adults, the off-set of the spinous processes verifies the presence of true subluxation.

Juvenile rheumatoid arthritis spares the lumbar and thoracic regions, and yet lower back pain was a prominent component of this 12 year old child's symptomatology (E10–5C). The lateral view of the thoracolumbar spine explains this inconsistency: there has been wedge collapse of several severely osteoporotic vertebral bodies. Generalized osteoporosis is often a prominent feature of juvenile rheumatoid arthritis, and fractures of any bone can occur.

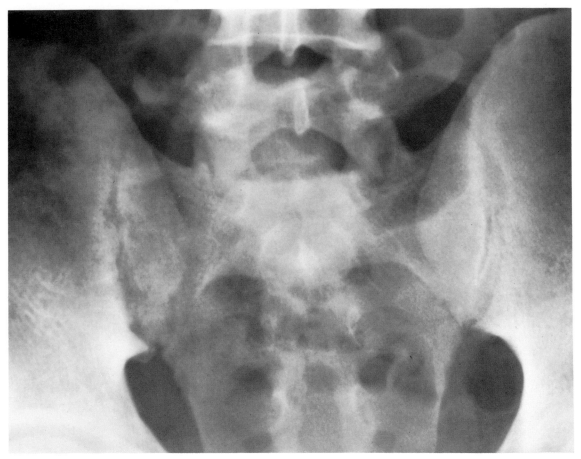

E10–6.

E10–6. Unilateral sacroiliitis must always be considered infectious until proven otherwise. Although blind biopsy of the right sacroiliac joint failed to capture an organism or to establish a diagnosis in this 22 year old man, a simultaneous blood culture revealed a Klebsiella septicemia. The incidence of gram negative infections is so high in patients with a history of intravenous drug abuse that the discovery frequently flags an unsuspected addict too reticent to reveal all sides of his past, and this individual with *Klebsiella sacroiliitis* was no exception.

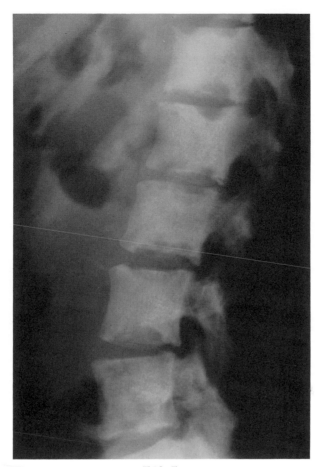

E10–7.

E10–7. Irregular patches of rarefaction involve each vertebral end plate, signifying disseminated infection and illustrating the bony origin of *infectious spondylitis.* Only later does herniation and secondary destruction of the avascular cartilaginous disc cause narrowing of the intervertebral space. This, again, is a heroin addict—as a matter of fact, the same man whose sacroiliac joint was illustrated in the previous exercise. Inadequate medication and poor follow-up of his infectious sacroiliitis resulted in dissemination of the Klebsiella infection within three months and a long, stormy hospitalization.

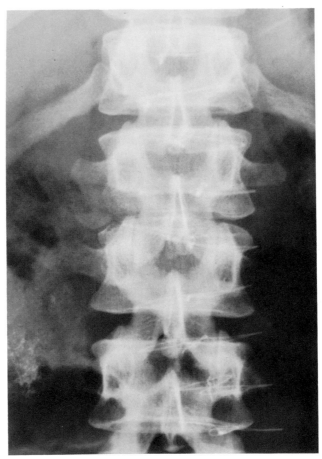

E10–8A.

E10–8. Metallic sutures and the faint spherical shadow of a colostomy stoma reveal only a fraction of this man's remembrances of a barroom brawl (E10–8A). A through-and-through knife wound at the level of the first lumbar vertebra skewered his organs in series. Complications began with a perforated transverse colon, lacerated liver and pancreas and ended with the findings on the second illustration. Unnoticed initially, the right lower corner of the first lumbar vertebra was also pierced by the knife, leaving a fragment of bone and an inoculum of mixed flora.

Confusing to the surgeons were a convalescent complaint of left side pain and a stooped posture two months later. The abdominal film revealed a huge left psoas abscess and rapid destruction of the first and second lumbar vertebrae, the signs of an *infectious spondylitis* (E10–8B). Only then was the original fracture seen and the unfortunate consequence of the oversight appreciated.

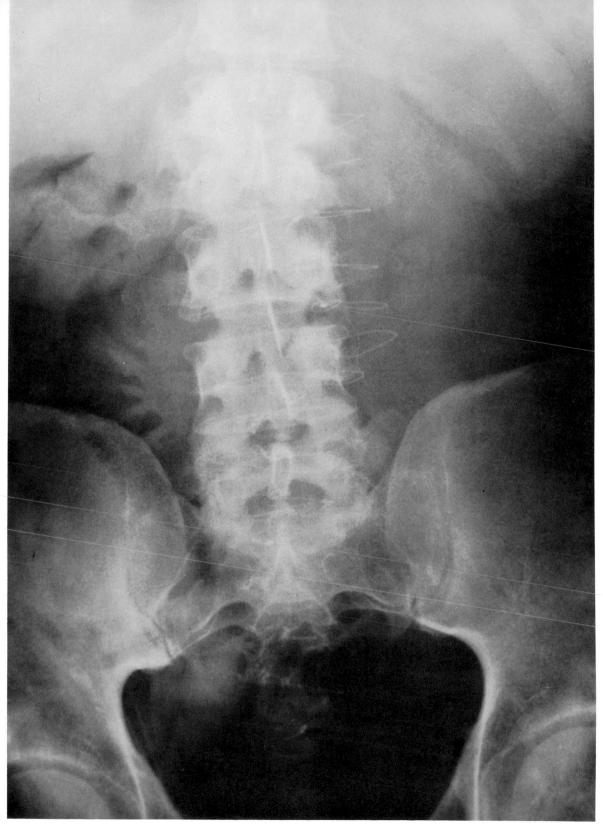

E10–8B. Two months later.

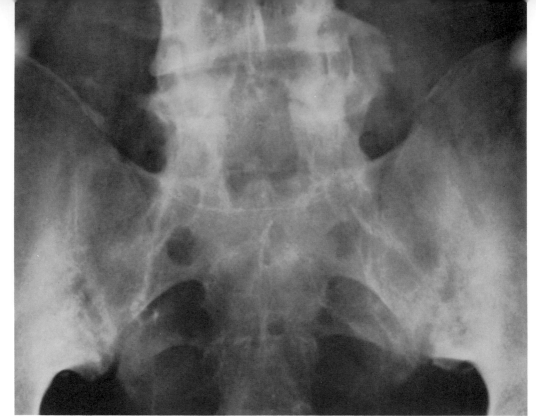

E10–9A.   (Patient A)

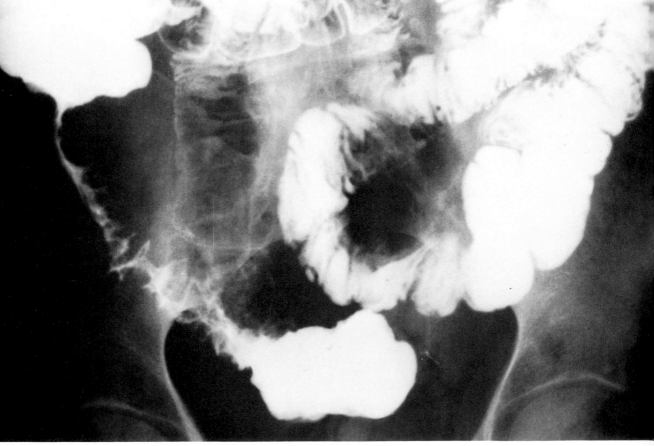

E10–9B.

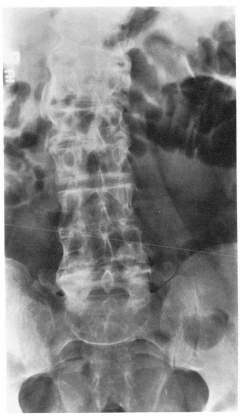

E10–9C. (Patient *B*)

E10–9. Bilateral sacroiliitis *symmetrically* involving both joints always suggests ankylosing spondylitis or the arthritis that accompanies ulcerative colitis and *Crohn's disease.* This is not an uncommon complication of Crohn's disease, and one must always be on guard for its development. Up to 20 per cent of patients may have sacroiliitis, and five per cent (or one quarter of these) develop an ankylosing spondylitis.

The sign of ill-defined back pain wrongly assessed is stamped indelibly on this man's film as a laminectomy defect of the last lumbar vertebra (E10–9A). Bridging syndesmophytes are beginning to unite the fourth and fifth lumbar vertebrae. Their bulkiness and the asymmetry of their development (the syndesmophytes to the left are far more pronounced than those on the right) are two criteria looked for to establish the spondylitis of Reiter's syndrome or psoriatic arthritis. Since they are present in this case of ankylosing spondylitis, the usefulness of these radiographic criteria is limited and such signs must be used with caution and consideration. The barium study (E10–9B) shows the narrowed terminal ileum typical of Crohn's disease.

A radiograph of the lumbar spine from a patient with Reiter's syndrome illustrates identical bulky syndesmophytes, asymmetry of their development and the tendency to skip intervertebral spaces (E10–9C). Although the presence of these distinguishing radiographic criteria suggest that one is dealing with a case of Reiter's syndrome or psoriatic arthritis rather than ankylosing spondylitis and a gastrointestinal disorder, the similarity of the preceding two illustrations suggests that the differences are not dependable. Far more important is the ability to recognize the earliest changes of any inflammatory spondylitis, no matter what rheumatoid variant is present.

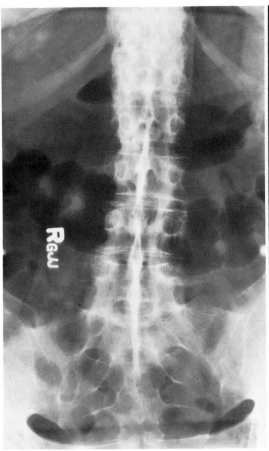

E10–10A.

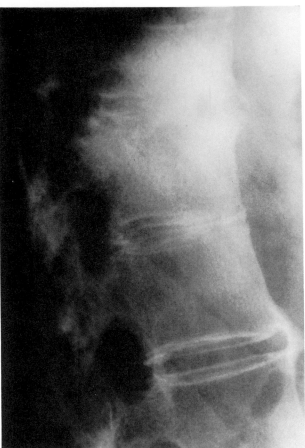

E10–10B.

E10–10. This patient is a 60 year old woman, but the gender should never dissuade one from the diagnosis of ankylosing spondylitis, as five to 10 per cent of patients with this disease will be female.

All of the classic changes of *ankylosing spondylitis* are present, and the radiologic diagnosis offers no difficulty: bilateral bony ankylosis of the sacroiliac joints, bony ankylosis of the apophyseal joints, syndesmophytes bridging the vertebral bodies and ossification fusing the spinous processes.

The diagnostic problem lies at the junction of the thoracic and lumbar spines (E10–10B). There is complete obliteration of the disc space anteriorly, loss of the sharp contours of the vertebral end plates and extensive reactive sclerosis of both vertebral bodies. In any other patient this would suggest an infectious spondylitis, but in ankylosing spondylitis the spine becomes vulnerable to fracture from minor trauma, and a reactive osteitis may mimic the changes of infection. Serial films to observe the sequence of changes or bone biopsy in an attempt to establish the presence of infection is necessary. In this case, despite a history of steroid medication and a high index of suspicion that her back pain was caused by infection, films over a 12 month period demonstrated the bony changes to be completely stable.

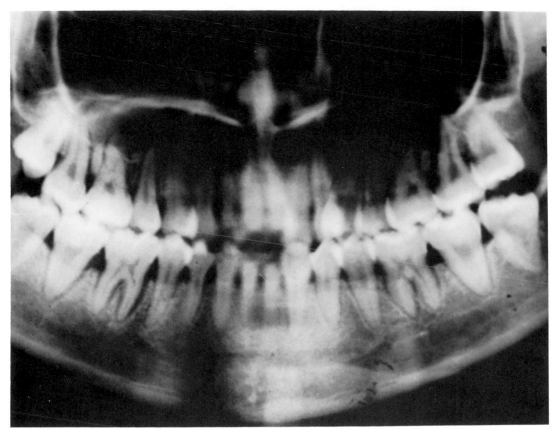

E10–11.

E10–11. Like the Cheshire cat from *Alice's Adventures in Wonderland* one is left at the end with a grin.

The panorex view of the mouth reveals wide black lines surrounding the roots of the teeth, and if periodontitis can be excluded, this periodontal membrane widening is diagnostic of *progressive systemic sclerosis.* It indicates resorption of the alveolar bone in addition to increased collagen in the periodontal membrane itself and results in loosening of the teeth. To compound the patient's problem, tightening of the skin around the mouth leaves little leeway for adequate dental care. Loss of teeth from infection can be prevented only by enthusiastic care on the part of both patient and physician.

"I think till I'm weary of thinking,"
    Said the sad-eyed Hindu King,
"And I see but shadows around me,
    Illusion in everything."

— Lyall

INDEX

Note: Page numbers in *italics* indicate illustrations.